Advancing Medical Education Through Strategic Instructional Design

Jill Stefaniak
Old Dominion University, USA

A volume in the Advances in Medical Education, Research, and Ethics (AMERE) Book Series

IGI GLOBAL
DISSEMINATOR OF KNOWLEDGE
www.igi-global.com

Published in the United States of America by
IGI Global
Medical Information Science Reference (an imprint of IGI Global)
701 E. Chocolate Avenue
Hershey PA, USA 17033
Tel: 717-533-8845
Fax: 717-533-8661
E-mail: cust@igi-global.com
Web site: http://www.igi-global.com

Copyright © 2017 by IGI Global. All rights reserved. No part of this publication may be reproduced, stored or distributed in any form or by any means, electronic or mechanical, including photocopying, without written permission from the publisher. Product or company names used in this set are for identification purposes only. Inclusion of the names of the products or companies does not indicate a claim of ownership by IGI Global of the trademark or registered trademark.

Library of Congress Cataloging-in-Publication Data

Names: Stefaniak, Jill E., 1984- editor.
Title: Advancing medical education through strategic instructional design / Jill Stefaniak, editor.
Description: Hershey, PA : Medical Information Science Reference, [2017] | Includes bibliographical references and index.
Identifiers: LCCN 2016053530| ISBN 9781522520986 (h/c) | ISBN 9781522520993 (ebook)
Subjects: | MESH: Education, Medical--methods | Learning | Educational Technology
Classification: LCC R834 | NLM W 18 | DDC 610.71--dc23 LC record available at https://lccn.loc.gov/2016053530

This book is published in the IGI Global book series Advances in Medical Education, Research, and Ethics (AMERE) (ISSN: Pending; eISSN: Pending)

British Cataloguing in Publication Data
A Cataloguing in Publication record for this book is available from the British Library.

All work contributed to this book is new, previously-unpublished material. The views expressed in this book are those of the authors, but not necessarily of the publisher.

For electronic access to this publication, please contact: eresources@igi-global.com.

Advances in Medical Education, Research, and Ethics (AMERE) Book Series

ISSN:Pending
EISSN:Pending

Mission

Humans are living longer now than ever as a result of advances in the medical field. Having the tools available to train knowledgeable and ethical future generations of doctors and medical researchers is essential to continuing to advance our understanding of the human body and develop new ways of treating and curing sickness and disease.

The **Advances in Medical Education, Research, and Ethics (AMERE)** book series highlights publications pertaining to advancements in pedagogical practice for developing future healthcare professionals, research methods, and advancements in 10 the medical field, as well as moral behavior and practice of healthcare professionals, students, and researchers. Featuring research-based book publications that are highly relevant to the healthcare community, this series is ideally designed for library inclusion at medical universities and research institutions as well as personal use by medical professionals, researchers, and upper-level students entering the field.

Coverage

- Clinical Research
- Conflicts of Interest
- Ethics in Medicine
- Healthcare Pedagogy
- Medical Curricula
- Medical Simulation
- Patient Data
- Professional Development
- Research Methods
- Scientific Misconduct

IGI Global is currently accepting manuscripts for publication within this series. To submit a proposal for a volume in this series, please contact our Acquisition Editors at Acquisitions@igi-global.com or visit: http://www.igi-global.com/publish/.

The Advances in Medical Education, Research, and Ethics (AMERE) Book Series (ISSN Pending) is published by IGI Global, 701 E. Chocolate Avenue, Hershey, PA 17033-1240, USA, www.igi-global.com. This series is composed of titles available for purchase individually; each title is edited to be contextually exclusive from any other title within the series. For pricing and ordering information please visit http://www.igi-global.com/book-series/advances-medical-education-research-ethics/132365. Postmaster: Send all address changes to above address.
Copyright © 2017 IGI Global. All rights, including translation in other languages reserved by the publisher. No part of this series may be reproduced or used in any form or by any means – graphics, electronic, or mechanical, including photocopying, recording, taping, or information and retrieval systems – without written permission from the publisher, except for non commercial, educational use, including classroom teaching purposes. The views expressed in this series are those of the authors, but not necessarily of IGI Global.

Titles in this Series

For a list of additional titles in this series, please visit: www.igi-global.com

Organizational Culture and Ethics in Modern Medicine
Anna Rosiek (Nicolaus Copernicus University in Toruń, Collegium Medicum in Bydgoszcz, Poland) and Krzysztof Leksowski (Nicolaus Copernicus University in Toruń, Collegium Medicum in Bydgoszcz, Poland)
Medical Information Science Reference • copyright 2016 • 448pp • H/C (ISBN: 9781466696587) • US $225.00 (our price)

Handbook of Research on Advancing Health Education through Technology
Victor C.X. Wang (Florida Atlantic University, USA)
Medical Information Science Reference • copyright 2016 • 588pp • H/C (ISBN: 9781466694941) • US $335.00 (our price)

Optimizing Medicine Residency Training Programs
Jayita Poduval (Pondicherry Institute of Medical Sciences, India)
Medical Information Science Reference • copyright 2016 • 300pp • H/C (ISBN: 9781466695276) • US $220.00 (our price)

IGI GLOBAL
DISSEMINATOR OF KNOWLEDGE
www.igi-global.com

701 E. Chocolate Ave., Hershey, PA 17033
Order online at www.igi-global.com or call 717-533-8845 x100
To place a standing order for titles released in this series, contact: cust@igi-global.com
Mon-Fri 8:00 am - 5:00 pm (est) or fax 24 hours a day 717-533-8661

Editorial Advisory Board

Jennifer Banas, *Northeastern Illinois University, USA*
Barbara Joyce, *Oakland University William Beaumont School of Medicine, USA*
Patricia Slagter van Tryon, *East Carolina University, USA*
Andrew Tawfik, *Northern Illinois University, USA*

Table of Contents

Preface xv

Chapter 1
Understanding Your Learner: Conducting a Learner Analysis 1
Tina M. Souders, University of North Carolina at Chapel Hill, USA

Chapter 2
Instructional Strategies and Sequencing 30
Thomas W. Lamey, University of South Alabama, USA
Gayle V. Davidson-Shivers, University of South Alabama, USA

Chapter 3
Using Backward Design for Competency-Based Undergraduate Medical Education 53
Barbara L. Joyce, Oakland University William Beaumont School of Medicine, USA
Stephanie M. Swanberg, Oakland University William Beaumont School of Medicine, USA

Chapter 4
Designing Simulated Learning Environments and Facilitating Authentic Learning Experiences in Medical Education 77
Xun Ge, University of Oklahoma, USA
Qian Wang, University of Oklahoma, USA
Kun Huang, Mississippi State University, USA
Victor Law, University of New Mexico, USA
Dominique C. Thomas, Cameron University, USA

Chapter 5
Medical Simulation as an Instructional Tool in Health Education: A Worked Example for Clinical Training 101
Anna Lerant, University of Mississippi Medical Center, USA
Oliver Jason Bates, University of Maryland Medical Center, USA
Michael G. Holder, University of Mississippi Medical Center, USA
Jeffrey D. Orledge, University of Mississippi Medical Center, USA
Robin (Rob) W. Rockhold, University of Mississippi Medical Center, USA
Richard Kyle, Independent Researcher, USA
Willie Bosseau Murray, Pennsylvania State University, USA

Chapter 6
The Nurse Educator's Role in Designing Instruction and Instructional Strategies for Academic and Clinical Settings 133
Patricia J. Slagter van Tryon, East Carolina University, USA

Chapter 7
Online Applied Learning in Nursing Education 150
Beth Oyarzun, University of North Carolina – Wilmington, USA
Elizabeth A. Gazza, University of North Carolina – Wilmington, USA

Chapter 8
Teaching Residents How to Teach 164
Heidi Kromrei, Detroit Medical Center, USA
William L. Solomonson, Oakland University, USA
Mark S. Juzych, Wayne State University, USA

Chapter 9
Interprofessional Education 186
Rebecca Moote, Regis University, USA

Chapter 10
Introducing Collaborative Care: Teaching Basics of Interprofessional Education in an Online Environment 208
Joy Doll, Creighton University, USA
Anna Maio, Creighton University, USA
Ann Ryan Haddad, Creighton University, USA
Margaret Jergenson, Creighton University, USA
Karen A. Paschal, Creighton University, USA
Katie Packard, Creighton University, USA
Meghan Potthoff, Creighton University, USA
Kathryn N. Huggett, University of Vermont, USA
Martha Todd, Creighton University, USA

Chapter 11
Informal Learning in Medical Education 225
Misa Mi, Oakland University William Beaumont School of Medicine, USA

Chapter 12
Virtual Patients in Health Professions Education 245
A. J. Kleinheksel, Shadow Health, Inc., USA

Chapter 13
Development and Evaluation of Neuroscience Computer-Based Modules for Medical Students: Instructional Design Principles and Effectiveness 262
Kathryn L. Lovell, Michigan State University, USA

Chapter 14
Faculty Development for Clinical Educators: A Competency Model for Continuous Improvement 277
Silvia Lizett Olivares Olivares, Tecnologico de Monterrey School of Medicine, Mexico
Mildred Vanessa López Cabrera, Tecnológico de Monterrey School of Medicine, Mexico
Martha Ruth Loyola Segura, Tecnologico de Monterrey School of Medicine, Mexico
Jorge Eugenio Valdez García, Tecnologico de Monterrey School of Medicine, Mexico

Compilation of References 301

About the Contributors 339

Index 346

Detailed Table of Contents

Preface xv

Chapter 1
Understanding Your Learner: Conducting a Learner Analysis 1
Tina M. Souders, University of North Carolina at Chapel Hill, USA

Now more than ever before, health care educators are being challenged to meet the complex and dynamic needs of an expanding health care workforce. Continuing education requirements as well as graduate and undergraduate programs are striving to keep pace with the demands for more highly skilled health care professionals. Likewise, technology and related instructional media have been evolving at an exponential pace. The confluence of these variables requires health care educators to be knowledgeable about the options and tools available to design and deliver instruction using a variety of platforms in more diverse settings. In order to ensure that instruction achieves its intended goals, it is imperative to fully assess the learner characteristics of the target audience. The purpose of this chapter is to discuss the rationale for conducting a learner analysis and utilizing learner characteristics in designing effective instruction.

Chapter 2
Instructional Strategies and Sequencing 30
Thomas W. Lamey, University of South Alabama, USA
Gayle V. Davidson-Shivers, University of South Alabama, USA

An instructional strategy is a designed course of action for an instructional goal framed by credible and realistic problems in order to activate prior knowledge and experiences in order to learn new knowledge and skills. In medical education, instructional strategies are designed as purposeful interventions to meet educational goals and achieve socio-cultural norms of medical practice. Reigeluth identified three major categories for instructional strategies: organizational, delivery, and management. The purpose of this chapter is to define and classify key concepts related to instructional strategies from an instructional design perspective and then apply them toward achieving medical education goals.

Chapter 3
Using Backward Design for Competency-Based Undergraduate Medical Education 53
Barbara L. Joyce, Oakland University William Beaumont School of Medicine, USA
Stephanie M. Swanberg, Oakland University William Beaumont School of Medicine, USA

This chapter focuses on strategies for approaching competency-based medical education (CBME) in the undergraduate medical curriculum (UME). CBME uses national professional standards, typically set by accrediting bodies or professional organizations, to shape curricular design and assessment of learner outcomes as well as to provide clarity to the learner about the knowledge, skills, and attitudes needed for successful practice. Wiggins and McTighe's Backward Design instructional design model provides a practical structure for approaching CBME since it proposes beginning with the national standards, defining outcomes and assessment methods, and then developing curricular content. The chapter will describe the backward design model, the history of CBME in the United States, current issues with CBME, and use of an integrated curriculum to successfully implement CBME. It will culminate with a discussion of creating action plans for individual programs to align assessment and outcome measures more directly to curriculum.

Chapter 4
Designing Simulated Learning Environments and Facilitating Authentic Learning Experiences in Medical Education 77
Xun Ge, University of Oklahoma, USA
Qian Wang, University of Oklahoma, USA
Kun Huang, Mississippi State University, USA
Victor Law, University of New Mexico, USA
Dominique C. Thomas, Cameron University, USA

The purpose of this chapter is to provide some practical guidance and theoretical basis on designing simulated learning environments to researchers and instructional designers, medical educators, instructional design students, and others who are committed to improving learning and instruction in medical education. This chapter will benefit those who are interested in designing simulated learning environments and facilitating simulated learning experiences in instructional settings. The chapter first defines various types of simulations and their cognitive functions in support of students' authentic learning experiences. Following this, the chapter highlights critical components for designing simulated learning environments, including identifying learning objectives, developing problem scenarios, and facilitating students' learning experiences. It is hoped that this chapter will be a useful tool and resource for medical educators, researchers and instructional designers, and graduate students who are pursuing an advanced degree in instructional design and technology.

Chapter 5
Medical Simulation as an Instructional Tool in Health Education: A Worked Example for Clinical Training 101
Anna Lerant, University of Mississippi Medical Center, USA
Oliver Jason Bates, University of Maryland Medical Center, USA
Michael G. Holder, University of Mississippi Medical Center, USA
Jeffrey D. Orledge, University of Mississippi Medical Center, USA
Robin (Rob) W. Rockhold, University of Mississippi Medical Center, USA
Richard Kyle, Independent Researcher, USA
Willie Bosseau Murray, Pennsylvania State University, USA

The purpose of this chapter is to provide a background and a worked example of using the Instructional Design System (ISD) as applied to a complex real life example. Specifically, the authors demonstrate the use of ADDIE (Analysis, Design, Development, Implementation, and Evaluation) for building the instruction curriculum of the skills of intubation. The majority of the planning time should be spent on the Needs Analysis and Design. The Learning Objectives, prepared during the Design phase, should be written as Objective Observable Behaviors, which can then serve as the assessments for Evaluation. The content includes two examples of the application of ADDIE: firstly a task that requires a large cognitive component and where simulators and mannequins are readily available. Secondly, a task that requires a high level of psychomotor skills where suitably realistic mannequins are not available, and virtual reality needs to be used as an additional educational modality.

Chapter 6
The Nurse Educator's Role in Designing Instruction and Instructional Strategies for Academic and Clinical Settings 133
Patricia J. Slagter van Tryon, East Carolina University, USA

Nursing education programs seeking to equip graduates with needed tools to integrate medical expertise with experience in the systematic design of instruction have the opportunity to better ensure positive learning outcomes in varied settings as graduates take on their new roles as nurse educators. The learning environment of the nurse educator is complex yet with skill in the reasoned approach to the design of instruction can progress into more knowable contexts for which to problem solve. Nurse educators possessing interdisciplinary skills in their field facilitated by expertise in instructional design will enhance their practice by developing and delivering precision instruction.

Chapter 7
Online Applied Learning in Nursing Education 150
Beth Oyarzun, University of North Carolina – Wilmington, USA
Elizabeth A. Gazza, University of North Carolina – Wilmington, USA

The instructional design process, Analyze, Design, Develop, Implement, and Evaluate (ADDIE), along with a pedagogical approach was applied to the design and implementation of an online applied learning activity. The activity was delivered in an accelerated nursing leadership asynchronous online course within the fully online RN-BSN program at the University of North Carolina Wilmington (UNCW). Research associated with online applied and experiential learning, particularly in the area of nursing education, that guided the design is presented. The design process and the evaluation results are discussed with future implications.

Chapter 8
Teaching Residents How to Teach 164
Heidi Kromrei, Detroit Medical Center, USA
William L. Solomonson, Oakland University, USA
Mark S. Juzych, Wayne State University, USA

In this chapter, the context of medical education is reviewed in terms of how to teach in the health care setting, commonly used instructional strategies, and the clinical learning environments of the medical student and resident trainees. Although accreditation bodies require residents to teach, and it is an activity that is assigned, it is often not delivered by the sponsoring institution. Key terms in education, learning theories, and instructional strategies are presented. In particular, strategies for medical educators to prepare residents to teach effectively in their residency program are provided. Finally, an instructional development plan for residents, with supporting worksheets and examples, is presented.

Chapter 9
Interprofessional Education 186
Rebecca Moote, Regis University, USA

Interprofessional education (IPE) is recognized as an important component in the education of healthcare students. The goal of bringing students together to learn with, from, and about each other is to ultimately impact collaborative practice and improve patient care. Over the last 20 years there has been increased focus on the design and implementation of IPE experiences. Several IPE collaborative organizations and IPE centers have been formed to provide evidence-based recommendations and guidelines. Strategies have been created for designing and implementing high quality IPE activities, developing faculty in IPE, overcoming student stereotypes, determining assessment strategies, and identifying barriers to IPE. This chapter will focus on each of these elements and provide specific recommendations on how to create and implement IPE that improves student learning.

Chapter 10
Introducing Collaborative Care: Teaching Basics of Interprofessional Education in an Online Environment 208
Joy Doll, Creighton University, USA
Anna Maio, Creighton University, USA
Ann Ryan Haddad, Creighton University, USA
Margaret Jergenson, Creighton University, USA
Karen A. Paschal, Creighton University, USA
Katie Packard, Creighton University, USA
Meghan Potthoff, Creighton University, USA
Kathryn N. Huggett, University of Vermont, USA
Martha Todd, Creighton University, USA

This chapter describes the development and implementation of an innovative course in interprofessional education (IPE), which ensures a large number and variety of health professions students have the appropriate foundations to collaborate. A description of the institution and the process of implementing interprofessional education is followed by a presentation of challenges and then solutions to address them in the creation of the course. Future research avenues in interprofessional education will be explored. This chapter will provide practical application of concepts for other institutions attempting to design and implement introductory interprofessional education for large numbers of students.

Chapter 11
Informal Learning in Medical Education 225
Misa Mi, Oakland University William Beaumont School of Medicine, USA

A great deal of valuable learning—informal learning—takes place within medicine's informal and hidden curriculum. It is this kind of informal learning that brings about more diverse and personal learning gains. Informal learning contributes to individuals' continuing professional development, personal mastery, and capacity building. Recognition of informal learning can be the key to the development of a strong lifelong learning orientation for learners as they go through the process of developing and forming their professional identity. Expanded insights into the informal learning process will contribute to the design and development of strategies, methods, and informal learning spaces that promote a broader spectrum of human learning within formal medical education settings. It is hoped that discussion on informal learning will also stimulate interest in investigating the impact of informal learning on learners across the spectrum of medical education.

Chapter 12
Virtual Patients in Health Professions Education 245
A. J. Kleinheksel, Shadow Health, Inc., USA

The field of health professions continues to struggle with the impact of increasing practitioner and educator shortages. Health professions education is also faced with the issues of limited clinical placements and an increasing demand for online education. To address these issues, health professions educators have increasingly turned to simulations to provide experiential learning in safe, controlled environments. One of the newest simulation technology innovations to emerge is that of virtual patient simulations. This chapter reviews the context in which virtual patients have emerged, the range of virtual patient technologies available, and the ways in which health professions educators currently use virtual patient simulations.

Chapter 13
Development and Evaluation of Neuroscience Computer-Based Modules for Medical Students: Instructional Design Principles and Effectiveness 262
Kathryn L. Lovell, Michigan State University, USA

Interactive neuropathology computer-based teaching modules and other neuroscience computer-based resources were developed to provide individualized self-paced content information accompanied by images and self-assessment questions with feedback, along with problem-solving cases to facilitate application of neuroanatomy, neurology, and neuropathology concepts to patient cases. Initial implementation occurred in three curricula for second-year medical students. Evaluation of the modules was conducted using quantitative and qualitative methods to determine features of the modules that were important for students. This chapter will describe the instructional design principles that evaluation results identified as important and effective for student learning, and compare those to current principles for effective multimedia instructional design identified in a variety of research. Especially important principles applied in the neuroscience modules included cognitive load theory, retrieval practice and self-assessment, feedback, and learner control.

Chapter 14
Faculty Development for Clinical Educators: A Competency Model for Continuous Improvement 277
Silvia Lizett Olivares Olivares, Tecnologico de Monterrey School of Medicine, Mexico
Mildred Vanessa López Cabrera, Tecnológico de Monterrey School of Medicine, Mexico
Martha Ruth Loyola Segura, Tecnologico de Monterrey School of Medicine, Mexico
Jorge Eugenio Valdez García, Tecnologico de Monterrey School of Medicine, Mexico

Since the Flexner report in the 20th century, teaching and learning process has evolved through: science learning, problem based learning, competency based learning and perspective learning. This evolution provides a consensus that educators need to develop competencies in their students to prepare them for an uncertain future. Competency refers not only to core knowledge or instrumental skills, but to interpersonal and systemic abilities required for lifelong learning. This transformation requires changes in both the educational model and faculty development programs. Previous research and proposals have defined important qualities and attributes; for clinical educators. The Faculty Development program presented here has been assessed with a mixed multiphase approach for continuous improvement process: 1) assessment of proposal, 2) assessment of implementation, 3) assessment of faculty experiences and 4) institutionalization of program. Results from this experience are presented, as well as other further challenges on this initiative.

Compilation of References 301

About the Contributors 339

Index 346

Preface

Technological innovations are changing the way education is delivered. With instructional media evolving at an exponential pace, instructional designers and educators have a variety of options when deciding what tools are best for delivering their instruction. Many healthcare programs and professional fields are increasing their instructional programming efforts to enhance faculty development and meet rising accreditation standards. Medical educators are responsible for creating instruction for a variety of learning audiences, managing the logistics involved with interprofessional team training and ensuring performance improvement across the healthcare system. Technological innovations now require educators to deliver instruction across a variety of platforms beyond the traditional classroom and include distance, mobile, and simulated learning environments. Regardless of the platform, it is imperative that educators adhere to sound instructional design principles in order to yield optimal learning outcomes.

"Instructional design is the science and art of creating detailed specifications for the development, evaluation, and maintenance of situations which facilitate learning and performance" (Richey, Klein, & Tracey, 2011, p. 3). The premise of this book is to provide individuals who work in the area of medical education with an instructional book that can serve as a tool kit for developing instruction in healthcare environments. The book covers topics related to conducting a needs assessment, analyzing performance, instructional theory, developing instructional materials, and tips for managing instructional projects. To date, there are very few resources that have addressed the foundational knowledge associated with instructional design for the field of medical education.

Topics addressed within the chapters include the following:

- Instructional theory.
- Performance analysis.
- Instructional strategies and sequencing.
- Informal learning.
- Online learning strategies.
- Medical simulation.
- Virtual patients.
- Instructional management.
- Interprofessional education.
- Noninstructional interventions.
- Faculty development.

BOOK OBJECTIVE

The overall mission of this book is to provide medical educators, who are involved with designing and delivering instructional to health care professionals, with an instructional design book that can provide them with the foundational knowledge needed to design effective instruction for a variety of audiences and learning contexts. This book includes 14 chapters from instructional design experts and medical educators and professionals who are responsible for delivering instruction to a variety of learners in the health care field. Each chapter highlights learning theory, instructional strategies, and suggestions for ensuring a successful implementation.

To date, there is increasing attention placed on curricular programs in health care at the undergraduate, graduate, and continuing medical education levels. While medical institutions are beginning to hire instructional designers and medical educators to ensure adherence to instructional design principles, many medical educators have been appointed to lead instructional interventions based on their subject-matter expertise. Few have received formal instructional relative to designing instruction. In order to maintain accreditation, many medical institutions are required to provide documentation on a regular basis of the various types of curricular projects they are embarking on as well as any scholarly activity/research that is emerging out of their organizations. This book provides individuals with the necessary foundational knowledge to design and implement sound instructional programs in the medical field.

AUDIENCE

The target audience for this book consists of educators, physicians, nurses, and allied health professionals who are responsible for designing instructional activities. Many of these educators have not had any formal training in pedagogy or instructional design. This book is intended to serve as a toolkit to aid them with curriculum development and to align activities with their desired learning objectives. Chapters in this book have been written to provide contextual examples for a variety of health care disciplines. Emphasis is placed on learning theory, instructional design principles, instructional strategies, and evaluative methods. In addition, authors have carefully identified challenges and constraints faced while implementing various instructional practices due to the unique nuances of health care.

ORGANIZATION

This book contains 14 chapters that span across a variety of health care disciplines including medical education, nursing, and allied health. Topics range from pedagogical strategies employed to teach a variety of different tasks, both procedural and cognitive. Each chapter presents strategies for how instructional design principles can be applied to achieve learning outcomes and facilitate improved performance. In addition to the emphasis on instructional theory, the chapters provide information for, how to integrate multimedia tools and technology to leverage desired learning goals and outcomes. Examples of technological integrations include, but are not limited to medical simulation, in situ simulation, task trainers, virtual patients, social media, and online learning applications.

Chapter 1 provides a detailed account of how to conduct a learner analysis With the multitude of technological tools and mediums to develop instructional design, health care educators can easily lose sight of the learner. Recognizing that learners vary considerably, a complete understanding of the target learning audience is a crucial step in developing and delivering quality instruction. Neglecting to understand or anticipate the educational needs of students can result in ineffective instruction and ultimately poor learning outcomes. This chapter will discuss the rationale for conducting a learner analysis, explore key learner characteristics, and examine the implications these characteristics may have on developing and teaching a course. Strategies for conducting a learner analysis are also provided.

Chapter 2 provides a rich account of how to sequence instruction with appropriate instructional strategies. Emphasis is placed on taking a systematic and systemic approach to instructional design. The authors provide an overview of learning and instructional theory and demonstrate alignment among various instructional strategies. Heuristics are provided to assist educators with delivering instruction using a variety of different methods. In addition to overview of several different types of instructional strategies, the authors explain the necessity of appropriate sequencing of instruction. An overview is provided in terms how elaboration theory can be applied to any learning environment to provide learners with the necessary scaffolded support to improve their clinical performance.

Chapter 3 provides a rich account of how backward design can be applied to develop competency-based medical education. Health care professionals and trainees across many disciplines are tasked with mastering a large number of professional competencies in a relatively short about of time. Due to the nature of health education, many of these competencies require learners to synthesize a lot of information to solve complex patient problems. Backward Design is an instructional design model that proposes instructors start with outcomes and work backward to design appropriate assessment tools and curricular content. Adapted from K-12 learning environments, this model tasks educators to sequence instruction in a particular way that begins with the end in mind. This allows students to gain a better understanding of the content and the desired learning outcomes so that they can strategize ways to arrive at the particular learning goal. Backward design can be applied to medical education by beginning with the national standards or competencies for medical education, defining outcomes and assessment methods, and then defining curricular content.

This chapter will cover the history of competency-based medical education in the United States. Examples of how the backward design model can be applied in clinical settings will also be discussed. The chapter will culminate with a discussion of creating action plans for individual programs to align assessment and outcome measures more directly to curriculum.

Chapter 4 moves us into the use of various instructional media and technology that can be used to enhance learning outcomes. During this past decade, there has been continuous emphasis placed on integrating medical simulation into health education curricula. Medical simulation presents many advantages to the traditional methods of clinical teaching in that it provides learners with an opportunity to learn and practice new skills in a safe environment, whilst protecting the patient. Medical simulation environments can be designed to reach a variety of fidelity levels to meet desired learning outcomes. The authors provide us with an overview of the various types of medical simulation tools available for health education, advantages and disadvantages with various simulated learning environments, and instructional strategies for delivering and facilitating simulated learning activities. Strategies are also provided to assist educators with identifying opportunities to leverage the learning experience by aligning simulated learning activities with sound instructional design principles.

Chapter 5 continues the discussion of how medical simulation can be used to enhance learning in the health professions. The authors provide a detailed account of how worked examples can be woven into the instructional design of clinical learning exercises to provide a scaffolded approach to instruction. The chapter provides a variety of examples to demonstrate how health educators can use worked examples to teach a variety of clinical competencies. Emphasis is placed on using a scaffolded approach to sequence and deliver instruction. Specific attention is placed on communicating the need for educators to anticipate challenges that their learners often face when tasked with learning new clinical procedures. The worked example approach allows educators to gradually increase the level of complexity when teaching new concepts.

Chapter 6 shifts the focus to instructional design considerations for the nurse educator. While many nurse educator programs include course work in curriculum development, it is important to note that curriculum development is not synonymous with instructional design. The design of instruction is a systematic approach to the development of instruction and instructional materials focused on solving educational problems where a reasoned assessment of the need for the instruction is determined up front and the evaluation of the instruction is precisely aligned with the assessment of learning outcomes. To support nurse educators in their design efforts, this chapter aligns a concise guide for an integration of principles from the field of instructional design to scaffold the core competencies for nurse educators in the realm of curriculum development.

Chapter 7 continues the discussion of nursing education as it relates to designing applied online learning experiences. While the context discussed in the chapter is on nursing, the instructional strategies discussed for designing and facilitating interactive online learning experiences can be applied to any health care discipline. Emphasis is placed on designing learning activities that promote interaction between the learner and the content, the learner and instructor, and the learner with their fellow peers. The authors provide insights as to how students can apply what they are learning when faculty are not physically present to assess their application of skills. Using a case study approach, the chapter includes a description of a theory-based pedagogical approach and the instructional design process that integrated applied learning experiences into an accelerated online asynchronous course in an RN-BSN program.

Chapter 8 shifts focus to training resident physicians how to teach. Medical education has embraced the use of peer coaching and mentoring throughout the post-graduate training experience. A core task of residency is to teach medical students as well as patients, families, students, and other health professionals. To this end, foundational concepts, instructional models, and instructional strategies for use in a residency teaching setting are presented. The authors provide medical educators, such as program directors, faculty, and chief residents, with basic instructional frameworks and tools to develop the teaching competencies of residents. Strategies are also provided to assist with reviewing the contextual setting of medical education, recognizing effective instructional strategies, and developing or assisting in the development of a plan that prepares resident physicians to teach.

Chapter 9 explores the instructional implications associated with interprofessional education. Continued emphasis has been placed on providing learning opportunities for different health care professionals to train together. A highly recognized performance challenge faced by many healthcare institutions involves team training. Most health care professionals are trained within their discipline with very little interaction with trainees outside of their field. Upon graduation, they are then expected to be able to perform their clinical tasks in a team-based setting. When designing interprofessional instructional activities, instructors must consideration several factors: the various disciplines involved, the unique nuances associated with each discipline, medical topics, and how to integrate with established curricula. This chapter provides an overview of different teaching frameworks that promote interprofessional education as well as suggestions for how these can be applied to different health scenarios and contexts.

Chapter 10 continues the discussion of interprofessional education and the impact that it can have on the quality of patient care. The authors present a case study highlighting how an online course was developed to promote interprofessional education and collaborative practice to a large number of learners from across multiple professions. Contextual factors are identified and discussed in terms of the influence they have on the design of interprofessional education. Challenges to consider when training learners across multiple disciplines are also discussed in addition to instructional strategies that can be used to design a meaningful learning experience for all involved. Emphasis is placed on planning and project management as it relates to facilitating interprofessional education and coordinating project logistics when working with multiple disciplines.

Chapter 11 shifts the focus to take into consideration various instructional strategies and opportunities that can be presented to learners within informal learning environments. While a lot of health education is formalized in terms of delivery and assessment, a lot of learning takes place ongoing. This chapter identifies various instructional frameworks as they relate to informal learning in medical education as well as strategies to identify and assess these learning experiences. Recognizing informal learning and creating a culture for the organizational learning that embraces informal learning will likely develop an enabling condition for developing master or expert lifelong learners who engage in continuing professional development and professional socialization. Specific examples of informal learning experiences as they relate to teaching evidence-based medicine are provided. In addition, contextual factors are also discussed to assist educators with providing the necessary support to learners during these learning opportunities.

Chapter 12 explores the use of virtual patients and the impact they can have on the learning experience. The purpose of this chapter is to document the emergence of virtual patient simulation in health professions education, and to define the range of technologies within this category of clinical simulation. Varying levels of fidelity are discussed and aligned with instructional design principles. Emphasis is placed on assisting educators with the ability to determine the needs and justification related to incorporating virtual patients into a health discipline curriculum. Examples of how virtual patients have been incorporated in various clinical disciplines are also discussed.

Chapter 13 expands on the discussion pertaining to self-paced instruction in an online learning environmental. The author provides an overview of how a curriculum can be developed to provide individualized, self-paced content information accompanied by images and self-testing questions with feedback, along with problem-solving cases to facilitate application of clinical concepts. Emphasis is placed on the design and development aspects of instructional design with careful consideration given to produce instruction, conducting usability tests to determine student perceptions of technical and instructional effectiveness, and revisions based on student input. Additional discussion is provided to align scaffolding techniques for instructional sequencing with multimedia and message design principles.

Chapter 14 provides an overview of competency models that can assist with facilitating faculty development programs within healthcare institutions. The authors explore various instructional strategies that can be used to prepare clinical faculty with the ability to use innovative pedagogical tools in their daily practice. Specific attention is given to contextual factors that support or hinder faculty acceptance and performance as it relates to integrating instructional design practices.

CLOSING REMARKS

Healthcare institutions and medical professionals are in a never-ending search to improve performance and improve the delivery of patient care. With the unique contextual factors associated with many health professions, it is important that educators are equipped with the necessary pedagogical tools to facilitate learning. This book focuses on the design of instructional solutions, grounded in learning theory, to deliver instruction to a variety of learners using different learning platforms such as face-to-face, blended, synchronous and asynchronous online instruction. Additional insights are also provided to address the noninstructional strategies needed to support the delivery and sustainability of instructional interventions.

Jill E. Stefaniak
Old Dominion University, USA

REFERENCES

Richey, R. C., Klein, J. D., & Tracey, M. W. (2011). *The instructional design knowledge base: Theory, research, and practice*. New York: Routledge.

Chapter 1
Understanding Your Learner:
Conducting a Learner Analysis

Tina M. Souders
University of North Carolina at Chapel Hill, USA

ABSTRACT

Now more than ever before, health care educators are being challenged to meet the complex and dynamic needs of an expanding health care workforce. Continuing education requirements as well as graduate and undergraduate programs are striving to keep pace with the demands for more highly skilled health care professionals. Likewise, technology and related instructional media have been evolving at an exponential pace. The confluence of these variables requires health care educators to be knowledgeable about the options and tools available to design and deliver instruction using a variety of platforms in more diverse settings. In order to ensure that instruction achieves its intended goals, it is imperative to fully assess the learner characteristics of the target audience. The purpose of this chapter is to discuss the rationale for conducting a learner analysis and utilizing learner characteristics in designing effective instruction.

INTRODUCTION

Healthcare professionals recognize that in order to provide quality medical care to patients, thorough and ongoing patient assessments are required. A complete patient history, along with an appraisal of current symptoms is necessary before diagnosis and treatment can occur. Similarly, counselors and therapists must first conduct a comprehensive mental health and substance use assessment with each client before determining the most effective treatment approach. Likewise, health care educators must assess and understand the unique characteristics of learners in order to design, develop, and deliver quality instruction. As we know, students enter the health care profession for a multitude of reasons and at dissimilar phases in their professional careers. Some adults return to school after many years of professional practice in an effort to acquire advanced skills, while others may be novices to the health care field. In either case, it is clear that learner populations vary considerably, yet most instructional faculty fail to assess the relevant characteristics of the target learning audience. Neglecting to understand or anticipate the educational needs of students can result in ineffective instruction and ultimately poor

DOI: 10.4018/978-1-5225-2098-6.ch001

Copyright © 2017, IGI Global. Copying or distributing in print or electronic forms without written permission of IGI Global is prohibited.

learning outcomes for students. Therefore, a complete understanding the target learning audience is a crucial step in developing and delivering quality instruction.

Conducting a comprehensive learner analysis is the most effective way to assess the plethora of learner variables that may affect instructional content and delivery. A learner analysis is a basic function of instructional development and results in specifications for effective and efficient instruction (Schwen, 1973). Considerations such as prior experience in the health care field, familiarity with technology, and motivation to learn are just a few of the many factors that may impact the development and delivery of instruction. Conducting a learner analysis should not be confused with assessing student learning styles. Research has consistently shown that learning style instruments are neither valid nor reliable (Dembo & Howard, 2007), thus, there is no evidence that matching instruction to learning preferences such as visual, auditory, or kinesthetic learners improves learning outcomes. In fact, a recent study of pre-clinical undergraduate medical students found learning preferences did not significantly contribute to improved learning outcomes and recommended strategies such as simulations and problem-based debates to promote deep and strategic learning (Liew, Sidhu, & Barua, 2015). Similarly, Cook (2012) noted that assessing prior knowledge and focusing on robust instructional methods are better options for influencing learning than attention to learning styles.

While a comprehensive learner analysis may be cost prohibitive or too time intensive for every course, attention to the most critical attributes of the target learning audience can significantly inform the design and delivery of a new or existing course. This chapter will discuss the rationale for conducting a learner analysis, explore key learner characteristics, and examine the implications these characteristics may have on developing and teaching a course.

BACKGROUND

Behavioral Learning Theory

The earliest theories of learning grew out of behavioral psychology. Behaviorism, as an educational learning theory, suggests that learning results in observable changes in behavior (Ertmer & Newby, 1993). Some of the most well-known behaviorists include Edward L. Thorndike, Ivan Pavlov, and B. F. Skinner. Their contributions to understanding learning focused on the observation of behavior and the predictable link between stimulus and response. Moreover, these early learning theorists argued that observing behavior was the most reliable way to research psychological and mental processes. Behaviorist theory posits that learners should be assessed prior to instruction in order to determine where instruction should begin (Ertmer & Newby, 1993). Limitations associated with behaviorism emerged in the late 1970s as researchers began to explore unobservable phenomena such as memory. As a result, a new theory of cognitive science, where memory, schema formation, and mental processes, was introduced and studied (Winn, 2004).

Cognitive Learning Theory

Cognitive theories of learning focus on how information is received, stored, retrieved, and transferred in memory (Sweller, 2008). From a cognitive perspective, learning is a change in knowledge. The learner is actively engaged in acquiring new knowledge and using that new knowledge to form internal mental structures that build on prior knowledge. An essential component of cognitivism is how the learner links existing knowledge with new knowledge and the ability to encode, store, and retrieve this knowledge when needed (Martinez, 2010). Short-term, working, and long-term memory are key components to learning. Cognitive theories of learning stress the need to make knowledge meaningful to the learner so that the learner can relate new knowledge to existing knowledge, making it harder to forget, and easier to recall and recode with new meaning (Sweller, van Merrienboer, & Paas, 1998). In order to facilitate this process, the learning environment should encourage frequent recall of prior knowledge, abilities, and skills among learners. Cognitivists explore learner characteristics in an effort to determine how to activate, maintain, and direct learning as well as how to structure, organize, and sequence material to facilitate optimal processing (Ertmer & Newby, 1993).

Learner Characteristics and Instruction

As these theories of learning evolved over the last century so did the notion that not all learners were alike. The origins of assessing individuals in order to develop instruction for a specific target audience dates back to World War II when educators and psychologists assessed military trainees in order to select individuals who would most benefit from specific training programs (Reiser, 2001). In an effort to improve the completion rate of a flight training program, psychologists assessed individuals who were able to perform the required skills and developed tests that would measure the necessary traits, such as intellectual ability, psychomotor skills, and perceptual skills (Reiser, 2001). These tests identified acceptable candidates for the flight training program and referred other candidates to more appropriate training programs.

In 1949, Ralph Tyler noted the importance of student specific information when formulating learning objectives and outcomes (Parks, 2010). Tyler noted that information about student's interests and needs was critical to identifying learning experiences that would be most effective for learning outcomes. Information about student's prior knowledge and level of development was fundamental to creating satisfying learning experiences for students.

In 1963, John B. Carroll proposed a model of learning that highlighted five major variables and three of them, (1) perseverance, (2) aptitude, and (3) ability, were specifically related to student characteristics (Carroll, 1989). According to Carroll (1989), perseverance refers to the amount of time a student may be willing to spend on a learning task and is often associated with student motivation for learning. Aptitude refers to the amount of time it may take a student to master the content or instruction. Thus, students with high aptitude may require less time to learn or complete a task as compared to students with low aptitude. Finally, the ability to understand instruction refers to the student's general intelligence, language comprehension, and verbal ability.

Jerome Bruner's views on culture added yet another dimension to the importance of learner characteristics (Takaya, 2008). Bruner specifically noted that student predispositions to learning greatly impact the desire to learn. Factors such as motivation to learn, cultivation of a learning culture, and individual learner traits significantly influence the learning process.

Benjamin Bloom examined the importance of learner characteristics in the mid 1970's. He noted that learner characteristics, such as cognitive and affective entry behaviors, would have an effect on whether a student was able to master the objectives of a learning task (Bloom, 1976). Cognitive entry characteristics, such as prerequisite knowledge and skills related to the instructional content, influence the level and rate of learning. Affective entry behaviors, such as attitudes toward school or learning, are equally important because these impact a student's desire to learn, general interest in the material, and self-confidence in mastering course content.

Malcolm Knowles introduced the concept of andragogy (Knowles, 1970). According to Knowles, andragogy is the theory and practice of teaching adults, and it differs from pedagogy, the theory and practice of teaching children. Knowles emphasized the connection between learner characteristics and the learning process and noted that these characteristics play a major role in adult learning experiences (Carpenter-Aeby & Aeby, 2013). Successful application of adult learning principles can result in collaborative learning opportunities, mutual negotiation, and planning between teacher and students, as well as the use of student prior life and work experiences to enrich the learning environment (Carpenter-Aeby & Aeby, 2013).

Today, researchers and instructional designers devote considerable attention to the assessment of learner characteristics and its importance toward developing effective instruction. Dick, Carey, and Carey (2015) target eight specific areas when conducting a learner analysis. These include assessing the learner's

1. Entry skills,
2. Prior knowledge,
3. Attitudes toward content and delivery system,
4. Academic motivation,
5. Educational and ability levels,
6. General learning preferences,
7. Attitudes toward the organization providing the instruction, and
8. Group characteristics.

Likewise, Morrison, Ross, Kalman, and Kemp (2013) identified eight types of learner characteristics. Many of these characteristics are similar however; Morrison et al. (2013) also suggest considerations such as gender and age, learning styles, academic performance, personal and social characteristics, culture, and disabilities. As these instructional design experts have highlighted, conducting a learner analysis, in an effort to better understanding the target audience, is an essential step in developing and delivering instruction that optimizes student learning outcomes.

FOCUS OF THE CHAPTER

The focus of the chapter is to provide health care educators with a basic understanding of the rationale for conducting a learner analysis and the implications of specific learner characteristics when developing and delivering instruction. A simple approach to conducting a learner analysis will be introduced based on the six key questions. For the learner analysis, the six key questions are:

- Who are my learners?
- What prior experiences and knowledge do my learners possess?
- When will the instruction occur?
- Where will the instruction be delivered?
- How will learners be expected to use the material?
- Why is the learning important?

These six key questions and related learner characteristics, along with methods for assessing the characteristics, and strategies for course design and delivery will be discussed in this chapter.

Rationale for Conducting a Learner Analysis

Students interested in the health care profession enter the educational arena with a wide variety of backgrounds, prior learning experiences, diverse levels of expertise in the field, and so forth. Moreover, educational programs in the health care field vary dramatically in terms of the size of the classroom to the delivery method of instruction. Conducting a learner analysis is a critical step in course development and delivery because it clarifies the target audience, including prior knowledge about the topic as well as attitudes toward learning. Attention to these learner characteristics ensures that the selection of content and instructional strategies are most appropriate for the learning audience, much like conducting a patient assessment before determining a diagnosis and treatment plan. Although there are a vast number of traits that differentiate learners from one another, attention to the most relevant characteristics is a feasible and necessary task.

The primary goal of conducting a learner analysis is to aid in the identification of essential instructional content based on the unique characteristics of the learners (Schwen, 1973). Consider the individuality of students entering a course of study or certificate program. Some students may begin the program directly after completing undergraduate studies, while some may have worked professionally for several years before deciding to return to school to earn advanced degrees. Yet others may be making a significant career change later in life. Each type of student described above will enter the educational system with considerable differences in age, health, motivation, and even anxiety about continued schooling. There will also be substantial differences in prior knowledge, expertise with using technology in an educational setting, and the ability to work cooperatively with others. Assessing and understanding these differences can help inform the selection of course content as well as the structure and pacing of course materials and assignments. Decisions regarding the number and complexity of examples provided, the amount of time devoted to instruction, and the type of feedback given to learners are all related to the unique characteristics of the target audience. Without a thorough analysis of learner characteristics, educators may develop and deliver instruction that is ultimately ineffective or inefficient for the specific learning audience.

SOLUTIONS AND RECOMMENDATIONS

The breadth and depth of the learner analysis may vary depending on a multitude of factors including available time and resources to conduct the analysis. Ideally, the scope of the learner analysis should be broad and comprehensive, yet this is not always feasible. Minimally, a learner analysis should reveal important considerations about the learning audience, prior knowledge and skills, along with learner goals and motivation.

A simple, yet usable framework from which to conduct the learner analysis harkens back to the information gathering questions learned early in our academic careers. Asking six basic questions about learners will yield useful information about the target audience that will aid in developing and delivering instruction. These six questions are:

- Who are my learners?
- What prior experiences and knowledge do my learners possess?
- When will the instruction occur?
- Where (or in what setting) will the instruction be delivered?
- How will learners be expected to use the material?
- Why is the content important to the learners?

Who Are My Learners?

One of the most important considerations in developing instructional material for health care professionals is having a thorough understanding of the target audience. Gaining basic demographic information about learners and detailed knowledge about the learner's social, psychological, and affective characteristics is critical to understanding the target learning audience but also ensures that instruction is relevant to the learners.

Demographic Characteristics

Demographic characteristics such as age, gender, socio-economic status, preferred language, and culture/ethnicity are key factors in understanding the learning audience (Rogers, Graham, & Mayes, 2007). Today's learners reflect increasingly diverse characteristics and educators should attend to these differences in the learning environment (Yukselturk & Top, 2013). Having this information will lead to the selection and use of relevant examples or case studies in the classroom. Furthermore, learners enter the educational system with varying levels of reading, writing, and general academic abilities.

Armed with a better understanding of the current skill level of students, instructors can determine the amount of reading, length of assignments, and the type of feedback students may need in order to grasp the content completely. Furthermore, students with previously diagnosed disabilities may require alternative testing formats, adaptive technologies, or tutoring services in order to participate in the educational environment. Demographic information is typically available through an academic department or college as well as through general admissions material. Reviewing this material in advance of instruction allows instructors to modify course materials to include relevant and culturally diverse examples and activities.

Social Characteristics

Social characteristics include considerations related to relationships learners have toward their peers and may include whether learners prefer to work collaboratively or competitively with one another. In general, collaborative learners tend to divide work among group members and collectively contribute to the end product (Arnold, Ducate, & Kost, 2012). Competitive learners, on the other hand, are more individually motivated and may be willing to stretch beyond their own expected potential (Sheridan & Williams, 2011). An example of how this impacts course design may prove informative. Suppose you are developing a course that requires learners to work in small groups to analyze a complex case study. Learners who prefer a more competitive educational environment may not fully engage with the material or their peers as compared to learners who thrive in a more cooperative situation. Individuals who are motivated by competition may be more strategic in group decision making activities and even withhold information for individual gain (Toma & Butera, 2015).

Knowing the social characteristics of the target audience, both individually and as a group, can help inform decisions related to classroom activities and course projects. Instructors can assess social characteristics such as preferences for cooperation or competition through a short survey of learner preferences or by careful attention to the dialogue that occurs in the classroom.

Depending on the course of study, students may enter a classroom with pre-existing relationships with one another as a result of taking previous classes together. These prior relationships can influence small group work or other aspects of course delivery, in both positive and negative ways. Establishing classroom rules may be necessary to effectively process activities or discuss sensitive topics. Instructors can establish rules on the first day of class by actively engaging students in discussions regarding the behavioral and social expectations of the classroom. These classroom rules may include how students behave toward one another, how group decisions are made, whether cell phones or other electronic devices should be used, and how to share discussion time so all classmates can participate. Agreed upon classroom rules can be recorded and referenced throughout the semester.

It is critical to remember that learning does not end at the classroom doors. Attention to the informal connections students make outside the classroom can have a significant impact on learning. A study exploring the importance of social networks among first year medical students found that informal social interaction, such as what occurs in collaborative learning assignments, significantly increased student learning (Hommes et al., 2012). Outside of the classroom, students frequently seek each other out for advice, help with completing assignments, or to form study groups, and these encounters provide opportunities for learners to reflect on their thoughts and experiences. These interactions contribute to peer collaboration and informal learning. Implications from this research suggests that instructors may want to increase the frequency in which learners work in small groups and refrain from frequently changing student group membership to strengthen collaborative relationships.

Psychological and Affective Characteristics

In addition to social characteristics, instructors should also consider psychological and affective characteristics of learners. Psychological characteristics may include students' ability to tolerate ambiguity and take risks. For instance, using the Socratic Method (asking and answering questions to stimulate critical thinking) may cause great anxiety for some students, but others may relish the opportunity to engage the instructor in this manner. Similarly, a problem or assignment that does not come with one correct solution may frustrate a learner who is less comfortable with uncertainty. One way instructors can assess psychological characteristics is by simply asking students to describe a previous, positive or negative learning experience and how that experience did or did not meet their learning needs. Thoughtful attention to the psychological characteristics of learners can enhance classroom discussions, lead to more productive group assignments, and increase successful learning experiences.

Affective characteristics such as student attitudes toward the subject matter and their beliefs about learning can influence the design and delivery of a course (De La Harpe & Radloff, 2000). Students' preconceived attitudes about a course such as – it's too hard, I'll never use it, or why do we have to take this- can greatly influence the general atmosphere of the class and student success in the academic environment. Some students even believe that there is no way to learn or benefit from the material, regardless of instructor competence (Mangels, Butterfield, Lamb, Good, & Dweck, 2006). Instructors facing these types of challenges can build frequent success experiences throughout the course and provide positively framed feedback in order to boost student self-confidence and promote optimal learning (Mangels et al.,

2006). Instructors teaching a course for the first time may also want to consult with more veteran faculty regarding typical student opinions about the course as well as previous course evaluations for further insight into student experiences with the course.

Other Learner Characteristics

There are additional learner characteristics to consider when developing instruction for health care professionals. In a six-year longitudinal study, researchers found that conducting an inventory of student approaches to learning, such as study habits, use of logic, and intrinsic interest in the material, were important determinants of performance in medical school (Arnold & Feighny, 1995). Likewise, a more recent study explored learner characteristics that were associated with residents being placed on probation during their academic career (Guerrasio, Brooks, Rumack, Christensen, & Aagaard, 2016). The ten year study found that characteristics such as being married, not Caucasian, older, transferring from another graduate program, and having taken time off between medical school and residency were more likely to result in being placed on probation as compared to the control group (Guerrasio et al., 2016).

Other considerations regarding learner characteristics include the number of students within the target audience, the geographic location of the students, and student mobility issues. The number of students taking a particular class can greatly impact course design and overall instructor workload for the course. Designing a ten-person seminar class on medical ethics will differ greatly from a seventy plus introductory biology course delivered in a large auditorium. Likewise, the geographic location of the students and the chosen course delivery method should be considered. Some students may travel a great distance to attend a face-to-face classroom while others may be live near the institution. In the event of inclement weather or some other disruption to the educational process, will the content or delivery method change? Similarly, it is important to know whether students are located within the same time zone or whether students live in multiple time zones, such as may occur with an online or distance course. Armed with this knowledge, an instructor can circumvent unnecessary questions from students by noting the applicable time zone on assignment due dates and proactively addressing how disruptions to the class schedule will be handled.

In summary, conducting a learner analysis that includes basic information about the target audience is an important consideration when developing and delivering instructional material. Seeking information regarding the target audience's basic demographics, as well as social, psychological, and affective characteristics can improve the final educational product and enhance learning outcomes. Table 1 provides a summary of the learner characteristics discussed in this section along with suggestions for assessing the characteristics and strategies for instruction.

What Prior Experiences and Knowledge Do My Learners Possess?

Another critical aspect related to understanding the learner is determining the breadth and depth of prior knowledge and work experiences the learner has before entering the classroom. Adult learners, in particular, enter the educational environment with a plethora of life, educational, and other relevant experiences. It would be unwise and counterproductive to overlook the prior knowledge and experiences adults have accumulated before entering the classroom. In addition, instructors should also be cognizant of the specific entry behaviors and knowledge students need in order to be successful in the course so that any gaps in knowledge or experience can be adequately addressed.

Table 1. Who are my learners?

Characteristic or Attribute	Method for Assessing	Strategies for Instruction
Demographics such as age, gender, socio-economic status, preferred language, culture	Review admissions material or student records	Use relevant and culturally diverse case examples and activities
General academic abilities including reading and writing	• Review admissions material or student records • Conduct brief pre-test of reading and writing abilities	• Vary the amount and complexity of assigned readings to conform to academic abilities • Vary the length of assignments – may need to use shorter and more frequent assignments • Provide regular feedback to learners including specifics on areas of strength and weakness
Social characteristics such as learner tendencies toward cooperation, collaboration, and competition	Conduct a brief survey of learner preferences, such as preference for working in small groups or working independently	Select instructional methods or strategies that reflect student preferences (e.g. game versus group project)
Psychological and affective characteristics including risk taking and attitudes toward learning	Ask students to describe a previous learning experience that was positive and why it contributed to learning or a negative experience and why it did not contribute to learning	• Provide opportunities for students to engage with one another • Develop in-class activities that promote positive learning • Provide positive feedback when students take risks in class or on assignments
Other characteristics including class size and geographic location	• Review University or college records • Review enrollment statistics	• Instructor workload for large classes should be addressed including ability to provide timely feedback • Ensure adequate physical space for classroom activities • Prepare in advance for disruptions to class schedule

Prior Knowledge

It is essential to assess the degree of prior knowledge students have about the course content or topic area because creating learning activities that build on prior knowledge leads to improved learning outcomes (Ertmer & Newby, 1993). If students enter the classroom with gaps in their knowledge base, then it is necessary to either remediate the knowledge gaps within the course itself or refer students to other resources where they can independently fill the gap. Moreover, it is also important to assess whether their prior knowledge is accurate. Building new schema on inaccurate prior knowledge complicates the learning process. For example, a recent study examined the differences in disinfection protocols for root canal treatment between general dentists and endodontists (de Gregorio, Arias, Navarrete, Cisneros, & Cohenca, 2015).

Results showed that disinfection protocols differed between the two groups, in that general dentists used protocols learned during their initial training but endodontists incorporated recently published protocols into their practice. Thus, dental students who gained prior knowledge and experience by working alongside a general dentist may be acting on outdated and inaccurate information, requiring the instructor to provide supplemental information that remediates an inaccurate knowledge base.

Moreover, an analysis of student's prior knowledge may reveal substantial gaps in knowledge. In fact, most learners have limited abilities to identify and remediate their own knowledge gaps, requiring instructors and learners to share this responsibility (Schumacher, Englander, & Carraccio, 2013). If learning gaps exist, then additional decisions must be made regarding how to address these knowledge gaps. For critical content, it may be necessary to include the missing information in the course itself and even devote some portion of class time to the material. In other courses, it may be desirable to provide refresher opportunities outside of classroom time. In either case, instructors should create a culture of safety in the classroom so that students and instructors can work as partners to address and remediate knowledge and skill deficits as well as attend to the reciprocal impact each has on the learning environment (Schumacher et al., 2013).

Attention to key learner attributes, such as prior knowledge and experience, can be used to activate learning as well. Advance organizers set the stage for upcoming learning and may include a preview of an upcoming lesson or an outline of the main points at the beginning of a new unit of instruction. The use of relevant examples that build on previous learning should be employed whenever feasible. In health care education particularly, the use of example based learning can improve learner's ability to organize and access information (Dyer et al., 2015). Additional strategies that build on the use of prior knowledge include outlines, analogies, and concept maps. Concept maps are graphic representations of knowledge that are used to explain relationships between concepts and help learners organize information. The use of concept maps have been shown to promote deep and meaningful learning (Dyer et al., 2015). Cutrer, Castro, Roy, and Turner (2012) found that using a concept map improved resident physician's ability to organize and integrate medical knowledge. Other learning strategies, such as elaboration and summaries, engage learners in actively processing information and facilitate meaningful learning as well (Grabowski, 2004).

Instructors should also consider the learner's ability to handle the volume and complexity of the material presented. New information ought to challenge learners, but it should not exceed their capacity to comprehend the information. Cognitive load, the mental energy needed to think about and understand new information, should be monitored and reduced if too much new information is presented at one time (Schumacher et al., 2013). Furthermore, information about learner's prior knowledge should inform the level and type of feedback given throughout the course. In short, instructors should be able to assess prior knowledge with three basic questions: is it active, is it accurate, and is it sufficient.

In order to avoid excessive or unnecessary cognitive load, it is equally important to eliminate non-essential information, competing activities, or confusing explanations from the instruction (Sweller et al., 1998). Piloting a new or redesigned course with several students from the target audience and conducting formative evaluations throughout the course development process should address these issues (Morrison et al., 2013). Feedback from these processes will ultimately improve the course design and delivery. Lastly, chunking instruction into smaller units to reduce demand on working memory and creating bridges between new knowledge and existing schema can help students make the material meaningful (Martinez, 2010). These are but a few specific strategies that help structure, sequence, and organize prior knowledge for optimal learning.

Prior Experience

While it is critical to know the extent of prior knowledge students bring to the course, it is equally important to explore their prior work experiences. Some students may have many years of relevant health care experience while others may be changing careers and have no experience in the health care field at all. Consider this example. Suppose you are teaching a class on clinical assessment and diagnosis. You may encounter students with little to no previous experience working in a clinical health care setting. Contrast this with a student who has been actively involved in conducting clinical assessments as part of the treatment process and participated in treatment team meetings where clinical diagnoses have been discussed. A student with extensive work experience will perform differently than the student who has never set foot in a clinical setting, read an assessment, or even discussed a patient history. Thus, knowing the degree of prior work experience can aid in developing instructional materials that meet students where they are. Studies have repeatedly shown that novice learners benefit from different instructional methods and strategies than do expert learners. For example, Jordan et al. (2013) found a mismatch between the educational methods used to teach topics related to acute care with novice and expert learners. Novice learners benefited from didactic instruction in acute care topics, and the use of asynchronous instruction as a compliment to traditional classroom instruction, more so than expert learners (Jordan et al., 2013).

Assessing learners' prior knowledge and experience will ensure the instructional material is best suited for the specific learning audience. If all students enter the classroom with a high degree of relevant experience, the learning outcomes and instructional strategies should be constructed around these prior experiences to challenge learners beyond their current knowledge and skill level. On the other hand, if students lack prior experience and knowledge, the learning outcomes and instructional strategies should reflect that difference. In most settings, instructors will get a mixed group, in that some students will enter with some degree of relevant experience and others will not. In this case, the instructor should carefully craft the learning goals and instructional strategies to meet the needs of this varied group. One strategy to address a group of students exhibiting a range of prior knowledge and experience may include having students with expert knowledge serve as mentors or consultants to novice students.

Prior Technology Experience

Most higher education institutions utilize learning management systems or other more sophisticated means to manage course content. In an effort to be efficient and productive, adult learners want to easily access and navigate through course content. The course delivery method (covered later in this chapter) will impact the degree of technology sophistication learners must possess in order to be successful in the course. For course content delivered asynchronously, or for content that utilizes multiple media platforms, students must have current hardware and software capabilities to access the content reliably. Furthermore, for the less technologically sophisticated students, ongoing help and tutorial services should be readily available. Instructors can assess student's technology experience in several ways, including a skills demonstration or a brief survey regarding student proficiency with specific technologies.

Considering learner characteristics such as prior knowledge, prior experience, and attitudes toward technology can greatly influence the success of a course or training module. Instructors may need to engage in a variety of activities in order to assess prior knowledge and experience. Some of these activities may include pre-course testing on important concepts or knowledge related to course material, reviewing employment histories and work experiences of students, and surveying students' previous experience with technology and attitudes toward using it educationally. Table 2 provides a summary of the characteristics described in this section, along with methods for assessing the characteristics and strategies for instruction.

Table 2. What prior experiences and knowledge do my learners possess?

Characteristic or Attribute	Method for Assessing	Strategies for Instruction
Prior knowledge of learner including accuracy, gaps, and depth	• Conduct pre-course assessment of major course concepts or procedures • Ask students to write a brief reflection on prior learning experiences	• Develop supplemental learning material for knowledge gaps or include a course review • Use advance organizers and concept maps as scaffolding strategies for difficult material
Prior work experience	• Review employment history and work experience • Have students complete a brief survey of prior work experience	• Select instructional methods and strategies that benefit both novice and expert learners
Prior technology experience	• Conduct a survey of student experiences and proficiency with learning management systems and specific technologies • Conduct skill based assessment in class or online • Review help desk data regarding frequency of use	• Provide links to tutorials or help services • Test multimedia files before classes begin • Consult with Information Technology department for assistance as needed

When Will the Instruction Occur?

Another important factor when conducting a learner analysis is to consider when the instruction will occur, specifically in relation to the overall curriculum and sequencing of other required courses. Typically, sequencing of learning activities within a course is addressed during the design phase of instruction, but early attention to the broader issues related to the sequencing of a particular course within an entire curriculum can be very valuable. For example, a typical course of study for medical students includes medical school, internship, residency, fellowship, and board certification. Similarly, a Master's degree in Social Work requires students to complete coursework along with two field practicums, before seeking clinical licensure. The sequencing of coursework along with internships requires careful attention to how skills and knowledge are integrated from one course to the next. It is crucial that students grasp content from each course in the curriculum sequence. Problems can arise if courses are offered out of sequence or if a required course was not taken as a pre-requisite.

Similarly, the time span between course offerings must also be considered. In some cases, students may proceed immediately from one course to the next, without any lapse in time. In other cases, there may be significant gaps in time due to a student taking a leave of absence from the program or a course not being offered on a regular basis. Instructors may need to examine student transcripts in order to assess whether students completed pre-requisite courses and whether courses were sequenced properly within the curriculum. It is advisable to not only review the course syllabus along with required readings and assignments, but if possible, speak to other teaching faculty and practitioners in the field. This way, you will have more confidence that your assessment of pre-requisite knowledge and skills is accurate. Further, instructors should consult with other teaching faculty to review course outcomes. Periodic reviews ensure vertical and horizontal alignment with curriculum goals and course goals. Adjustments to both can be made as needed.

As we know, the health care field is changing rapidly. Educational goals and course content should be revised to align with these changes. Considering when a particular course is offered within a speci-

Table 3. When will the instruction occur?

Characteristic or Attribute	Method for Assessing	Strategies for Instruction
Sequence of courses in overall program curriculum	• Review curriculum handbook • Consult faculty, administrators, and practitioners in the field	• Identify pre-requisite content and material needed for course • Align course goals with curriculum goals
Time span between pre-requisite courses	• Review curriculum handbook • Review student transcripts (if accessible) or seek student feedback on when courses were taken	• Provide review of pre-requisite course content, if needed • Develop supplemental material for student reference as needed

fied curriculum as well as amount of time between courses can impact an instructor's ability to build on learner's prior knowledge and skills. In instances where students lack pre-requisite knowledge or a large time span between courses exists, supplemental material or course reviews may be required. Table 3 provides a summary of the characteristics and attributes described in this section, along with methods for assessment and strategies for instruction.

Where (Or in What Setting) Will the Instruction be Delivered?

Another consideration in conducting a learner analysis is where, or in what setting, the instruction will be delivered. The delivery method, whether it is synchronous or asynchronous, online or face-to-face, requires special attention to ensure it is available and accessible by all learners as well as ensuring it is the most effective and efficient delivery method. Factors such as the type of media used to convey course content, tools that foster socialization, platforms for accessing the material, and other support systems must be addressed.

Face-To-Face or Synchronous Instruction

For instruction that occurs in a face-to-face environment, the physical space where learning will occur must be evaluated. For example, in a CPR class, students will need adequate floor space for the inflatable manikins along with access to necessary protection and safety equipment such as kneel pads, face masks, and manikin wipes. In addition to considerations regarding the physical environment and necessary equipment, it is important to know whether students have ever worked in this type of simulated environment before. Students with physical disabilities or severe allergic reactions to synthetic materials may have difficulty performing the life-saving skills. Additional accommodations may effectively address these concerns, but only if the instructor gathers this information in advance of the class.

Similarly, suppose a small group, face-to-face seminar is the chosen delivery setting and method for a clinical studies course. In this instance, a large lecture style classroom with non-movable desks and chairs would be inappropriate and counterproductive for students to engage in small group discussion. On the other hand, a large, lecture style course delivered in a 200 seat auditorium would provide adequate physical space to comfortably accommodate a large number of students. In addition to the physical space, the use of technology to enhance learning and engage students should also be explored. Personal response systems or clickers to gauge student learning in real time may be effective with a large group, but will also require classroom technology that supports this. Furthermore, students must have the technological capability to effectively utilize advanced technology.

For instruction that occurs synchronously, but remotely, such as via web conferencing, interactive television, or other media, it is equally important to assess student familiarity with the learning platforms and determine whether necessary technology and/or supports to access the media are available. Nothing frustrates a student more than being ready for class to begin and not being able to log in. In addition, it would be appropriate to consider the technological sophistication of learners. For learners who lack experience or skill with an identified technology, training or remediation may be required before students are able to participate successfully using this type of delivery method. To address this issue, it may be advisable to create an introductory week to the course in an effort to address technological glitches or student fears regarding their competency in using the required technology.

Online or Asynchronous Instruction

A similar argument can be made for asynchronous or online instruction. Online learners must have the necessary knowledge and tools to utilize the online learning technologies. Some of the technology related skills that online learners must now possess include the ability to use search engines and browsers, download and install plugins to access multimedia content, and the ability to use synchronous and asynchronous communication tools for collaborative learning activities (Dabbagh & Bannan-Ritland, 2005). This simple, but necessary component of online learning is often overlooked when planning instruction. It is best to assume that learners do not have up to date computers or software, or may not even know how to update software without technical assistance. Access to tutorials and other technology supports should be readily available for all students.

Furthermore, when designing internet-based courses, it may be helpful to consider the learners thoughts and experiences about the use of technology in education. Prospective learners will want to know how the technology will increase their access to learning, save them money and time, or be a convenient and consistent way to receive instruction (Wong, Greenhalgh, & Pawson, 2010). There are many advantages to using instructional multimedia during a course or lesson, including the option to repeat instructional content as often as needed and student ability to control the pacing of the material (Smith, Cavanaugh, & Moore, 2011). More importantly, research supports higher cognitive level interactions among students who utilize instructional multimedia and students report a heightened sense of autonomy (Smith et al., 2011). Pedagogically sound course design is a key factor in Internet-based instruction. The fit between the learners' needs and priorities, along with the technical attributes of the Internet based course or use of multimedia, should be assessed and addressed during the design of instruction.

Self-Regulation

Asynchronous, online instruction is best accomplished with self-regulated and self-directed learners, that is, learners who are able to regulate and monitor their academic learning. In an online or asynchronous environment, learners must be able accurately assess their strengths and weaknesses and expend sufficient effort on tasks to ensure academic success. This self-directed approach to learning may be difficult for students who do not possess the skills, discipline, and responsibility to independently monitor their learning (Jordan et al., 2013).

Successful online learners are able to manage their own learning process, which is a critical skill for academic success (Zimmerman, 2002), and measuring learning characteristics, such as self-regulation, significantly informs course development and learning outcomes. While it may not be feasible for all students to complete a self-regulated learning inventory before each asynchronous class, it may be advisable for all students to complete one upon entering an online program. For example, Song, Kalet, and Plass (2011) developed the Self-Regulation Measure for Computer-based learning (SRMC) tool which was designed with medical students in mind. The SMRC categorizes ten types of self-regulatory behavior, including self-evaluation, organizing and transforming, goal setting and planning, seeking information, keeping records and monitoring, environmental structuring, self-consequences, rehearsing and memorizing, seeking social assistance, and reviewing records (Song, Kalet, & Plass, 2011).

The setting in which instruction is delivered is a critical factor to consider when planning and delivering instruction. Online learning affords a great deal of flexibility for students because the educational content can be accessed when it is convenient for the learner. To be successful, learners must have the technological and psychological ability to navigate this type of learning environment successfully. Synchronous and asynchronous instructional environments vary considerably and specific learner characteristics may influence individual success or failure in these different settings. Table 4 summarizes the characteristics and attributes discussed in this section, along with methods for assessment and strategies for instruction.

How Will Learners be Expected to Use the Information?

One of the most important goals of higher education is for students to not only perform well in the classroom, but to ensure that students are able to transfer what they have learned in the classroom to real world situations and problems. Both students and society invest much in the notion that classroom education will result in directly relevant skills in the work environment and lead to lifelong contributions as productive citizens. But how do educators promote both knowledge acquisition in the classroom and the transferability and application of that information to circumstances and events outside of the classroom?

By far the most common terminology used to describe transfer of learning is near and far transfer. *Near transfer* refers to the ability of a learner to apply previously learned knowledge in a similar or identical manner to how it was initially taught (Hung, 2013). *Far transfer*, on the other hand, requires more complex cognitive abilities in that the learner must apply previously learned knowledge to dissimilar or

Table 4. Where (or in what setting) will the instruction be delivered?

Characteristic or Attribute	Method for Assessing	Strategies for Instruction
Face-to-face or synchronous instruction	• Inspect physical environment to ensure adequate space for classroom activities • Evaluate available technology in classroom including student's ability to access it	• Select activities that conform to physical space of the classroom • Use technology to support, enhance, or supplement instruction
Online or asynchronous instruction	• Have students complete a brief poll or survey prior to class beginning regarding previous experiences with online or asynchronous instruction • Have students demonstrate skills in advance of course beginning	• Provide students with hardware and software requirements well in advance of class start date • Provide links to IT support • Ensure tutorials and help services are available throughout course
Self-regulation and self-directed learners	• Conduct a student survey or inventory of learning habits, such reading, outlining, summarizing • Ask students to self-report most successful learning habits	• Provide clear learning goals and deadlines • Assess student progress frequently and use a variety of assessment methods

unrelated situations from how the knowledge was originally acquired (Hung, 2013). Barnett and Ceci (2002) developed a unique taxonomy that addresses transfer of learning. Their framework explains how transfer occurs and under what conditions. According to Barnett and Ceci (2002), two important factors associated with near and far transfer are *content*, which relates to what is being transferred, and *context*, which relates to the time and place the learning is being transferred.

Content

The first factor to consider is the type of content that is being transferred. This could range from mere facts to more complex concepts and sophisticated procedures. An example may prove informative. Consider students in a phlebotomy class. There are many facts that students must learn before drawing blood from a patient, such as the proper procedures for ensuring a sterile environment and drawing samples in the correct order. To teach the proper procedure for drawing blood, students may first be required to memorize and recognize the steps in the correct order. Then students may recall the steps without any additional cues, and finally, students would perform each step in the procedure correctly. As students become more experienced and proficient in executing the procedure, then other factors such as speed and accuracy can be addressed, along with patient interaction. As the example illustrates, students are expected to master a great deal of content related to drawing blood, from what constitutes a sterile environment to the order in which blood samples should be drawn.

Context

Another, more robust, factor related to transfer of learning is the context in which the transfer will occur. According to Barnett and Ceci (2002), there are six different dimensions from which learning may be transferred. These are (1) knowledge domain, (2) physical context, (3) temporal context, (4) functional context, (5) social context, and (6) modality. When considering these six dimensions, think of them as falling along a continuum, with near transfer on one end of the continuum and far transfer on the other.

Context: Knowledge Domain

The first dimension, *knowledge domain*, refers to the knowledge base from which the initial learning occurred to where the learning is being transferred. For example, transferring basic concepts, such as the scientific method and testing hypotheses, from a physics class to a chemistry class seems related and would naturally fall very close to the near transfer end on the continuum. On the other hand, transferring these same concepts and knowledge to an art class seems unrelated and would fall near the far transfer end of the continuum. For this type of far transfer to occur, students may need additional instruction or more examples in order to make the necessary connections.

Furthermore, it is advisable to provide as many practice contexts as possible in order to promote transfer of learning. Consider two different ways to teach complex physiology concepts, such as fluid dynamics, Laplace's law, and Starling's law. One instructional strategy is to use blocked practice, which typically involves learning a concept, followed by practice with multiple examples of the same concept (Kulasegaram et al., 2015). In the physiology example, instruction using blocked practice would result in each of the three concepts being taught independently and providing multiple examples of each concept. Mixed practice, on the other hand, occurs when students are practicing examples of all three concepts at the same time. Mixed practice has repeatedly been shown to promote transfer (Kulasegaram et al., 2015). In general, blocked practice teaches students how to recognize a concept, whereas mixed practice teaches students to discern which concept is most applicable.

Context: Physical Context

The second dimension related to transfer is *physical context*. This refers to the actual physical location of the learning and potential transfer settings. For example, students in a phlebotomy class will demonstrate each discrete skill in a classroom setting, under the watchful eye of an instructor, before drawing blood in a hospital clinic. Consequently, students who are able to execute the skill in the classroom where the skill was taught would be demonstrating near transfer, since there is no variation in the physical context when executing the skill. Contrast this with students who are performing the skill in a busy hospital environment. This is far transfer, and ultimately what students would be expected to do after completing the class. Therefore, when developing instruction, it is important to consider how changes to the physical surroundings may influence the success or failure of student transfer and performance.

Context: Temporal Context

The third dimension, *temporal context*, is related to the amount of time that passes between the initial training or learning event and the testing phase, which can span moments to years. Imagine that students are required to perform one-step of a complex procedure, such as identifying the median cubital vein, immediately following a demonstration by the instructor. The temporal context in this example is very short. Alternatively, consider students who have learned how to deal with a patient who faints while giving blood. The opportunity to apply that knowledge may not occur for many years. This example illustrates that continued education may be necessary for skills and knowledge that are not accessed or demonstrated on a regular basis.

Context: Functional Context

The fourth dimension is related to the *functional context* of the particular skill and how alike or dissimilar it is from its intended purpose. Continuing with the phlebotomy example, suppose students are asked to read about the proper technique for drawing blood and then watch a video demonstration. An instructor may require students to complete a written test, listing all steps the proper order while noting associated safety protocols. While the proper steps and safety protocols for drawing blood are very important, it is not the same as actually drawing blood from a real patient. Therefore, from a functional context, the written test is very dissimilar from the actual intended purpose, which is the ability to draw blood from a living human being. With this in mind, instructors should consider how student knowledge and performance will be assessed during instruction and how closely these align with the intended purpose.

Context: Social Context

The fifth dimension is referred to as the *social context*. More specifically, the social context reflects the degree to which learners work with others to learn and transfer the skill or task, or whether they work independently. Health care settings are often fast-paced and multi-disciplinary, requiring ongoing collaboration to meet patient and client needs. Students exposed to a learning environment which requires working collaboratively with others will likely be more successful in a work setting which requires teamwork and coordination. With this in mind, instructors can design activities, projects, and assignments so that the social context of the classroom closely resembles the expected transfer environment. As an example, having students shadow hospital phlebotomists will expose novice learners to a practice setting and allows experts to monitor student interactions.

Context: Modality

The final dimension, *modality*, is related to how learning is assessed. Suppose students are required to read an article on successfully working with patients who are anxious about giving blood. In formulating an assessment of student knowledge, one modality to assess the content would be a written essay asking students to note what they would say to a patient who was nervous about giving blood and any actions they would take to calm the patient. On the other hand, an assessment that promotes far transfer would require the students to respond orally to the same type of questions through the use of a role play or demonstration. While the specific words and actions that students write in an essay are informative, factors such as voice tone, touch, and genuineness are difficult to assess from a piece of paper alone. This example illustrates how the modality of assessment can differ from the modality in which the material was first acquired. Taken together, understanding the conditions under which the learner will be required to apply and demonstrate classroom learning as well as the final performance context are critical factors when developing course learning activities and assessment methods.

Obviously, one of the goals of education is for learners to use and apply the knowledge and skills acquired in the classroom in real practice settings. Understanding the circumstances in which students are able to successfully transfer classroom learning to real life contexts is one of the main goals of education. Table 5 summarizes the characteristics and attributes discussed in this section, along with methods for assessment and strategies for instruction.

Table 5. How will learners be expected to use the information?

Characteristic or Attribute	Method for Assessing	Strategies for Instruction
Content transfer	• Review course syllabi for key concepts and skills • Review learning goals	• Develop course content and assessments that build on previous material • Provide frequent opportunities to practice skills • Include additional examples for students to review
Context transfer	• Review course syllabi • Review learning goals • Consider various practice settings • Observe students in practice setting • Ask students to demonstrate skills	• Select instructional strategies that promote far transfer of learning such as mixed practice • Allow students to demonstrate skills in multiple settings • Incorporate diverse scenarios or case studies • Use a variety of assessment methods • Provide continuing education opportunities for less frequently used skills or knowledge

Why is the Learning Important?

Understanding and assessing a learner's motivation to learn is another key step in the learner analysis. Some argue that the instructor is most responsible for student learning. Others take a contrasting view and argue that students have the most to gain from the educational endeavor and therefore, students are responsible for their own learning. Likely, the responsibility for learning is shared and understanding student motivation to learn will aid in developing instructional material that assists students in meeting their educational and professional goals.

Historically, motivation has been categorized into two types, *intrinsic motivation* and *extrinsic motivation*. Intrinsic motivation typically refers to circumstances when learners engage in tasks for which there is no apparent reward. Examples may include playing a game for the mere challenge associated with competing against others or writing poetry to express feelings. Extrinsic motivation, on the other hand, refers to tasks learners engage in with the anticipation of rewards for successful completion. This may include earning a degree, a raise, or praise from a valued colleague. Misch (2002) identified the concept of secondary gain in relation to medical student's motivation to learn.

A host of secondary benefits, such as prestige, power, and respect, often result with the achievement of a medical degree, thus arguing that a student's internal and external motivation to learn may be more complex, nuanced, and interrelated than previously understood (Misch, 2002). According to Keller, (2010), motivation to learn is promoted when a learner perceives a gap in knowledge and a desire to close the gap is aroused. Keller (1979) is credited with developing the ARCS model of motivation (attention, relevance, confidence, and satisfaction), which is still widely used today.

Attention

Gaining the learners attention, building curiosity around the subject matter, and actively engaging the learner in activities that promote learning are necessary components of motivation. Curiosity can be aroused in a variety of ways, such as using games or roleplays to involve learners in the material, posing problems for learners to solve, or using visual stimuli to evoke excitement (Keller, 2008). Likewise, it is essential to explore the dynamics around boredom as it relates to learners. While boredom is not necessarily the reverse of curiosity, learners can become disinterested in a topic because of the physical stimuli (such as a classroom that is too warm) or by a long lecture that does not include variations to instructional tactics, voice tone, or activities.

Relevance

Relevance refers to the meaningfulness of the learning as related to learning goals. Learners can have multiple goals or reasons for being in the classroom (Mann, 1999). Some may be motivated by earning an advanced degree in order seek more fulfilling professional employment while others seek to engage in activities that meet more personal or emotional needs. Course content and instructional strategies should connect to learner's goals and experiences in an effort to promote the relevance of the material and pique motivation. For adult learners in particular, engaging in realistic activities that are clearly connected to the instructional content will increase student motivation to learn (Means, Jonassen, & Dwyer, 1997).

Confidence

Confidence refers to the notion that learners believe they can be successful in mastering specific content or a learning task. In order to promote feelings of confidence, learners must experience academic achievement and success as directly resulting from their own efforts and abilities, rather than from chance or fate (Keller, 2008). Allowing learners to control some elements of goal setting and goal achievement increase confidence as well. In addition, offering students choices in regard to assignments and activities can greatly influence motivation and confidence (Malone, 1981), although advance preparation may be necessary to ensure that all alternatives are viable and will result in achieving similar learning outcomes (deCharms, 1977).

Satisfaction

Satisfaction refers to the positive and fulfilling feelings generated from achieving a learning outcome. The satisfaction that results from earning a high grade for a difficult assignment or from receiving public recognition for completing a task can sustain student motivation. Furthermore, satisfaction may also result from the opportunity to use particular skills or knowledge in a real life situation, such as during an internship or field placement. In a classroom situation, instructors can reinforce student satisfaction by praising student performance, providing awards or privileges, and treating all students in a fair and consistent manner (Keller, 2008).

Volition

Recently, Keller (2008) noted a fifth concept related to motivation. Volition, or the cognitive willpower to commit to a course of action, requires learners to employ self-regulatory strategies throughout their educational endeavors. In short, learners who are motivated to achieve a goal must persist in light of many obstacles and distractions that can occur (Keller, 2008). Adult learners, in particular, often juggle multiple responsibilities such as work, school, and family life. Likewise, learners who do not possess sufficient learning self-efficacy may be highly interested in acquiring new knowledge and skills but lack the persistence of effort to complete the tasks.

Student motivation to learn is a complex topic which requires continued study. In this section, variables related to intrinsic and extrinsic motivation were described along with numerous examples. There are many formal and informal options available to assess student motivation and self-regulation. Self-report is a simple way to learn more about what motivates students in the classroom. Surveys and questionnaires related to desired goals and previous successful learning experiences may shed light on student motivation as well. More formal measures include the motivation regulation assessment developed by Wolters and Benzon (2013) and the Healthcare Learning and Studying Inventory (HLSI) developed by Baxter, Mattick, and Kuyken (2013). Table 6 summarizes the attributes discussed in this section, along with methods for assessment and strategies for instruction.

Table 6. Why is learning important?

Characteristic or Attribute	Method for Assessing	Strategies for Instruction
Gaining student attention	• Observe students verbal and non-verbal responses to instruction • Student self-report • Ask students to rate interest in material	• Use interactive activities such as games and roleplays to increase student attention • Ask provocative questions • Vary instructor stimuli such as changing voice tone or moving around the classroom • Change physical setting, such as field trips
Relevance of learning	Ask students to describe personal and professional goals	• Use learning activities that mirror real world application • Connect learning activities to learning goals
Student confidence	• Observe students in classroom • Ask students to rate level of confidence with procedure or task using a simple scale or other form of measurement	• Allow learners to set goals when appropriate • Offer choices in assignments and activities • Praise student performance • Provide certificates or other tangible rewards for major accomplishments
Student satisfaction	Conduct weekly or bi-weekly student surveys	Provide multiple opportunities to use knowledge and skills
Student volition	• Seek feedback from students on barriers to learning • Review previous coursework • Inquire about personal and professional learning goals	• Refer to course learning goals frequently • Offer additional office hours throughout the semester

PUTTING IT ALL TOGETHER

Without question, conducting a comprehensive learner analysis is the most efficient and effective way to identify relevant learner characteristics. Understanding learner characteristics such as prior knowledge and skills, demographics, and motivation are just a few variables that should be considered when developing a course or other instructional material. Instruction, whether it is delivered synchronously or asynchronously, should be developed using sound instructional design principles with attention to the specific learning audience. Students in the health care field will not always be students. Eventually, these students will become nurses, doctors, phlebotomists, x-ray techs, or clinical social workers, attending to complex and critical patient needs in the health care setting. Assessing the specific learner characteristics addressed in this chapter will lead to the development and delivery of efficient and effective instruction, which ultimately results in quality patient care in a variety of health care settings.

This chapter provided a framework for conducting a learner analysis and the implications specific learner characteristics may have on the development and delivery of course material. The six key questions for conducting a learner analysis (who, what, when, where, how, and why) aid in identifying unique characteristics of learners so that effective instructional strategies are selected and educational goals are achieved. A comprehensive Learner Analysis Worksheet, which can be used when planning a new course or revising an existing course, is provided in the Appendix. The Learner Analysis Worksheet summarizes the learner characteristics or attributes associated with each of the six key questions, identifies common methods for assessing the characteristics, and suggests specific strategies for instruction based on the particular needs of the learner.

FUTURE RESEARCH DIRECTIONS

While much is already known regarding the importance of conducting a learner analysis and the rationale for doing so, unanswered questions still remain. In general, additional research is needed to determine the relative importance of specific learner characteristics. For example, assessing the degree of prior knowledge is a critical factor in conducting a learner analysis; however, questions remain regarding the depth and breadth of domain specific knowledge that is required for students to achieve learning goals successfully. Valid and reliable measures to assess these characteristics are also required. Additional research must be conducted to verify the effectiveness of specific instructional strategies to patient care such as saving time, fewer errors, and reduced readmissions.

As noted previously, technological innovations are occurring swiftly. Health care providers are using mobile devices to monitor patients such as the use of wearable ECG devices that provide real time information to doctors (Hii & Chung, 2011). Likewise, students are using mobile devices for many purposes, including formal education. Most of the research conducted on the use of mobile devices in the classroom involves K-12 age students. More research on the use of mobile devices by adult learners and in domain specific areas, such as nursing, medicine, dentistry, and other allied health disciplines, must be conducted. Likewise, the use of simulation games are becoming very popular in health care education, however, more research is needed on the relationship between case-fidelity, learner motivation, and skill development (Dankbaar et al., 2015). The use of new and emerging technologies, such as personal response systems or clickers, needs to be explored. While studies have shown that students feel engaged and energized when using clickers, more research is needed to determine whether these types of devices lead to increased knowledge and the most effective approaches for using this technology (Sternberger, 2012).

Student motivation is critical to successful learning. Adults pursue post-secondary education, advanced certificates, and other continuing education for a variety of reasons and at different times in their adult lives. Several surveys and assessment instruments were noted in this chapter; however, further testing is needed to evaluate the validity and reliability of these tools, particularly in the health care field. A more nuanced understanding of the motivational factors in adult learners will result in better instruction and improved learning outcomes. Similarly, more research is needed regarding successful self-regulating and self-directing behaviors in adult learners. Nothnagle, Anandarajah, Goldman, and Reis (2011) found that graduating residents lacked confidence in their ability to evaluate their learning in clinical settings. Ongoing research regarding the necessity and acquisition of critical self-regulating behaviors, particularly among non-traditional learners, would inform the development of instructional supports for students and provide guidance to curriculum developers.

Finally, understanding how learning is transferred from the classroom to the hospital or clinic setting requires further exploration. Barnett and Ceci (2002) provide a succinct framework to discuss near and far transfer, however, there has been little research conducted regarding the effects of collaborative learning on far transfer. Most healthcare professionals work in multi-disciplinary teams, yet the efficacy of collaborative educational environments on eventual practice is an area ripe for further research.

CONCLUSION

Health care educators are uniquely positioned to meet the increasing demands for qualified and competent health care professionals. Developing and delivering instruction that meets the needs of a diverse learning audience is challenging, however, conducting a comprehensive learner analysis will inform a multitude of decisions that will ultimately lead to optimal learning outcomes for students. This chapter provided the reader with six key questions to ask when conducting a learner analysis, methods for assessing these characteristics, and specific strategies for instruction based on the needs of the learner. While it may not be feasible to conduct a comprehensive learner analysis for every course, attention to key attributes of the learning audience can significantly inform the development of sound instructional activities, which leads to optimal learning outcomes for students, and improved patient care for us all.

REFERENCES

Arnold, L., & Feighny, K. M. (1995). Students general learning approaches and performances in medical school: A longitudinal study. *Academic Medicine*, *70*(8), 715–722. doi:10.1097/00001888-199508000-00016 PMID:7646748

Arnold, N., Ducate, L., & Kost, C. (2012). Collaboration or cooperation? Analyzing group dynamics and revision processes in wikis. *CALICO Journal*, *29*(3), 431–448. doi:10.11139/cj.29.3.431-448

Barnett, S. M., & Ceci, S. J. (2002). When and where do we apply what we learn?: A taxonomy for far transfer. *Psychological Bulletin*, *128*(4), 612–637. doi:10.1037/0033-2909.128.4.612 PMID:12081085

Baxter, L., Mattick, K., & Kuyken, W. (2013). Assessing health care students intentions and motivations for learning: The Healthcare Learning and Studying Inventory (HLSI). *Advances in Health Sciences Education: Theory and Practice*, *18*(3), 451–462. doi:10.1007/s10459-012-9383-y PMID:22717990

Bloom, B. S. (1976). *Human characteristics and school learning*. New York: McGraw-Hill.

Carpenter-Aeby, T., & Aeby, V. G. (2013). Application of andragogy to instruction in an MSW practice class. *Journal of Instructional Psychology*, *40*(1-4), 3–13.

Carroll, J. B. (1989). The Carroll Model: A 25-Year retrospective and prospective view. *Educational Researcher*, *18*(1), 26–31. doi:10.3102/0013189X018001026

Cook, D. A. (2012). Revisiting cognitive and learning styles in computer-assisted instruction: Not so useful after all. *Academic Medicine*, *87*(6), 778–784. doi:10.1097/ACM.0b013e3182541286 PMID:22534603

Cutrer, W. B., Castro, D., Roy, K. M., & Turner, T. L. (2011). Use of an expert concept map as an advance organizer to improve understanding of respiratory failure. *Medical Teacher*, *33*(12), 1018–1026. doi:10.3109/0142159X.2010.531159 PMID:22225439

Dabbagh, N., & Bannan-Ritland, B. (2005). *Online Learning: Concepts, Strategies, and Application*. Upper Saddle River, NJ: Pearson Education, Inc.

Dankbaar, M. E. W., Alsma, J., Jansen, E. E. H., van Merrienboer, J. J. G., van Saase, J. L. C. M., & Schuit, S. C. E. (2015). An experimental study on the effects of a simulation game on students' clinical cognitive skills and motivation. *Advances in Health Sciences Education: Theory and Practice*, 1–17. doi:10.1007/s10459-015-9641-x PMID:26433730

de Gregorio, C., Arias, A., Navarrete, N., Cisneros, R., & Cohenca, N. (2015). Differences in disinfection protocols for root canal treatments between general dentists and endodontists: A Web-based survey. *The Journal of the American Dental Association*, *146*(7), 536–543. doi:10.1016/j.adaj.2015.01.027 PMID:26113101

De La Harpe, B., & Radloff, A. (2000). Informed teachers and learners: The importance of assessing the characteristics needed for lifelong learning. *Studies in Continuing Education*, *22*(2), 169–182. doi:10.1080/713695729

deCharms, R. (1977). Students need not be pawns. *Theory into Practice*, *16*(4), 296–301. doi:10.1080/00405847709542716

Dembo, M. H., & Howard, K. (2007). Advice about the use of learning styles: A major myth in education. *Journal of College Reading and Learning*, *37*(2), 101–109. doi:10.1080/10790195.2007.10850200

Dick, W., Carey, L., & Carey, J. O. (2015). *The Systematic Design of Instruction*. Upper Saddle River, NJ: Pearson.

Dyer, J.-O., Hudon, A., Montpetit-Tourangeau, K., Charlin, B., Mamede, S., & van Gog, T. (2015). Example-based learning: Comparing the effects of additionally providing three different integrative learning activities on physiotherapy intervention knowledge. *BMC Medical Education*, *15*(1), 1–16. doi:10.1186/s12909-015-0308-3 PMID:25889066

Ertmer, P. A., & Newby, T. J. (1993). Behaviorism, cognitivism, constructivism: Comparing critical features from an instructional design perspective. *Performance Improvement Quarterly*, *6*(4), 50–72. doi:10.1111/j.1937-8327.1993.tb00605.x

Grabowski, B. L. (2004). Generative learning contributions to the design of instruction and learning. In D. H. Jonassen (Ed.), *Handbook of Research on Educational Communications and Technology* (2nd ed.; pp. 719–743). Lawrence Earlbaum.

Guerrasio, J., Brooks, E., Rumack, C. M., Christensen, A., & Aagaard, E. M. (2016). Association of characteristics, deficits, and outcomes of residents placed on probation at one institution, 20022012. *Academic Medicine*, *91*(3), 382–387. doi:10.1097/ACM.0000000000000879 PMID:26352762

Hii, P.-C., & Chung, W.-Y. (2011). A comprehensive ubiquitous healthcare solution on an Android™ mobile device. *Sensors (Basel, Switzerland)*, *11*(7), 6799–6815. doi:10.3390/s110706799 PMID:22163986

Hommes, J., Rienties, B., de Grave, W., Bos, G., Schuwirth, L., & Scherpbier, A. (2012). Visualising the invisible: A network approach to reveal the informal social side of student learning. *Advances in Health Sciences Education: Theory and Practice*, *17*(5), 743–757. doi:10.1007/s10459-012-9349-0 PMID:22294429

Hung, W. (2013). Problem-based learning: A learning environment for enhancing learning transfer. *New Directions for Adult and Continuing Education, 2013*(137), 27–38. doi:10.1002/ace.20042

Jordan, J., Jalali, A., Clarke, S., Dyne, P., Spector, T., & Coates, W. (2013). Asynchronous vs didactic education: Its too early to throw in the towel on tradition. *BMC Medical Education, 13*(1), 105–105. doi:10.1186/1472-6920-13-105 PMID:23927420

Keller, J. M. (1979). Motivation and instructional design: A theoretical perspective. *Journal of Instructional Development*, 2(4), 26–34. doi:10.1007/BF02904345

Keller, J. M. (2008). First principles of motivation to learn and e3-learning. *Distance Education, 29*(2), 175–185. doi:10.1080/01587910802154970

Keller, J. M. (2010). *Motivational Design for Learning and Performance: The ARCS Model Approach.* NY: Springer. doi:10.1007/978-1-4419-1250-3

Knowles, M. S. (1970). *The modern practice of adult education: Andragogy versus pedagogy.* New York: Association Press.

Kulasegaram, K., Min, C., Howey, E., Neville, A., Woods, N., Dore, K., & Norman, G. (2015). The mediating effect of context variation in mixed practice for transfer of basic science. *Advances in Health Sciences Education: Theory and Practice*, *20*(4), 953–968. doi:10.1007/s10459-014-9574-9 PMID:25524224

Liew, S.-C., Sidhu, J., & Barua, A. (2015). The relationship between learning preferences (styles and approaches) and learning outcomes among pre-clinical undergraduate medical students. *BMC Medical Education*, *15*(1), 44. doi:10.1186/s12909-015-0327-0 PMID:25889887

Malone, T. W. (1981). Toward a theory of intrinsically motivating instruction. *Cognitive Science*, *5*(4), 333–369. doi:10.1207/s15516709cog0504_2

Mangels, J. A., Butterfield, B., Lamb, J., Good, C., & Dweck, C. S. (2006). Why do beliefs about intelligence influence learning success? A social cognitive neuroscience model. *Social Cognitive and Affective Neuroscience*, *1*(2), 75–86. doi:10.1093/scan/nsl013 PMID:17392928

Mann, K. V. (1999). Motivation in medical education: How theory can inform our practice. *Academic Medicine*, *74*(3), 237–239. doi:10.1097/00001888-199903000-00011 PMID:10099642

Martinez, M. E. (2010). *Learning and Cognition: The design of the mind.* Upper Saddle River, NJ: Pearson Education, Inc.

Means, T. B., Jonassen, D. H., & Dwyer, F. M. (1997). Enhancing relevance: Embedded ARCS strategies vs. purpose. *Educational Technology Research and Development*, *45*(1), 5–17. doi:10.1007/BF02299610

Misch, D. A. (2002). Andragogy and medical education: Are medical students internally motivated to learn? *Advances in Health Sciences Education: Theory and Practice*, *7*(2), 153–160. doi:10.1023/A:1015790318032 PMID:12075147

Morrison, G. R., Ross, S. M., Kalman, H. K., & Kemp, J. E. (2013). *Designing Effective Instruction* (7th ed.). Hoboken, NJ: John Wiley & Sons, Inc.

Nothnagle, M., Anandarajah, G., Goldman, R. E., & Reis, S. (2011). Struggling to be self-directed: Residents paradoxical beliefs about learning. *Academic Medicine*, *86*(12), 1539–1544. doi:10.1097/ACM.0b013e3182359476 PMID:22030764

Parks, D. J. (2010). Lest we forget our past: A leader in curriculum development—Ralph Winfred Tyler. *The Educational Forum*, *75*(1), 80–86. doi:10.1080/00131725.2010.528549

Reiser, R. A. (2001). A history of instructional design and technology: Part II: A history of instructional design. *Educational Technology Research and Development*, *49*(2), 57–67. doi:10.1007/BF02504928

Rogers, P. C., Graham, C. R., & Mayes, C. T. (2007). Cultural competence and instructional design: Exploration research into the delivery of online instruction cross-culturally. *Educational Technology Research and Development*, *55*(2), 197–217. doi:10.1007/s11423-007-9033-x

Schumacher, D. J., Englander, R., & Carraccio, C. (2013). Developing the master learner: Applying learning theory to the learner, the teacher, and the learning environment. *Academic Medicine*, *88*(11), 1635–1645. doi:10.1097/ACM.0b013e3182a6e8f8 PMID:24072107

Schwen, T. M. (1973). Learner analysis. *AV Communication Review*, *21*(1), 44–72. doi:10.1007/bf02770828

Sheridan, S., & Williams, P. (2011). Developing individual goals, shared goals, and the goals of others: Dimensions of constructive competition in learning contexts. *Scandinavian Journal of Educational Research*, *55*(2), 145–164. doi:10.1080/00313831.2011.554694

Smith, A. R., Cavanaugh, C., & Moore, W. A. (2011). Instructional multimedia: An investigation of student and instructor attitudes and student study behavior. *BMC Medical Education*, *11*(1), 38–38. doi:10.1186/1472-6920-11-38 PMID:21693058

Song, H. S., Kalet, A. L., & Plass, J. L. (2011). Assessing medical students self-regulation as aptitude in computer-based learning. *Advances in Health Sciences Education: Theory and Practice*, *16*(1), 97–107. doi:10.1007/s10459-010-9248-1 PMID:20872071

Sternberger, C. S. (2012). Interactive learning environment: Engaging students using clickers. *Nursing Education Perspectives*, *33*(2), 121–124. doi:10.5480/1536-5026-33.2.121 PMID:22616412

Sweller, J. (2008). Human cognitive architecture. In J. M. Spector, M. D. Merrill, J. van Merrienboer, & M. P. Driscoll (Eds.), *Handbook of Research on Educational Communications and Technology* (3rd ed.; pp. 369–381). New York: Lawrence Erlbaum Associates.

Sweller, J., van Merrienboer, J. J. G., & Paas, F. G. W. C. (1998). Cognitive architecture and instructional design. *Educational Psychology Review*, *10*(3), 251–296. doi:10.1023/A:1022193728205

Takaya, K. (2008). Jerome Bruners theory of education: From early Bruner to later Bruner. *Interchange*, *39*(1), 1–19. doi:10.1007/s10780-008-9039-2

Toma, C., & Butera, F. (2015). Cooperation versus competition effects on information sharing and use in group decision-making. *Social and Personality Psychology Compass*, *9*(9), 455–467. doi:10.1111/spc3.12191

Winn, W. (2004). Cognitive perspective in psychology. In D. H. Jonassen (Ed.), *Handbook of Research on Educational Communications and Technology* (2nd ed.; pp. 79–112). Lawrence Earlbaum.

Wolters, C. A., & Benzon, M. B. (2013). Assessing and predicting college students use of strategies for the self-regulation of motivation. *Journal of Experimental Education*, *81*(2), 199–221. doi:10.1080/00220973.2012.699901

Wong, G., Greenhalgh, T., & Pawson, R. (2010). Internet-based medical education: A realist review of what works, for whom and in what circumstances. *BMC Medical Education*, *10*(1), 12–12. doi:10.1186/1472-6920-10-12 PMID:20122253

Yukselturk, E., & Top, E. (2013). Exploring the link among entry characteristics, participation behaviors and course outcomes of online learners: An examination of learner profile using cluster analysis. *British Journal of Educational Technology*, *44*(5), 716–728. doi:10.1111/j.1467-8535.2012.01339.x

Zimmerman, B. J. (2002). Becoming a self-regulated learner: An overview. *Theory into Practice*, *41*(2), 64–72. doi:10.1207/s15430421tip4102_2

KEY TERMS AND DEFINITIONS

Advance Organizers: An instructional tool provided by the instructor to assist learners with understanding the relationships between instructional content.

Asynchronous Learning: Learning that does not involve instructors and learners interacting with one another in real time.

Cognitive Load: The mental energy needed to think about and understand new information, should be monitored and reduced if too much new information is presented at one time.

Concept Maps: A visual representation that is used to help individuals organize content and make connections when learning new concepts.

Extrinsic Motivation: Motivation that refers to tasks learners engage in with the anticipation of rewards for successful completion. This may include earning a degree, a raise, or praise from a valued colleague.

Intrinsic Motivation: Motivation that typically refers to circumstances when learners engage in tasks for which there is no apparent reward.

Learner Analysis: An analysis that assesses the plethora of learner variables that may affect instructional content and delivery.

Prior Knowledge: Information that a learner knows prior to embarking on a new lesson.

Self-Regulated Learning: The ability to monitor and control our behavior as it relates to learning.

Synchronous Instruction: Learning that involves instructors and learners interacting with one another in real time.

Volition: The cognitive willpower to commit to a course of action.

APPENDIX

Learner Analysis Worksheet

Instructions: When you begin planning a new course or need to revise an existing course, consider your target learning audience and how that will affect your course design and delivery. This worksheet serves as a quick reference for each of the six questions in the learner analysis. There are three simple steps to completing this worksheet.

1. Review each question along with the specific learner characteristics or attributes. Consider what you know or do not know about your own learners and make notes in the blank space provided.
2. Review the methods for assessing the specific learner characteristics and note what you may need to do to gather more information about your learners.
3. Reflect on the sample strategies for instruction and note what strategies you might use when developing and delivering your course, based on the specific characteristics or attributes of your learners.

Table 7.

Who Are My Learners?	
Characteristics or attributes	Consider basic learner demographics, general academic abilities, social characteristics, psychological and affective characteristics, class size, geographic location of class and students
What do I know about my learners?	
Method for assessing	Review admissions material, student records, conduct brief pre-tests, learner preference surveys, describe previous learning experiences, review enrollment statistics
How will I get more information?	
Strategies for instruction	Use culturally diverse case examples and activities, vary the amount and complexity of readings and assignments, provide regular feedback to students
What strategies will I use?	
What Prior Experiences and Knowledge do my Learners Possess?	
Characteristics or attributes	Consider prior knowledge of learner, prior work experience, and prior technology experience
What do I know about my learners?	
Method for assessing	Conduct pre-course assessment of major concepts or procedures, seek feedback on prior experiences, review employment and work history, conduct survey of student experiences with learning technology, conduct skill based assessment, review data from help desk
How will I get more information?	
Strategies for instruction	Develop supplemental material for knowledge gaps, include a course review, use advance organizers and concept maps, select instructional strategies that benefit novice and expert learners such as mixed practice, provide links to tutorials and help surveys, test media files before class begins
What strategies will I use?	

continued on following page

Table 7. Continued

	When Will the Instruction Occur?
Characteristics or attributes	Consider sequencing of your course in overall program curriculum and time span between pre-requisite courses
What do I know about my learners?	
Method for assessing	Review curriculum handbook, consult administrators and faculty, review student transcripts, seek student feedback on when courses were taken
How will I get more information?	
Strategies for instruction	Identify pre-requisite content, provide review of content and/or develop supplemental material for student reference, align course goals with curriculum goals
What strategies will I use?	
	Where (Or in What Setting) Will the Instruction be Delivered?
Characteristics or attributes	Consider course delivery methods including face-to-face, synchronous with technology, online or asynchronous, as well as learners self-regulation skills
What do I know about my learners?	
Method for assessing	Inspect physical environment, evaluate available technology, have students complete brief poll regarding previous experience with online instruction, have students demonstrate skills, conduct survey or have students self-report learning habits
How will I get more information?	
Strategies for instruction	Select activities that conform to physical space, use technology to support or enhance instruction, provides students with technology requirements prior to class, provide links to IT support, ensure tutorials and help services are readily available, provide clear learning goals, assess student progress frequently
What strategies will I use?	
	How Will Learners be Expected to Use the Information?
Characteristics or attributes	Consider content transfer and context transfer including complexity of material, practice contexts and settings, time between practice sessions, assessment methods, and learning environment
What do I know about my learners?	
Method for assessing	Review course syllabi for key concepts and skills, review learning goals, observe students in practice setting, ask students to demonstrate skills
How will I get more information?	
Strategies for instruction	Develop course content that builds on previous material, provide frequent opportunities to practice skills, include multiple examples for review, incorporate diverse case studies, use a variety of assessment methods, allow students to demonstrate skills in multiple settings
What strategies will I use?	
	Why is the Learning Important?
Characteristics or attributes	Consider gaining student's attention, relevance of the material, student confidence in learning, student satisfaction, and student ability to persevere
What do I know about my learners?	
Method for assessing	Ask students to rate interest in material, observe verbal and non-verbal responses to instruction, observe students, have students rate level of confidence with procedure or task, solicit student feedback frequently, inquire about personal and professional goals
How will I get more information?	
Strategies for instruction	Use interactive activities, ask provocative questions, vary instructor stimuli, connect learning activities to learning goals, use learning activities that mirror real world application, allow learners to set goals and offer choices when appropriate, praise student performance, provide rewards for major accomplishments, frequent opportunities to use knowledge and skills, refer to course learning goals frequently
What strategies will I use?	

Chapter 2
Instructional Strategies and Sequencing

Thomas W. Lamey
University of South Alabama, USA

Gayle V. Davidson-Shivers
University of South Alabama, USA

ABSTRACT

An instructional strategy is a designed course of action for an instructional goal framed by credible and realistic problems in order to activate prior knowledge and experiences in order to learn new knowledge and skills. In medical education, instructional strategies are designed as purposeful interventions to meet educational goals and achieve socio-cultural norms of medical practice. Reigeluth (1983) identified three major categories for instructional strategies: organizational, delivery, and management. The purpose of this chapter is to define and classify key concepts related to instructional strategies from an instructional design perspective and then apply them toward achieving medical education goals.

INTRODUCTION

Medical education, guided through a philosophy of modern science, has continuously re-analyzed the scientific explanation process to help communicate its social purpose (Tang, 2015) by: (a) *reporting* information through an organized classification, description, or comparison approach, (b) *explaining* processes and underlying causes, (c) *experimental reporting* through presented methodology, results, and discussion, and (d) *argument* of evidence to support a claim or position. The changing dynamics of medicine is not lost on medical educators, who establish and re-establish educational goals to align with evidence-based medicine practice expectations of modern society.

DOI: 10.4018/978-1-5225-2098-6.ch002

Copyright © 2017, IGI Global. Copying or distributing in print or electronic forms without written permission of IGI Global is prohibited.

Established medical educational goals might vary from one U.S. medical college to another, but there are over-arching commonalities. Common goals include (The University of Kentucky College of Medicine, 2016):

1. Providing patient care through demonstration of knowledge, skills and attitudes to effectively evaluate and treat common health problems and promote the health of patients.
2. Demonstrating medical knowledge through the application of fundamental biomedical, clinical, and social science to the care of patients.
3. Demonstrating practice-based learning and improvement through critically evaluating performance and identifying opportunities for improvement.
4. Providing interpersonal and communication skills that develop effective and appropriate relationships with patients, colleagues, and other health professionals.
5. Demonstrating professionalism through sensitivity and respect of patient individuality, accountability of clinical and educational activities, and interactions with family members as well as colleagues.
6. Applying a systems-based practice that incorporates the inter-professional healthcare team and protects organizational accountabilities of timeliness, patient-centeredness, and fiscal efficiency.

Reaching these goals can be heavily influenced by the medical educator's choice of instructional strategies throughout the classroom and clinic. The purpose of this chapter is to introduce strategic examples of instructional strategy implementation throughout the medical education environment in order to achieve instructional goals.

Foundations of Instructional Strategy

An *instructional strategy* is a designed course of action for an instructional goal framed by credible and realistic problems in order to activate prior knowledge and experiences in order to learn new knowledge and skills. In medical education, instructional strategies are designed as purposeful interventions to meet educational goals and meet best-practice guidelines of medical practice. This chapter highlights three categories of instructional strategies: organizational, delivery, and management (Reigeluth, 1983). Organizational strategies are intended to scope, sequence, or specify order to activities of small and large bodies of information as well as instructional events, or activities. Delivery strategies in medical education are intended to support decisions on readiness of learner transition between stages of education, training, and practice. Management strategies support structures to promote self-awareness of knowledge, skills, and attitudes necessary to guide development of a competent professional. This chapter largely emphasizes organizational and delivery instructional strategies in medical education: micro strategies, problem-based learning (PBL), and distance learning (DL). Practical applications for each are presented along with guiding theory and design principles leading up to implementation.

Instructional strategy is a preferred term used in the instructional design (ID) field instead of teaching methods or approaches for a variety of reason. One simple explanation is that instruction might not always be delivered by an instructor, but could be delivered through alternative means instead. The term, *instructional strategy*, is a combination of *strategy* and the adjective form of *instruction*. *Strategy* is a goal attainment approach developed through purposeful and intentional courses of action. *Instruction* engages learners through authentic problems in order to activate existing knowledge and provide a foundational framework for new knowledge (Merrill, 2002). The authors believe elements of ID theory and practice such as design, development, utilization, management, and evaluation of processes may further transform instructional quality in medical education. As the ID field emerged, instructional strategies were refined and categorized. One ID theorist, Charles Reigeluth (1983) identified three major categories for instructional strategies: *organizational, delivery, and management.*

Organizational strategies are classified into two categories: micro and macro (Reigeluth, 1999). *Micro strategies* are concerned with order sequencing of specific activities to facilitate various aspects of the learning process. Gagne's events of instruction is a well-known micro strategy (1985). It is based on his theory about internal and external factors within or outside the learner that contribute to and facilitate the learning process (Richey, Klein, & Tracey, 2011). Furthermore, his events of instruction also serve as "… guidelines for presenting the instructional information and framing [instruction] into a cohesive structure." (Davidson-Shivers & Rasmussen, 2006, p. 207). Although not emphasized in this chapter, *macro strategies* are concerned with organizational scope and sequence of content area(s) in order to assist the learner achieve an instructional goal.

Delivery strategies are those affecting the way information is conveyed to the learner (Reigeluth & Stein, 1983). Part of the delivery strategy is to determine how the instruction is to be conveyed. For instance, instruction could be delivered by an instructor or through various forms of media (including books) or by a combination of both instructor and media. A steady example of emergent delivery strategy are advances in DL utilizing internet-based technologies to deliver student-centered and flexible education at a distance from the resident medical instructor.

The reciprocal relationship of instructional strategies often de-emphasize the important role *management strategies* assist in developing course consistency, replicability, and access capabilities (Smith & Ragan, 2005). Organizational strategies are used to control and support the learning process while serving to coordinate resource distribution in medical education (Smith & Ragan, 2005).

Use of Organizational Instructional Strategies in Medical Education

Organizational strategies in medical education are intended to scope, sequence, or specify order to activities of small and large bodies of information. Organizational strategies in medical education are used to emphasize best-practice guidelines and encourage persistence. Gagne's (1985) events of instruction is a micro strategy medical instructors should be familiar with to help achieve instructional goals.

Micro Strategy: Gagne's Events of Instruction

Should lessons follow an organizational pattern? Can the instructor select strategies that effectively communicate a lesson while achieving learning objectives? The introduction, body, conclusion, and assessment of an instructional episode directed by the instructor can be organized while accommodating for mental operations of students through Robert Gagne's events of instruction (1985):

1. Gaining Attention.
2. Informing the learning of the objective.
3. Stimulating recall of prerequisite learning.
4. Presenting stimulus material.
5. Providing learner guidance.
6. Eliciting performance.

7. Providing feedback about performance correctness.
8. Assessing performance.
9. Enhancing retention and transfer.

Gaining Attention event involves focusing learner attention to the initial learning episode, primarily through interest arousal. Informing the learning of the objective event initiatives student expectancy and motivation through direct explanation of what they should be able to do at the end of instruction. Stimulating recall of prerequisite learning activates prior knowledge and skills necessitating linkage to information included in new material. Presenting stimulus material provides an organized and meaningful presentation for material and information included in the learning event. Providing learner guidance requires cues, hints, and suggested actions by the instructor to assist learner mastery performance. Eliciting performance enhances likelihood of retention through purposeful student demonstration, allowing for repetition and self-efficacy of performance. Providing feedback about performance correctness immediately informs learners about quality of performance, errors made, and question/answering guidance for subsequent performances. Assessing performance requires performance without aide to provide evidence of satisfactory learning occurring; in the medical field, this commonly requires a rubric, checklist, or flow-chart. Enhancing retention and transfer event provides for repeated practice attempts over time in order to retain the knowledge, or learning, into long-term memory and later transfer that knowledge to adjacent settings.

Gagne (1985) considered complete instruction to include all nine events; however, all events do not need to be included for some instructional situations. Richey (2000) further pointed out that the events of instruction do not need to be carried out in a linear fashion. In addition, the amount of instructional content and/or chunking of information can warrant events being combined or re-ordered (Smith & Ragan, 2005). Adequate learner, context, and instructional analyses prior to events of instruction should bring clarity to these considerations and mitigate inclusion of unnecessary steps (For more detail see: Dick, Carey, & Carey, 2014 or other books on instructional design). Although Gagne is not specific concerning scope of the learning event, medical educators commonly use the events of instruction in-full on a lessons plan level. Examples of this found in the medical literature are for subjects such as performing a peritoneal drain and interpretation of chest radiographs (Khadjooi, Rostami, & Ishaq, 2011; Belfield, 2010).

Practical Application of Gagne's Events of Instruction

Khadjooi, Rostami, and Ishaq (2011) utilized the events of instruction to design a lesson plan on the procedure of inserting of a peritoneal drain for junior physicians. Likewise, Belfield (2010) used the events of instruction for a lesson plan on interpretation of chest radiographs. The Belfield (2010) example arose from medical students having poor prior experience and exposure to radiological diagnosis and management during undergraduate training. The drive for better student outcomes was an immediate concern and component of the final course objective structured clinical exam (OSCE); also of note, a peripheral benefit from the instruction being a decrease reliance on radiologists for teaching chest radiographs over the long-term. Table 1 provides an overview and comparison of each study's utilization of the events of instruction.

Strategies to organize large and small bodies of information can be used to emphasize best-practice guidelines and boost persistence. However, organizational strategies are rendered useless without an

Table 1. Events of Instruction for Instruction on Peritoneal Drain Insertion & Chest Radiograph Interpretation

Events of Instruction	Peritoneal Drain Insertion	Chest Radiograph Interpretation
Gaining attention	Case scenario of patient with ascites with relevant investigations and images	Show students example of chest radiographs that are easy and difficult to interpret
Informing the learner of the objective	• List of learning objectives • "Upon completing this lesson you will be able to…"	Explain the learning objectives for interpreting a chest radiograph, present findings, and formulate a radiology report for the clinicians
Stimulating recall of prerequisite learning	• 20-30 minutes of interactive discussion • Previous observations and experiences • Indications of inserting a peritoneal drain and relevant anatomy	• Student explanation of chest radiograph interpretation • Subsequent anatomical questions • Establish prior knowledge thought heart and lung anatomy and physiology questions
Presenting stimulus material	• Broken into different steps of the procedure • Patient consent, monitoring, equipment, patient positioning, technique of drain insertion, and tests post procedure.	• Interactive teaching with discussions and questions • Students given a checklist of important structures to be evaluated
Providing learner guidance	• Instructor shows equipment and performs on mannequin, explaining step by step • Use of graphical representations, mnemonics, and case studies	• Instructor demonstrates own interpretation, findings, and report methodology • Instructor as role model or ego ideal
Eliciting performance	Each student gets familiar with equipment, demonstrates sterile technique, and performs procedure on mannequin under direct supervision	• Student in "hot seat" for chest radiograph interpretation • Valuable experience in non-threatening environment
Providing feedback about performance correctness	• Immediate individual feedback by the instructor • Questions from student answered • Feedback from learners observing performance answered	• Instructor comment on interpretation and presentation skills • Use of checklist to see areas for improvement
Assessing the performance	• Single demonstration on mannequin • Performance on "real patient" during on-calls and on wards under direct supervision multiple times	Student present one final chest radiograph and use checklist for objective feedback
Enhancing retention and transfer	• Repetition of procedure on mannequin • Suggestion of staggered or broken practice periods followed by rest is more effective in long-term transfer of knowledge and skills	• Students continue to interpret while on clinical • Instructor provides contact details for further questions

(Adapted from Khadjooi, Rostami, & Ishaq, 2011; Belfield, 2010)

effective delivery strategy for instructor-learner communication. Delivery strategies in medical education are an integral instructional strategy to support activities between planned instruction and student readiness to learn.

Use of Delivery Strategies in Medical Education

Delivery strategies in medical education are intended to support decisions on readiness of learner transition between stages of education, training, and practice. For the medical educator PBL and DL are delivery strategies commonly used in an instructional setting to effectively connect with students. The purpose of this section is to examine delivery strategies common to medical education and assist educator design, development, and implementation for each.

Foundations of Problem-Based Learning

Problem-Based learning is defined as a curricular level instructional delivery strategy facilitated by the instructor to stimulate self-directed learner relevancy, authenticity, and activity through ill-structured problem scenarios. Problem-based learning is not a new concept to medical education, as it's been around for 50 to 60 years and shows no sign fading. Problem-based learning methodology manifested from student disenchantment and boredom of exceedingly vast amounts educational content despite little *relevance* and *authenticity* to actual practice (Spaulding, 1991).

Howard Barrows, founding father of PBL, was quick to develop specific approaches that motivated student involvement, promoted independent learning and problem solving, reduced lecture hours, and reexamined the evaluation process (Barrows, 1996). Classical lecturing techniques that destroyed clinical reasoning skills and ability over time, mostly in-part to cognitive fading or decay, gave way to numerous PBL medical schools such as Southern Illinois University, Michigan State University, McMasters University, and University of New Mexico taking on PBL to stress authenticity and relevancy to their curriculum (Barrows, 1996). In the early 1980's PBL was established throughout the U.S. through a sponsored GPEP report by the Association of American Medical Colleges, titled *Report of the Panel on the General Professional Education of the Physician and College Preparation for Medicine* (Muller, 1984).

As medical colleges uniquely personalized PBL courses to reflect institutional rigor and excellence, four important PBL educational objectives were identified to unite the delivery strategy (Barrows, 1986 & 1996):

1. Focused structure of knowledge based on clinical context,
2. Development of knowledge hinging on cues and effective clinical reading process (CRP),
3. Development of team and self-directed learning skills, and
4. Motivational increase for learning through enmeshed problem solving used in clinical medicine.

Although PBL continues to evolve and change over time, these four intertwined educational objectives from Barrows represent critical design elements of which the student is expected to practice and perfect under the tutelage of a medical educator (1986).

A primary focus of PBL is to integrate knowledge structure by associating student tasks with clinical scenarios throughout the problem. Challenges in practice, integration, and reasoning of tasks in the problem scenario intentionally layers knowledge (think: less to more complex) through iterative cycles of clinical science knowledge, application, synthesis, and evaluation. Knowledge development structured around cues and effective CRP involve repetition and mastery learning through student-patient inquiry, data analysis, following of protocols, and clinical effectiveness of treatment. Self-directed learning skills is ideal in allowing preferred student learning approaches while maintaining an affiliation to a team that holds unique and vastly more resources of knowledge. Motivation through enmeshed problem solving used in clinical medicine hinges of scenarios being relevant, authentic, challenging, and inclusive of active clinical skills such as writing prescriptions, dialogues with patients and family members, and procedural techniques.

Curricular objectives of PBL determines what the medical instructor *wants students to learn and how they'll know they learned it* through clearly focused and defined assessment activities. In addition to defined curricular educational objectives, PBL presents unique principles and essential components necessary to cue students into natural learning areas of self-directed and group elaboration, discussion, activity, and meaning making.

Principles of Problem Based Learning

Reigeluth and Moore (1999) proposed that the PBL learning process takes place in two environments: the "problem space" where the learner is directly immersed and engaged with the problem and an "instructional space" where knowledge, skills, and attitudinal deficiencies are identified and improved on. The two PBL environments throughout the learning process assist interpretive and intellectual support systems for both medical instructor *and* student. An overview of seven principles found within PBL offering varying degrees of support and structure in the delivery of instruction is provided in Table 2.

The purpose of support and structure in the two environments is to *align* instructional contexts with training and performance contexts throughout the PBL scenario. Ebb and flow transitions in environments throughout the PBL assist in limiting cognitive load and stresses to proximal development. As evidence-based knowledge is advanced in the instructional environment requiring student application of content in a meaningful and emergent professional manner, integration of knowledge in the problem environment activates through medical educator facilitated advance organizers and is solidified through

Table 2. Problem-Based Learning Support & Structure Principles

	"Problem Space"	**"Instructional Space"**
Principle 1: Contents of case should adapt well to prior student knowledge	Learners construct explanatory models to assist knowledge processing and comprehension	Small group advanced organizer discussions and use of materials confronted in cases prior
Principle 2: Stimulate student elaboration through purposeful cues	Learners elaborate in various forms: discussions, answering questions, asking critical questions, and giving explanations	Cues should encourage students to research explanations to encourage clarify ideas, focus answers, and ask questions
Principle 3: Create professional relevancy to scenario through appropriate context	Activation of knowledge is better accessible for later use when the instructional contexts aligns with performance context	Cases that link future professional behavior demands rational decision making and understanding of underlying pathological processes by the student
Principle 4: Develop student relationship between clinical problem and basic science concepts to integrate knowledge	Biomedical and clinical knowledge integrate within a clinical setting scenario	The context of a clinical scenario presents to the learner all entry skills, knowledge, and abilities
Principle 5: Stimulate student interest in research and learning issues to shape self-directed learning	Student involvement of acquiring knowledge is activated through scenario relevancies and pre-designed learning issues	Self-generated learning issues encourages student research into questions that prepare for a more accomplished self-directed learner
Principle 6: Educator leads discussions and solution strategies to generate student interest in scenario	Student self-study dependency and intrinsic interest attention created through attentive solution strategy discussions and terms for underlying pathological processes	Multiple solution strategy iterations and discussions explore alternatives to current subject-matter while furthering student perceptual interest to current scenario environment
Principle 7: Instructor aligns curriculum objectives to corresponding case scenarios	Single scenario and curricular objectives are stated and clearly outlined prior to confronting student with a case	Medical educator analyzes cases and creates learning objectives to align with student negotiated research interests

(Adapted from Dolmans, Snellen-Balendong, Wolfhagen, & Van Der Vleuten, 1997)

patient-management problems, clinical reasoning exercises, and structured oral questioning (Wood, Cunningham, & Norman, 2000). Mentioned earlier, most medical schools have altered PBL to accommodate educator, student, and local environmental as well as ever evolving university standards. The authors believe it is important for medical educators to identify with an integrated and manageable PBL framework, using essential ID components representative of *most* PBL curriculums throughout the US.

Practical Application and Components of Problem-Based Learning

Problem-based learning originates from constructivist learning theory that utilizes cognitive tools, collaborative communities of learners, social negotiation, and authentic environmental tasks to facilitate knowledge construction (Jonassen, 1999). To promote higher order thinking skills Duffy and Cunningham (1996) identify five implementation purposes for PBL: illustrating principles, concepts, and procedures; testing; guiding; fostering content processing; and activity through purposeful stimuli. To the medical educator designing a PBL course can be a challenging, therefore the authors suggest using a fundamental question presented by Weiss (2003) to drive PBL design: "What is being accomplished by assigning this particular problem or set of problems?". From that point forward the effectiveness of designing a PBL course is based on precise interventions, relevant outcomes, relevant solution strategies, and purposeful manipulation of variables in the case scenario, instructional environment, and problem environment (Norman & Schmidt, 2000).

Although a significant amount of planning goes into creating PBL cases, the design element is procedurally straight-forward. All PBL models have six common characteristics across most curriculums (Barrows, 1996):

- A move to student centered learning.
- Small student grouping (5-8 per group).
- Medical educator as guide and facilitator.
- Focus and stimuli for learning originates from problem.
- Specific clinical problem solving skills are developed due to problem.
- Self-directed learning is primary mode of acquiring new information.

Table 3. identifies three PBL models in a progression from a general to more advanced and fleshed out model. Although there are numerous medical PBL models available in the literature, the authors believe these three adequately characterize the PBL framework from a general, intermediate, and modern perspective.

The design-heavy 3C3R PBL model by Hung (2009) utilizes intensive analysis for all aspects of content acquisition, problem solving skills, and self-directed learning to provide an integrated and comprehensive learning experience. It is a model mastered by instructional designers and used in joint fellowship with medical educators for ground-up PBL curriculum development. The general and intermediate PBL model designs are very much a "working in real-time classroom" process that medical educators can either fully or partially implement as standalone (entire course) or adjunct (week) instructional delivery strategy.

The authors believe there are steps within each model that intertwine and embody practical ID design, delivery, implementation, and evaluation processes for the common medical educator desiring to establish or refine a PBL curriculum. The authors offer an integrated 5-step PBL model (see Figure 1) that could produce a *manageable* instructional delivery method for medical educators.

Table 3. PBL Model Designs

	General (Hung, Jonassen, & Liu, 2006)	Intermediate (Schmidt, 1983)	Advanced 3C3R Model (Hung, 2009)
Step 1	Grouped students encounter and reason through problem	Clarify terms and concepts not available or comprehensible to student	Educator sets goals and objectives
Step 2	Individual students complete assignments during self-directed study	Define the problem	Educator conducts task and content analysis
Step 3	Student group sharing of hypotheses and discussion	Analyze the problem	Educator analyzes context specification
Step 4	Summary and integration of knowledge at end of complete problem solution strategy	Create inventory of possible explanations and solutions based on Step 3 analysis	Educator selects and generates the PBL problem
Step 5		Establish and negotiate learning objectives	Educator conducts PBL problem affordance analysis
Step 6		Self-directed collection of additional information	Educator conducts correspondence analysis
Step 7		Synthesize and examine newly acquired information	Educator conducts calibration processes
Step 8			Educator constructs reflection component
Step 9			Educator examines interrelationship of supporting components

(Adapted from Hung, Jonassen, & Liu, 2006; Schmidt, 1983; Hung, 2009)

Figure 1 Integrated medical problem-based learning model

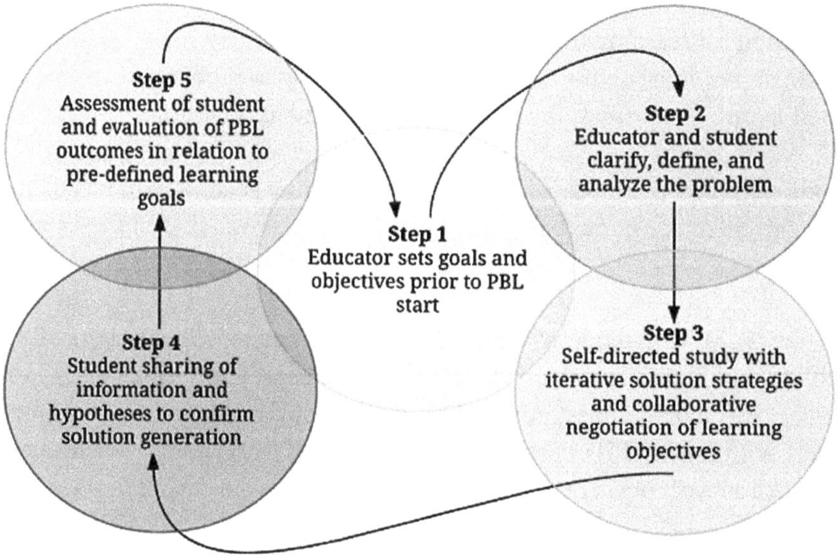

The first step requires the medical educator to establish learning goals and objectives for PBL prior to beginning the course. Established learning goals and objectives assist structuring and scoping the problem as well as alignment to university standards (Trafton & Midgett, 2001). Hung (2009) suggested the educator consider three aspects during this step: domain knowledge, problem solving skills, and self-directed learning skills. As higher-order intellectual efforts are demanded throughout PBL cases, the authors offer action verb word-clouds in Figures 2 through 7 for outcome levels in the cognitive domain based on Bloom's Taxonomy (1956).

Figure 2 Knowledge action verbs

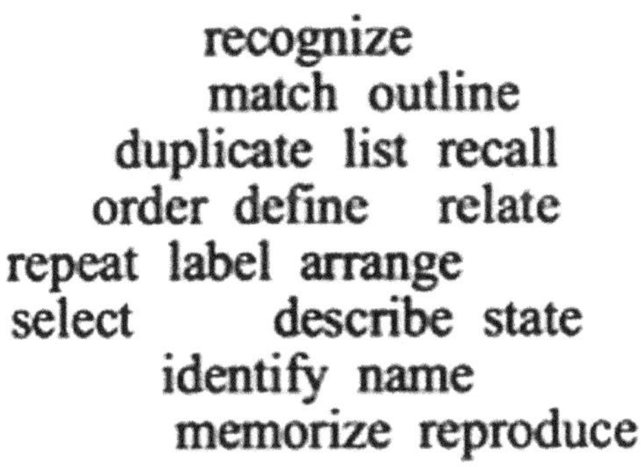

Figure 3 Comprehension action verbs

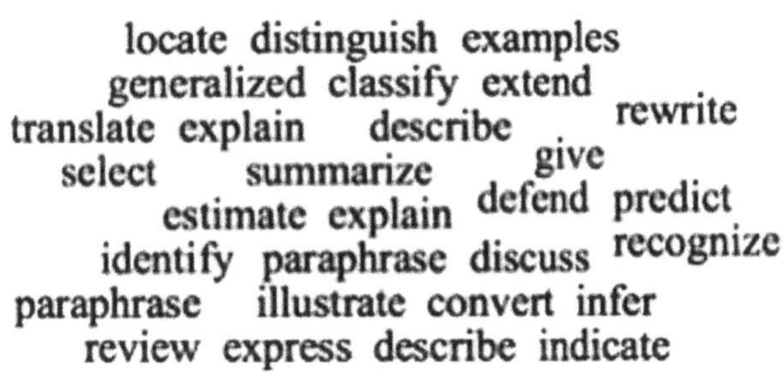

Figure 4 Application action verbs

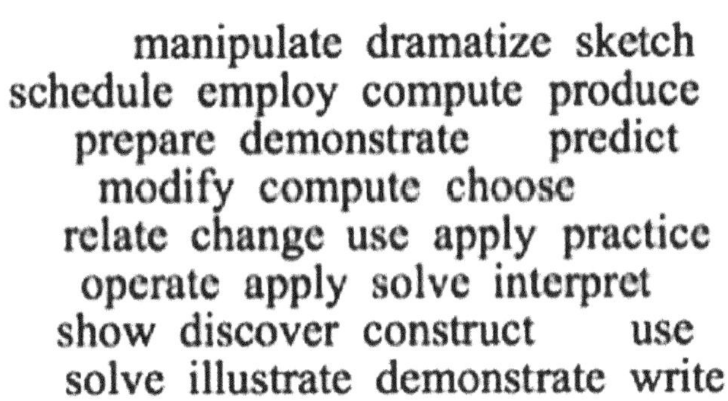

Figure 5 Analysis action verbs

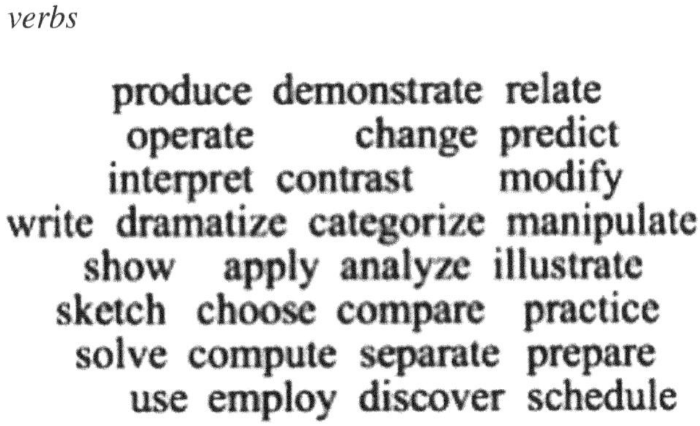

Figure 6 Synthesis action verbs

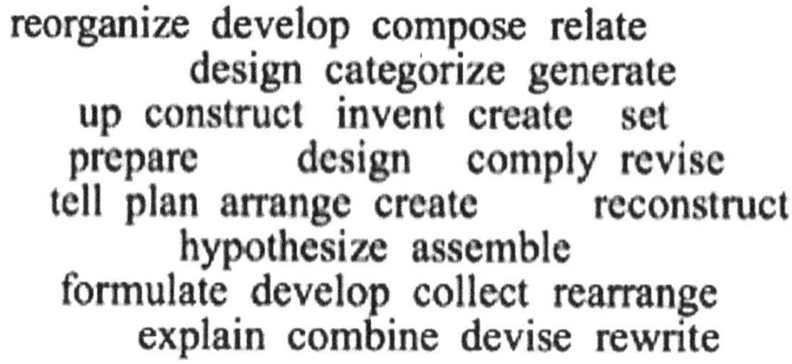

Figure 7 Evaluation action verbs

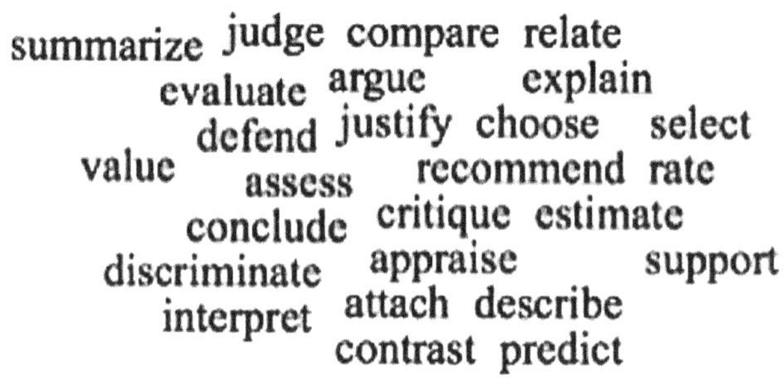

The second step involves collaboration between the student groups and educator to clarify, define, and analyze the problem. Primary, secondary, and tertiary phenomena pertaining to the case are identified, jointly agreed upon for relevancy, and explained prior to breaking for deeper self-directed study. Advanced organizers and cues by the educator help students analyze the situation and immediate resources help solidify ideas and suppositions about the structure of the problem (Schmidt, 1983). It is common to have a breakout "brainstorming" session during this step to freely share ideas and knowledge on the subject case. The end of the second step should result in initial hypotheses setting based on sound reasoning with a motivation to investigate underlying processes.

The third step permits student self-directed study to confirm, deny, and elaborate on initial hypotheses or ideas as well as negotiate learning objectives with their instructor upon return. This step is iterative, allowing the student to continually improve research through analysis of connections between hypotheses, potential solution strategies, and defined problem. Independent and group dialogue with the instructor offers time to clarify problem processes, producing emergent questions and objectives to concentrate on through further research or tasks. The authors believe independent learning time is crucial for the learner, as it allows for students' preferred learning style to dominate and motivation for self-discovery of solution strategy to emerge. The end of the third step are students holding unique and integrated knowledge of processes identifiable to the current problem and transferrable to adjacent cases (Schmidt, 1983).

The fourth step is a culminating dialogue among the group and instructor to share information and confirm hypotheses and ideas. Reflection of content, context, and connections made during the case is a feature of PBL. Hung (2009) advocated structuring reflection based on: (a) acquisition of prior and new knowledge, (b) depth of study to determine adequacy of knowledge, skills, and abilities advanced through problem solving, (c) reasoning processes based on effectiveness and logic of treatment, (d) research effectiveness and efficacy during self-directed study, (e) integration of knowledge on a conceptual level, and (f) solution strategy effectiveness over the life of the PBL case.

The final step targets student assessments to evaluate PBL case effectiveness in attaining the learning objectives and goals prescribed. Recall, Duffy and Cunningham (1996) identified five purposes for PBL: illustrate principles, concepts, and procedures; test; guide; foster content processing; and activity through purposeful stimuli. Assessment method is ultimately determined by the medical educator (It is up to you!), but the authors suggest answering five key questions prior to making that determination:

- What are we assessing?
- When are we going to assess?
- Who will be carrying out the assessment?
- Where will the assessment take place?
- What feedback will students receive?

Macdonald and Savin-Baden (2004) identified numerous assessment methods for PBL and the authors focus on methods easily identifiable to medical school curricula: portfolios, clinical reasoning examinations (CRE), and group presentations. A *portfolio* defined as a compilation of work and material unique to a case or series of cases. Clinical reasoning examinations requires student comparison and contrasts to hypothesis sets obtained through patient history, physical, and ancillary examinations (Nendaz & Tekian, 2009). *Group presentations* are defined as students working within an authentic context to perform, identify, explain, diagnose, and offer solution strategies unique to a case.

Portfolios should include evidence of student work such as flowcharts, path diagrams, clinical simulation laboratory performances, preceptor evaluations, guidelines for selecting the portfolio contents, and criteria for judging the quality of the work. Because portfolios lend themselves to be employed digitally, PBL resources and assignment tools could also be transferred to distance learning environments. Problem-based learning assessment in the distance learning environment is still a work in progress, with recent concerns over validity and reliability of collaborative demonstrations, work, and competency via artifacts created by students Barrows (2002).

Clinical reasoning examinations, developed at Southern Illinois University, require that students compare and contrast hypothesis sets obtained through patient history, physical, and ancillary examinations (Nendaz & Tekian, 2009). Unique to CRE, students are given multiple workbooks with the same problem to carry out iterative self-directed solution strategy and hypothesis testing, culminating in a final examination and end hypothesis to test the reasoning process. Nendaz and Tekian (2009) note that student self-directed study skills are secondarily assessed through a listing of learning issues and resources created from the case that are corrected, summarized, and evaluated throughout the lifecycle of the PBL case.

Along with end-year student questionnaires common to all universities, assessments serve to determine instructor and course effectiveness in facilitating learning goals and objectives. The authors suggest five summative evaluation questions to guide the assessment instrument(s):

- Did the purpose of the assessment align with needs and goals of the PBL course?
- Does the assessment truly measure the knowledge, skills, and abilities you are trying to capture?
- Are scores consistent over time (case by case, semester, school year)?

- Was the assessment practical to administer for both student and instructor?
- Could bias (cultural or gender) in the assessment influence scoring?

Problem-based learning effectiveness is determined by student change in knowledge, skills, and abilities (a gap was filled) and evaluations direct course revisions of learning goals, learning objectives, and materials essential to the instructional and problem environment.

Reflecting on Problem-Based Learning

Problem-based learning is a curricular level instructional delivery strategy used to stimulate self-directed learner relevancy, authenticity, and activity through ill-structured problem scenarios. It is not a new concept to medical education and has been around for 50 to 60 years. Core to PBL is student-centered learning, utilization of small groups of students, shift to educator as guide, and problem serving as stimuli for self-directed learning and motivation. Problem-based learning was developed to motivate student involvement, promote independent learning and problem solving, reduce lecture hours, and reexamine the evaluation process (Barrows, 1996). The authors provided an integrated view of PBL steps, suggesting a more manageable instructional delivery method for medical educators to provide a holistic and meaningful learning experience. While distance learning grows in popularity throughout universities PBL is experiencing difficulties accommodating valid and reliable assessment instruments. As PBL finds its niche in distance learning, a focal shift to emerging e-learning technology tools and social media communication as an instructional delivery strategy are discussed.

Distance Learning

Distance learning is an instructional delivery method utilizing web-based technologies that allows for flexibility and convenience for students at a distance from the resident medical instructor. Distance learning (DL) is synonymous with terms such as e-learning, web-based learning, and computer-managed learning. Geographically scattered and with variable working hours, medical students increasingly rely on DL for learning content and activities, resource materials, and social communication (Smaldino, 1999). To promote a balanced and interactive learning space in medical education, ID harmonizes these four essential components to produce outcome efficiency and effectiveness. Creating a fully online or blended course can be challenging to a medical educator; however, embedded instructional strategies guided by learning theory might provide guidance to reduce the stress of creating a DL environment.

Medical educators have increasingly relied on DL to provide increased student access, more accommodating and flexible scheduling, decreased time and fiscal demands of travel (by both sides), and increased individualized attention to students (Harris, Kutob, Surprenant, Maiuro, and Delate, 2002). The migration to DL is fueled by increased demands on medical faculty, changes in academic and community-based learning environment, and changes in traditionally offered healthcare delivery methods (Ruiz, Mintzer, and Leipzig, 2006). Increased connectivity speeds and authentic medical virtual learning environments have retooled DL design principles and components to specific target audiences, altering organization and distribution strategies once held by educators (Sherry, 1995). Distance learning environments as "knowledge dump" fixed bodies of information are giving way to constructivist learning theories of practice.

Distance Learning and Constructivist Theory in Medical Education

Constructivist theory is rooted in the works of Jean Piaget, who believed that knowledge is constructed by an individual and not simply transferred. Key assumptions to constructivism noted by Smith and Ragan (2005) are that: (a) knowledge is constructed through experience, (b) personal interpretations of learning experiences shape knowledge, and (c) learning is experiential and should be an active process. With DL and alternative forms of delivery there appears to be a shift from what is referred to as a "knowledge dump" of information, replaced by medical education environments that are complex, interactive, and ever evolving (Sherry, 2005). Virtual learning environments allow for closely authenticating the context of actual situations for medical students by providing a relevancy to everyday applications of practicing medicine. Distant and virtual learning environments often align with the constructivist assumption of *contextualization*, which is defined as placing a student in an authentic, complex, and realistic learning processes to practice, apply, and assess task and cognitive activities.

To meet shifting demand of DL and authentic cognitive and task activities, states and private universities have adopted standardized DL models. An example is the Iowa Model, which incorporate evidence-based practice into their healthcare system through two-way live classroom interactions and simultaneous engagement with problem identification and solution strategies (Steelman, 2016). A transition away from teacher-centered learning has placed responsibility on learners to discover the information, maintaining a high level of engagement to constructing their own solution strategy(ies) and bounded body of knowledge. The authors believe *engaging the learner* is the single most important design element to consider. Engaging the learner through principled ID delivery strategies can provide quality student reliance on authentic content, resource materials, activities, and communication.

Practical Application of Distance Learning in Medical Education

According to Ruiz et al. (2006), *content* in DL consists of learning objects in instructional material(s) constructed around learning objectives and embedded throughout lessons, modules, and complete courses. The scope of content and time involved in delivery are two important factors for the medical educator to consider. Smaldino (1999) suggested scoping content up to a minimal level of sufficiency in order to produce desired learning outcomes. Fieschi et al., (2002) have integrated concepts of evidence-based medicine with DL to produce unique educational objectives for medical courses:

- Understand information resources.
- Develop an ability to effectively research information.
- Develop an ability to effectively analyze and evaluate information.
- Develop information management skills essential to medical practice.
- Develop ability to turn problem into questions based on experience.

Smith, Roberts, and Partridge (2009) identified respiratory trainee preference for content that is easily downloadable to visual and listening devices as well as instruction on specific diseases, bronchoscopic anatomy, physiology, lung function, and spirometry. It is important for the educator to present instruction across a wide-range of presentations (i.e., videos, pictures, narrated slides, podcast, and blogs) to garner different student responses to instruction (Sherry, 1995). *The medical educator must decide where the minimum threshold of competency through readings and presentations lie, as a jumping off point should be instituted for student self-directed learning through finding additional information and resources on their own.* In order to maintain the integrity of instruction, the authors believe providing adequate resources, activities, and social communication prior to the jumping off point is important in transitioning the educator to a guide in this student-centered method.

Sherry (1995) recommended that activities in DL go beyond simple audio, video, and basic teacher-student online discussions. The authors believe DL medical educators should implement specific existing tools or design, develop, implement, and evaluate their own in order to improve the medical teaching process. with videoconferencing course, developed by Kavamoto et al., (2005) to introduce recent amputee rehabilitation and associated back pain to medical students. The first videoconference introduced learning strategies, objectives of the course, and tools used through the remaining six weeks of the course. The second phase required student participation of 3D modules (11 in all) with guided questions and links to supporting information throughout. The third phase included a second videoconference with short student presentations, questions, general discussion, and instructor feedback from prior 3D model performances. The last phase generated an open threaded discussion to promote student reflection and peer-feedback on critical subject matter.

Distance learning discussion and feedback in medical education are readily surpassing the confinements of threaded discussions in an LMS. Medical educators and medical students alike are communicating to one another in multiple ways with one thing in common: a move toward social and shareable online learning environments (Cheston, Flickinger, & Chisolm, 2013).

Use of Management Strategies in Medical Education

Management strategies guide orchestration of organization and delivery for implementation of instruction (Smith & Ragan, 2005). Management of instruction requires a coordination and harmonization of the instructional components of a course. In medical education, *management strategies* include controlling and managing resources so that they are ready and available for the educator and students to use at the point in time needed. A common management strategy could be the use of a learning management system (LMS). Learning management systems are characterized as a, "...web-based system designed to translate, facilitate, and support implementation functions (e.g., information delivery, communication, assessment, and feedback) to readily accessible online instruction." (Smith & Ragan, 2005, p 322). Instructional design professionals consider the various aspects of an LMS, viewing it as a system of components: the instructor, learners, material, and system (Simsonson, Smaldino, & Zvacek, 2015). A systems perspective of managing LMS workload time, material resource allocation, and current status of system is fundamental in the administration and operation of a smooth running online course (Gilbert, 2001).

Management in Medical Education

The complexity of LMS course design, implementation, and day-to-day operation requires the medical educator to purposefully plan and schedule instruction (Simonson et al., 2015). Coordinating tasks and identifying responsibilities for learners requires educator readiness preparation, as suggested by Pina & Mizell (2014):

- Mindfulness on previously taught traditional courses and the transition to visual presentations that require engaging material and timing considerations.

- New methods of illustrating key concepts and topics using multiple visual representations.
- Planned student interactions and activities that require group work and supportive environments.
- Awareness of possible LMS technical failures and planning of course communications, assignments, and instruction in case of failure.

The educator also needs to determine what course design structure is appropriate to achieve desired learning goals: fully online or blended learning. *Blended learning* is defined as a combination of online and on campus class activities for the instructional situation. Alternatively, fully online learning solely relies on the online course for all activities. Duque et al., (2013) suggested medical educators use a blended learning strategy in order to produce higher efficacy in terms of student learning and fulfillment.

Readiness preparation and LMS course structure jointly relies on established institutional support infrastructure and educator competency. Simonson et al., (2015) identified four institutional management functions: (a) providing leadership and direction for DL programs, (b) target student bodies ideal for DL programs, (c) ensure readily accessible DL support mechanisms, and (d) provide adequate training to educators and students prior to instruction. Through these institutional management functions educators were recognized as being managerially responsible in four areas: (a) coordinating DL program and individual course development, (b) meeting DL coursework and support accessibility standards, (c) certification of instructional readiness to teach DL courses, and (d) control quality of DL activities and program effectiveness (Simonson et al., 2015). Once operational readiness of educator and LMS infrastructure are established a focus on educator, learner, material, and technology management strategies throughout the medical course can support development of a competent professional.

Practical Application of Management Strategies in Medical Education

Day-to-day management of an LMS requires the educator to strategically manage their time and establish limits to activities and interactions within the learning environment (Davidson-Shivers & Rasmussen, 2006). Savery (2005) identified six successful strategic management characteristics found within an LMS:

- A visibility presence through multiple communication channels.
- An organization to instruction, sequence to content, and specific assessments and activities.
- A compassionate sense of trust to overcome student isolation of DL.
- Multiple analytical assessment types with defined learning outcomes.
- Demonstration of leadership through feedback and effective activities.

Additional and more specific LMS management strategies were offered by Davidson-Shivers and Rasmussen (2006):

1. Activating links,
2. Establishing deadlines,
3. Provide secure learner assessments,
4. Flexible backup pans to technology failures,
5. Track and organize learner participation, and
6. Self-monitor communication and activities.

Beyond simple "readiness checks" for learners, students must continually demonstrate an ability to manage their own time and workload (Gilbert, 2001). Managing their own schedule is dependent on concisely identifying class activities, participating in structured activities, and completing all assignments (Davidson-Shivers & Rasmussen, 2006, p. 303). Simonson et al., (2015, p. 284) identified expectant learner management strategies within an LMS:

- Equal access to support services within LMS as compared to on-campus.
- Unlimited access to information will be provided through LMS and supporting online structures.
- Instructor and student service contact information is easily accessible.
- Responses to student questions are delivered in a timely fashion.
- Customizability of instruction to student preference.

Immediate access to student support is an integral course management strategy, dependent upon concise instructions of technologies necessary to complete the course and instructions for accessing help hotlines, admission procedures, registration of courses, and obtaining transcripts (Simonson et al., 2015).

Material Management Strategies in Medical Education

Material management strategies within an LMS focuses on equal learner accessibility and distribution of printed and electronic media and resources required throughout a course. Examples are materials common to medical education are computer disks (CDs), workbooks, textbooks, video-logs (vlogs), and textbooks. Rienties, Toetenel, and Bryan (2015) noted that material managed within an LMS should identify with seven learning activities:

1. *Assimilative* activities that attend to information.
2. *Finding and handling information* through searched for and processed information.
3. *Communicative* activities that discuss model content with one-another and educator.
4. *Productive* activities requiring student creation of an online artifact.
5. *Experimental* activities of real-world application.
6. *Interactive* activities of virtual-world and simulated settings.
7. *Assessment* activities can be accomplished by formative and summative measures or be the student self-appraisals of their learning.

Material commonly embedded within an LMS course such as documents, flowcharts, and storyboards should be routinely accessed by the educator to ensure student usability. Coordinating material open/close dates and times are often time consuming endeavors for the educator, but must be carefully carried out. Likewise, notifying students of scheduled LMS upgrades and maintenance can limit material accessibility; therefore, a good strategy is to maintain all material files on a central computer (this means your computer!) for rapid alternative delivery via email or social media.

Systems Management Strategies in Medical Education

Systems management within an LMS is concerned with maintaining website, server, and software integrity throughout the course of instruction. Content can be easily updated within an LMS, but students must have equal technological capabilities for usability (Schank, 2002). Simonson et al., (2015) identified activities and strategies for managing the LMS:

- *Maintain website* through saved documentation, designs, and easily identifiable names to embedded tools.
- *Maintain server* by keeping up with most current file versions and network upgrades.
- *Maintain software* through continual testing of browsers and usability of embedded applications, activities, and instruction.
- *Maintain content changes* by continual testing of links and content under embedded files.

Managing the system moderates the preservation of up to date and accessible material. Prior mentioned strategies to accommodate for systems and technological failures are a matter of continual educator commitment and demonstration of leadership to producing effective instruction throughout the lifespan of an online course. An LMS manages learners, tracks progress, and provides learner activities and training performances on an equally accessible 24/7 basis. Maintaining LMS system integrity throughout the lifespan of a course is contingent on flexible retrieval of learning content and is an effective strategy for educator creation, storage, and delivery of instructional material.

REFERENCES

Barrows, H. S. (1986). A taxonomy of problem-based learning methods. *Medical Education*, *20*(6), 481–486. doi:10.1111/j.1365-2923.1986.tb01386.x PMID:3796328

Barrows, H. S. (1996). Problem-based learning in medicine and beyond: A brief overview. *New Directions for Teaching and Learning*, *1996*(68), 3–12. doi:10.1002/tl.37219966804

Barrows, H. S. (2002). Is it truly possible to have such a thing as dPBL? *Distance Education*, *23*(1), 119–122. doi:10.1080/01587910220124026

Barrows, H. S., & Tamblyn, R. M. (1980). *Problem-based learning: An approach to medical education.* New York, NY: Springer.

Belfield, J. (2010). Using Gagnes theory to teach chest X-ray interpretation. *The Clinical Teacher*, *7*(1), 5–8. doi:10.1111/j.1743-498X.2009.00329.x PMID:21134135

Bloom, B. S. (1956). Taxonomy of educational objectives: Vol. 1. *Cognitive domain*. New York, NY: McKay.

Cheston, C. C., Flickinger, T. E., & Chisolm, M. S. (2013). Social media use in medical education: A systematic review. *Academic Medicine*, *88*(6), 893–901. doi:10.1097/ACM.0b013e31828ffc23 PMID:23619071

Davidson-Shivers, G. V. (2015). Universal design. In J. M. Spector (Ed.), *The SAGE encyclopedia of educational technology* (pp. 799–802). Thousand Oaks, CA: Sage Publication.

Davidson-Shivers, G. V., & Rasmussen, K. L. (2006). *Web-based learning: Design, implementation, and evaluation*. Upper Saddle River, NJ: Prentice Hall.

Davis, R., & Surajballi, V. (2014). Successful implementation and use of a learning management system. *Journal of Continuing Education in Nursing*, *45*(9), 379–381. doi:10.3928/00220124-20140825-12 PMID:25198116

Denton, J. J., Armstrong, D. G., & Savage, T. V. (1980). Matching events of instruction to objectives. *Theory into Practice*, *19*(1), 10–14. doi:10.1080/00405848009542866

Dolmans, D. H., Snellen-Balendong, H., & van der Vleuten, C. P. (1997). Seven principles of effective case design for a problem-based curriculum. *Medical Teacher*, *19*(3), 185–189. doi:10.3109/01421599709019379

Duffy, T. M., & Cunningham, D. J. (1996). Constructivism: Implications for the design and delivery of instruction. In D. J. Jonassen (Ed.), *Handbook of research for educational communication and technology* (pp. 170–198). New York, NY: McMillan.

Duque, G., Demontiero, O., Whereat, S., Gunawardene, P., Leung, O., Webster, P., & Sharma, A. (2013). Evaluation of a blended learning model in geriatric medicine: A successful learning experience for medical students. *Australasian Journal on Ageing*, *32*(2), 103–109. doi:10.1111/j.1741-6612.2012.00620.x PMID:23773249

Fieschi, M., Soula, G., Giorgi, R., Gouvernet, J., Fieschi, D., Botti, G., & Berland, Y. (2002). Experimenting with new paradigms for medical education and the emergence of a distance learning degree using the internet: Teaching evidence-based medicine. *Medical Informatics and the Internet in Medicine*, *27*(1), 1–11. doi:10.1080/14639230110105301 PMID:12509118

Gagne, R. M. (1985). *The conditions of learning and theory of instruction*. New York, NY: Holt, Rinehart and Winston.

Gilbert, S. D. (2001). *How to be a successful online student*. New York, NY: McGraw-Hill.

Harris, J. M., Kutob, R. M., Surprenant, Z. J., Maiuro, R. D., & Delate, T. A. (2002). Can internet-based education improve physician confidence in dealing with domestic violence? *Family Medicine*, *34*(4), 287–292. PMID:12017143

Hung, W. (2009). The 9-step problem design process for problem-based learning: Application of the 3C3R model. *Educational Research Review*, *4*(2), 118–141. doi:10.1016/j.edurev.2008.12.001

Jonassen, D. H. (1999). Designing constructivist learning environments. In C. M. Reigeluth (Ed.), *Instructional design theories and models: A new paradigm of instructional theory* (Vol. 2, pp. 215–239). Mahwah, NJ: Lawrence Erlbaum Associates.

Kavamoto, C. A., Wen, C. L., Battistella, L. R., & Bohm, G. M. (2005). A Brazilian model of distance education in physical medicine and rehabilitation based on videoconferencing and internet learning. *Journal of Telemedicine and Telecare, 11*(Supplementary 1), 80-82.

Khadjooi, K., Rostami, K., & Ishaq, S. (2011). How to use Gagne's model of instructional design in teaching psychomotor skills. *Gastroenterology and Hepatology from Bed to Bench, 4*(3), 116. PMID:24834168

Macdonald, R., & Savin-Baden, M. (2004). *A briefing on assessment in problem-based learning*. LTSN Generic Centre Assessment Series No 7. York, England: LTSN Generic Centre. Retrieved from http://www.ltsn.ac.uk/application.asp?app=resources.asp&process=full_ record&section=generic&id=349

Merrill, M. D. (2002). First principles of instruction. *Educational Technology Research and Development, 50*(3), 43–59. doi:10.1007/BF02505024

Muller, S. (1984). Physicians for the twenty-first century: Report of the project panel on the general professional education of the physician and college preparation for medicine. *Journal of Medical Education, 59*, 1–208. PMID:6492116

Nendaz, M. R., & Tekian, A. (1999). Assessment in problem-based learning medical schools: A literature review. *Teaching and Learning in Medicine, 11*(4), 232–243. doi:10.1207/S15328015TLM110408

Norman, G. R., & Schmidt, H. G. (2000). Effectiveness of problem-based learning curricula: Theory, practice and paper darts. *Medical Education, 34*(9), 721–728. doi:10.1046/j.1365-2923.2000.00749.x PMID:10972750

Pina, A. A., & Mizell, A. P. (2014). *Real-life distance education: Case studies in practice*. Charlotte, NC: Information Age.

Reigeluth, C. M. (1983). Meaningfulness and instruction: Relating what is being learned to what a student knows. *Instructional Science, 12*(3), 197–218. doi:10.1007/BF00051745

Reigeluth, C. M. (1999). *The elaboration theory: Guidance for scope and sequence decisions. In Instructional design theories and models: A new paradigm of instructional theory* (Vol. 2, pp. 425–453). Mahwah, NJ: Lawrence Erlbaum Associates.

Reigeluth, C. M., & Moore, J. (1999). Cognitive education and the cognitive domain. In C. M. Reigeluth (Ed.), *Instructional design theories and models: A new paradigm of instructional theory* (Vol. 2, pp. 51–68). Mahwah, NJ: Lawrence Erlbaum Associates.

Richey, R. C. (2000). *The legacy of Robert M. Gagne*. Syracuse, NY: ERIC Clearinghouse on Information & Technology.

Richey, R. C., Klein, J. D., & Tracey, M. W. (2010). *The instructional design knowledge base: Theory, research, and practice*. New York, NY: Routledge.

Rienties, B., Toetenel, L., & Bryan, A. (2015, March). Scaling up learning design: Impact of learning design activities on LMS behavior and performance. In *Proceedings of the Fifth International Conference on Learning Analytics And Knowledge* (pp. 315-319). ACM. doi:10.1145/2723576.2723600

Ruiz, J. G., Mintzer, M. J., & Leipzig, R. M. (2006). The impact of e-learning in medical education. *Academic Medicine, 81*(3), 207–212. doi:10.1097/00001888-200603000-00002 PMID:16501260

Saettler, P. (1990). *The evolution of American educational technology*. Englewood Cliffs, NJ: Libraries Unlimited.

Savery, J. (2005). Be VOCAL: Characteristics of successful online instructors. *Journal of Interactive Online Learning*, *4*(2), 141–152.

Schank, R. (2002). *Designing world-class e-learning*. New York, NY: McGraw-Hill.

Schmidt, H. G. (1983). Problem-based learning: Rationale and description. *Medical Education*, *17*(1), 11–16. doi:10.1111/j.1365-2923.1983.tb01086.x PMID:6823214

Sherry, L. (1995). Issues in distance learning. *International Journal of Educational Telecommunications*, *1*(4), 337–365.

Smaldino, S. (1999). Instructional design for distance education. *TechTrends*, *43*(5), 9–13. doi:10.1007/BF02818158

Smith, P. L., & Ragan, T. J. (1999). *Instructional design*. New York, NY: Wiley.

Smith, S. F., Roberts, N. J., & Partridge, M. R. (2009). UK respiratory trainees' views about implementing e-learning into postgraduate training. *THORAX, 64*(Supplementary 4). doi:10.1136/thx.2009.127191z

Spaulding, W. B. (1991). *Revitalizing medical education, McMaster medical school: The early years, 1965–1974*. Hamilton, Canada: Decker.

Steelman, V. M. (2016). The Iowa model. *AORN Journal*, *103*(1), 5. doi:10.1016/j.aorn.2015.11.020 PMID:26746021

Tang, K. S. (2015). The PRO instructional strategy in the construction of scientific explanations. *Teaching Science: The Journal of the Australian Science Teachers Association*, *61*(4), 14–24.

Trafton, P. R., & Midgett, C. (2001). Learning through problems: A powerful approach to teaching mathematics. *Teaching Children Mathematics*, *7*(9), 532–536.

University of Kentucky Office of Medical Education. (2016. April 22). *Medical Education Goals*. Retrieved from http://www.meded.med.uky.edu/medical-education-goals

Wagner, N. L., Wagner, P. J., & Jayachandran, P. (2005). Distance learning courses in occupational medicine: Methods and good practice. *Indian Journal of Occupational and Environmental Medicine*, *9*(2), 57. doi:10.4103/0019-5278.16742

Weiss, R. E. (2003). Designing problems to promote higher-order thinking. In D. S. Knowlton & D. C. Sharp (Eds.), *Problem-based learning in the information age* (pp. 25–31). San Francisco, CA: Jossey-Bass.

Wood, T. J., Cunnington, J. P. W., & Norman, G. R. (2000). Assessing the measurement properties of a clinical reasoning exercise. *Teaching and Learning in Medicine*, *12*(4), 196–200. doi:10.1207/S15328015TLM1204_6 PMID:11273369

ADDITIONAL READING

Barrows, H. S. (1996). Problem-based learning in medicine and beyond: A brief overview. *New Directions for Teaching and Learning*, *1996*(68), 3–12. doi:10.1002/tl.37219966804

Barrows, H. S., & Tamblyn, R. M. (1980). *Problem-based learning: An approach to medical education.* New York, NY: Springer.

Belfield, J. (2010). Using Gagnes theory to teach chest X-ray interpretation. *The Clinical Teacher*, *7*(1), 5–8. doi:10.1111/j.1743-498X.2009.00329.x PMID:21134135

Peek, H. S., Richards, M., Muir, O., Chan, S. R., Caton, M., & MacMillan, C. (2015). Blogging and social media for mental health education and advocacy: A review for psychiatrists. *Current Psychiatry Reports*, *17*(11), 1–8. doi:10.1007/s11920-015-0629-2 PMID:26377948

Reigeluth, C. M. (1999). *The elaboration theory: Guidance for scope and sequence decisions. Instructional design theories and models: A new paradigm of instructional theory* (Vol. 2, pp. 425–453). Mahwah, NJ: Lawrence Erlbaum Associates.

Smith, P. L., & Ragan, T. J. (2005). *Instructional design* (3rd Ed.). New York, NY: Wiley.

KEY DEFINITIONS

Blended Learning: A combination of online and on campus class activities for the instructional situation.

Contextualization: Student placement to authentic, complex, and realistic learning processes in order to practice, apply, and assess task and cognitive activities.

Delivery Strategies: Strategies intended to support decisions on readiness of learner transition between stages of education, training, and practice.

Distance Learning: Instructional method utilizing internet-based technologies to deliver student-centered, self-directed, flexible, and direct education to students at a distance.

Elaboration Theory: A scoping and sequencing strategy for large units of instruction that allows for meaning-making by students throughout the learning process.

Epitome: The simplest form of a task that embodies the whole task.

Group Presentation: Students working within an authentic context to perform, identify, explain, diagnose, and offer solution strategies unique to a case.

Instructional Strategies: Course of action for an instructional goal framed by credible and realistic problems in order to activate prior knowledge and experiences in order to learn new knowledge and skills.

Learner Analysis: Identification of student entry-level knowledge, skills, and demographics.

Macro Strategies: Strategies concerned with organizational scope and sequence of content area(s) in order to assist the learner achieve an instructional goal.

Management Strategies: Controlling and managing resources so that they are ready and available for the educator and students to use at the point in time needed.

Micro Strategies: Strategies concerned with order sequencing of specific activities to facilitate various aspects of the learning process.

Organizational Strategies: Strategies intended to scope, sequence, or specify order to activities of small and large bodies of information.

Portfolio: A compilation of work and material unique to a case or series of cases.

Problem-Based Learning: A curricular level instructional delivery strategy facilitated by the instructor to stimulate self-directed learner relevancy, authenticity, and activity through ill-structured problem scenarios.

Scope: Generic skills and attitudes that should be covered, the "what to teach" decisions that are normally determined through a content analysis.

Sequence: Regulation of superordinate, coordinate, and subordinate relationships into a conceptual relationship utilizing a hierarchical-topical or spiral-topical method.

Social Media: An online space for talking, participating, networking, and fact-finding through discussions, feedback, and information sharing.

Chapter 3
Using Backward Design for Competency-Based Undergraduate Medical Education

Barbara L. Joyce
Oakland University William Beaumont School of Medicine, USA

Stephanie M. Swanberg
Oakland University William Beaumont School of Medicine, USA

ABSTRACT

This chapter focuses on strategies for approaching competency-based medical education (CBME) in the undergraduate medical curriculum (UME). CBME uses national professional standards, typically set by accrediting bodies or professional organizations, to shape curricular design and assessment of learner outcomes as well as to provide clarity to the learner about the knowledge, skills, and attitudes needed for successful practice. Wiggins and McTighe's (2015) Backward Design instructional design model provides a practical structure for approaching CBME since it proposes beginning with the national standards, defining outcomes and assessment methods, and then developing curricular content. The chapter will describe the backward design model, the history of CBME in the United States, current issues with CBME, and use of an integrated curriculum to successfully implement CBME. It will culminate with a discussion of creating action plans for individual programs to align assessment and outcome measures more directly to curriculum.

INTRODUCTION

Competency-based medical education (CBME), organized around a set of national competencies and learner outcomes, has inspired a transformational shift in our conversations about what it means to educate learners in medicine (Accreditation Council Graduate Medical Education [ACGME], 2016; Carraccio, Wolfstal, Englander, Ferentz, & Martin, 2002; Carraccio and Englander, 2013; Harden,

DOI: 10.4018/978-1-5225-2098-6.ch003

Copyright © 2017, IGI Global. Copying or distributing in print or electronic forms without written permission of IGI Global is prohibited.

1999). This transformational shift required medical education programs to re-examine curricular content and outcome measures used to determine whether graduates have acquired the knowledge, skills, and attitudes necessary for independent practice. During the 1990's, the transition to CBME was prompted by The Accreditation Council of Graduate Medical Education (ACGME) to improve physician training, and address the skills necessary for the practice of medicine in the 21st century. Following an extensive stakeholder review, the accrediting body identified the need to focus on educational outcomes, increase the rigor in process requirements, and the need to build a learning community across many specialties focused on implementing CBME (Bataldan, Leach, Swing 2002). All specialties were required to begin implementing CBME over the next ten years (Bataldan, Leach, Swing 2002).

The impact on curricular design and assessment measures was significant, and many programs struggled with designing curricula that leads to the desired outcomes. Competency-based outcomes, in the form of national standards, have been added to existing curriculum without determining whether the curriculum directly relates to the desired outcomes. Learners may find this approach confusing since there can be a disconnect between what they are learning and what they are expected to know or do. Competency-based standards for a profession are meant to shape curricular design and measurement of outcomes, and to provide clarity to the learner about knowledge, skills, and attitudes needed for successful practice.

Backward Design is an instructional design model that proposes instructors start with outcomes and work backward to design appropriate assessment tools and curricular content (Wiggins & McTighe, 2005). This model is used in K-12 education to align curriculum and assessment with national standards. "To begin with the end in mind means to start with a clear understanding of your destination. It means to know where you're going so that you better understand where you are now, so the steps you take are always in the right direction" (Covey, 1989, p. 98). Backward design can be applied to medical education by beginning with the national standards or competencies for medical education, defining outcomes and assessment methods, and then defining curricular content.

There are three components to the Backward Design model. The first component is 'Identify Desired Results.' This component encourages educators to define what criteria or performance standards are necessary for students to demonstrate the required knowledge and skills for independent practice. The second component is 'Determine Acceptable Evidence.' What is the evidence the learner has achieved the desired skill? This component encourages the medical educator to operationalize the learning outcomes and identify appropriate assessment methods to determine whether the learner possess the desired skill set. The third component is 'Plan Learning Experiences and Instruction' Careful planning of curricular experiences encourages educators to analyze what is "enduring knowledge" (the key concepts necessary for practice), "important to know or do" (prerequisite knowledge), and "worth being familiar with" (detail). Lastly, teaching strategies are considered. These three categories can help educators align their curriculum with key components of national standards for medical education and hone in on content that is essential for independent practice (Wiggins & McTighe, 2005).

Medical educators may find backward design a useful instructional design methodology as they begin to shift their curriculum to competency-based outcomes. It provides a framework and strategy for thinking through measurement of competency as well as for identifying key curricular content and linking it to outcomes. The net result of a curricular revision using this model is likely to result in learners having clearer expectations of what they need to learn and outcomes related to national standards.

This chapter will cover the history of CBME in the United States. A review of the backward design model, with examples of application to CBME, will be discussed. Opportunities to use this curriculum design model for curricular integration will also be discussed. The chapter will culminate with a discussion of creating action plans for individual programs to align assessment and outcome measures more directly to curriculum.

BACKGROUND

History of Competency-Based Medical Education in the U.S.

Graduate Medical Education (GME)

CBME was discussed in the 1970's and 1980's but did not gain traction as a framework for designing medical education curricula (Carraccio et al., 2002). By the late 1990's, however, external factors, such as increasing public and government pressure to train and certify competent physicians, led the ACGME and American Board of Medical Specialties (ABMS) to adopt a set of six competencies in 1999 as a framework for graduate physician training and board certification. These six core competency domains were: Medical Knowledge (MK), Patient Care (PC), Interpersonal and Communication Skills (ICP), Professionalism (PC), Systems-based Practice (SBP), and Practice-based Learning and Improvement (PBLI). Each competency domain reflected an integration of knowledge, skills, and attitudes, and had a set of sub-competencies that more explicitly defined each competency domain (Swing, 2007). Table 1 provides a definition of each competency domain and an adapted list of the sub-competencies associated with it. The ACGME created the Outcome Project in 2001 and phased in regulatory requirements requiring graduate medical education training programs in the U.S. to develop competency-based curricula and measure the educational outcomes of training (Swing, 2007). The paradigm shift from a process and content structure of residency training to a competency-based structure with defined outcomes was challenging for the medical education community to develop and implement. Assessment of educational outcomes of the six competency domains for residency training programs proved equally daunting.

Some progress was seen in the implementation of curricula in the competency domains following the Outcome Project and in the development of assessment tools, largely due to: regulatory bodies requiring implementation, increasingly widespread adoption of CBME worldwide, and alignment of competency domains with broader health care quality aims (Australian Medical Council Limited, 2010; Frank & Danoff, 2007; Royal College of General Practitioners, 2016; Simpson et al., 2002; Swing, 2007). Assessment of an individual resident's competence remained overwhelming, despite the fervor of the CBME movement. Experts recommended using multiple assessment methods, including direct observation and multisource feedback, over the course of training but these methods were challenging to implement given the structure of residency training.

In 2010, the International Competency-based Medical Educator Collaborators met to discuss pertinent issues related to CBME in medical education in an effort to provide consensus around a shared definition, review progress to date, and explore future directions (Frank et al., 2010b). Frank et al. (2010), after a thorough review of the literature, proposed the following definition of competency-based education: "Competency-based education (CBE) is an approach to preparing physicians for practice that is fundamentally oriented to graduate outcome abilities and organized around competencies derived from an analysis of societal and patient needs. It de-emphasizes time-based training and promises greater accountability, flexibility and learner-centeredness" (Frank et al., 2010a, p. 636). This definition became the standard description for CBME (Frank et al., 2010b). The curricular implications of this descrip-

Table 1.

ACGME Competencies	Definition	Subcompetency
Medical Knowledge	Demonstrate knowledge of established and evolving biomedical, clinical, epidemiological and social-behavioral sciences, as well as the application of this knowledge to patient care	Determined by specialty
Patient Care and Procedural Skills	Provide care that is compassionate, appropriate and effective for treatment of health problems and promotion of health	Perform diagnostic, medical and surgical procedures essential to specialty
Practice-based Learning and Improvement	Investigate and evaluate care of patients	Utilize quality improvement techniques to improve practice
	Critically appraise and integrate scientific evidence	Use and apply evidence from research studies Use information technology to increase learning Educate patients, families and other health professionals
	Use self-evaluation and life-long learning to improve patient care	Accurately assessment limits of one's own expertise Set goals for future learning and self-improvement Identify appropriate self-directed learning activities Utilize formative feedback from peers and mentors
Interpersonal and Communication Skills	Ability to communicate effective with patients, families and other healthcare professionals	Demonstrate effective communication with patients Demonstrate effective communication with physicians and other members of healthcare team Participate effectively as a team member or leader Provide consultations to colleagues and members of the team Maintain accurate medical records
Professionalism	Commitment to professional responsibilities and ethical principles	Demonstrate compassion, integrity and respect Patient needs come before self-interest Protect patient privacy and autonomy Skills in cultural diversity
Systems-based Practice	Awareness of the broad health care system and ability to utilize resources	Be able to work in different healthcare settings Coordinate patient care Understand cost awareness and risk-benefit analysis Advocate for better systems of patient care Advocate for patient Be a member of an interprofessional team Identify system errors and determine solutions

tion are striking. The educational outcomes for physician training are based on the acquisition and demonstration of broad domains of knowledge, skill, and attitudes (competencies) that progress along a developmental continuum from novice to expert (milestones) rather than on time spent in training. In competency-based education, the focus is on the learner reaching a specific level of performance in each of the broad competency domains. Albanese, Mejicano, Mullan, Kokotailo, and Gruppen (2008) articulated the following characteristics of competencies:

1. A competency reflects expectations determined, in large part, by external stakeholders;
2. A competency reflects measurable behavior;
3. A competency uses explicit criteria for determining whether or not a learner has obtained a required level of performance; and
4. A competency is transparent and outlines expectations to the learner and external stakeholders (Albanese, Mejicano, Mullan, Kokotailo, & Gruppen, 2010).

But, were the ACGME/ABMS competencies enough? Were learners able to construct an explicit roadmap of their learning and were faculty able to provide appropriate feedback at specific points in that journey? Were curriculum designers and those tasked with developing assessment tools able to explicitly define outcomes?

In 2013, a key element of the ACGME Next Accreditation System was the development of specialty-specific educational milestones for each of the competencies and sub-competencies. Milestones provided a series of developmental benchmarks for each sub-competency resulting in more accurate assessment of educational outcomes and resident performance. Milestones also provided trainees with an explicit roadmap for learning and encouraged faculty to target specific developmental feedback (Nasca, Philibert, Brigham, & Flynn, 2012). Achievement of a milestone was rated on a scale of 1-5, following the Dreyfus model, to provide a snapshot of a resident's developmental progression from novice to expert (an aspirational goal) (Batalden, Leach, Swing, Dreyfus, & Dreyfus, 2002; Swing et al., 2013). The Dreyfus model identifies five stages of adult skills acquisition beginning with novice learners, and progressing through additional stages of advanced beginner, competent, proficient, and expert (Dreyfus, 2004). This model of skill acquisition represents a pattern that aligns with graduate medical education training, and provides benchmarks (milestones) to enable learners to progress along the developmental continuum

Assessment of milestones required use of multiple assessment methods, such as direct observation and multisource feedback, and the aggregation of assessment data. A committee of expert faculty reviewed the assessment data to determine whether a resident was acquiring the necessary knowledge, skills, and attitudes particular to a milestone. The aggregation of this data has proved challenging for many residencies, given the lack of technological resources and adequate personnel. Direct observations of resident performance and multi-source feedback are resource intensive and were challenging to implement (Swing et al., 2013). Residency programs continued to struggle to implement the necessary assessment tools, aggregate data, provide feedback to trainees, and make decisions about where an individual resident falls on a developmental continuum.

In response to the challenges associated with assessing competencies, ten Cate and Scheele (2007) introduced Entrustable Professional Activities (EPAs). These researchers argued that assessing competencies was difficult and the assessment of competence, in many programs, consisted of a series of checklists, making assessment of competencies reductionistic. This reductionistic approach diluted the original meaning of competency-based education. Ten Cate and Scheele further proposed that competency-based curriculum should be constructed to reflect the critical clinical activities of a profession. "EPAs are those professional activities that together constitute the mass of critical elements that operationally define a profession" (ten Cate & Scheele, 2007, p. 544). EPAs contain multiple competency domains and sit at the top of the hierarchy for CBME. EPAs are core professional activities that contain multiple competency domains with concomitant sub-competencies and milestones. See Figure 1 for a representation of this hierarchy. Faculty review the performance of the trainee, using aggregate assessment data, and make decisions about whether the learner can be trusted to perform a clinical task without direct supervision. The expert judgment of the faculty serves as a focal point for determining entrustment. Varying levels of supervision ranging from direct supervision to independent practice can be accorded to trainees based on these entrustment decisions. Hauer et al. (2014) clearly defined the distinction between assessment of competencies and milestones compared to EPAs. "Assessment of competencies and milestones captures the range of trainee behaviors that are foundational for entrustment…EPAs exemplify assessment based on trust, as an emerging strategy for supervision grounded in the trust a supervisor holds in a trainee to perform a given activity" (Hauer et al., 2014, p. 451).

Figure 1. Representation of hierarchy

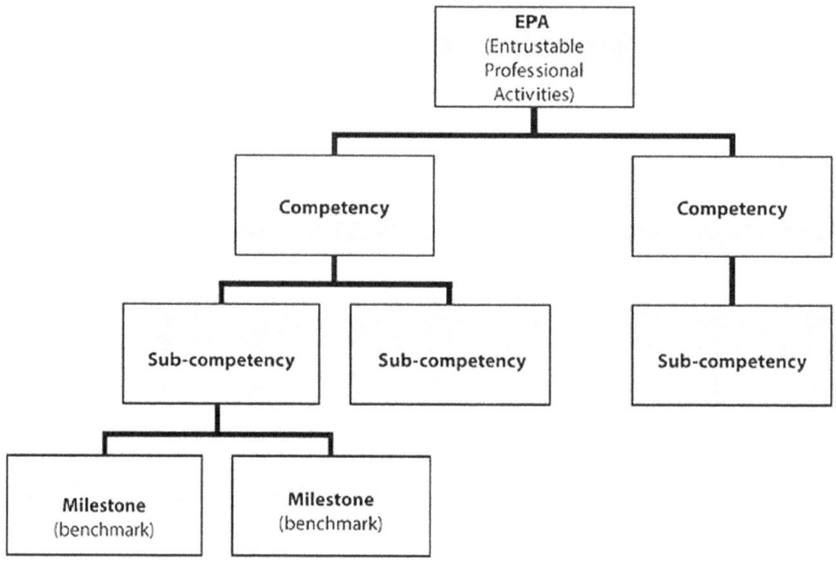

EPAs, therefore, become an overarching assessment framework for a training program whereas competencies and milestones capture the developmental progression of the trainee and provide a more complete and granular picture of resident performance (Englander & Carraccio, 2014). Some specialties in graduate medical education have embraced EPAs while others have not yet done so.

Since 1999 there has been an attempt to embed CBME into GME. It began with the ACGME/ABMS outlining six competency domains containing sub-competencies and adding specialty specific milestones or benchmarks for each competency in 2013.

EPAs were introduced in some specialties. Assessment of competencies, milestones, and EPAs remains challenging, and difficulties persist in implementing authentic assessments, such as direct observation and multisource feedback. Curriculum design, for the most part, has focused primarily on defining objectives for each rotation or educational experience, which may not make explicit links to assessment tools or outcomes.

Undergraduate Medical Education (UME)

CBME has been slower to catch on in UME due, in large part, to lack of a consistent national competency framework from which to design curricula and assessment systems. In addition, the Liaison Committee on Medical Education (LCME), the accrediting body for UME, has not identified what the specific educational outcomes should be for UME, and individual schools are expected to determine their own desired educational outcomes (Liaison Committee on Medical Education [LCME], 2016). To fill this gap, Englander et al. (2013) developed a competency framework for UME that could be used across all health professions training. This competency framework drew upon the work of ACGME and included the six competency domains from GME, but added an additional two domains, Interprofessional Collaboration (IC) and Personal and Professional Development (PPD), to reflect a set of competency domains that would be inclusive of all health professions training. The taxonomy was named the Physician

Competency Reference Set (PCRS). The eight competency domains are reflected in Table 2. Table 3 also lists an example of the subcompetencies for Interpersonal and Communication Skills. Each medical school was encouraged to link its overall educational objectives to these eight competency domains and corresponding sub-competencies (Englander et al., 2013). UME competency domains can serve as a curricular framework shaping both content and assessment for medical schools. For further information on the competency domains and subcompetencies associated with each domain, please consult Core Entrustable Professional Activities for Entering Residency: Teachers and Learners Guide (Association of American Medical Colleges [AAMC], 2014).

In 2013, the AAMC convened an expert panel of medical educators to further refine the conceptual framework for UME outcomes so that educational outcomes could be linked across the UME-GME continuum. The panel took into consideration the prior work done on competencies and milestones, existing competency frameworks, as well as the more recently introduced concept of EPAs (AAMC, 2014; ten Cate, 2005). The panel drafted 13 core EPAs and encouraged medical schools to adopt these as outcome measures. UME competencies could be mapped to EPAs in such a manner that both clinical skills and more domain-specific competencies could be identified and measured. Englander et al. (2016) recently articulated the milestones for UME were behavioral descriptors of "pre-entrustable" vs. "entrustable" learners who could perform a particular EPA without supervision. An example of a UME Milestone is outlined in Table 4. Each subcompetency had a series of milestones or behavioral descriptors identifying behaviors expected for entrustment. The hierarchical representation of EPAs, competencies, and milestones proposed for UME are similar to GME (See Figure 1). The document *Core Entrustable Professional Activities for Entering Residency* contains more detailed descriptions of each of the EPAs, competencies and sub-competencies, and milestones (AAMC, 2014).

Table 2. Physician Competence Reference Set (PCRS)- Eight Domains of Physician Competence AAMC (Englander et al., 2013)

1.	Patient care
2.	Knowledge for practice
3.	Practice-based learning and improvement
4.	Professionalism
5.	Interpersonal and communication skills
6.	Systems-based practice
7.	Interprofessional collaboration
8.	Personal and professional development

Table 3. Example of sub-competencies for Interpersonal and Communication Skills (Englander et al., 2013)

Demonstrate interpersonal and communication skills with patients, their families, and health professionals	
1.	Communicate effectively with patients, families, and the public across a broad range of socioeconomic and cultural backgrounds
2.	Communicate effectively with colleagues, other health professionals and health related agencies
3.	Work effectively on a health care team
4.	Act in a consultative role to other health professionals
5.	Maintain comprehensive, timely, and legible medical records
6.	Demonstrate sensitivity, honesty, and compassion in difficult conversations
7.	Demonstrate insight and understanding about emotions and their impact on human responses that allow one to manage interpersonal interactions.

Table 4. EPAs for Entering Residency (AAMC, 2013)

1.	Gather a history and perform a physical examination
2.	Prioritize a differential diagnosis following a clinical encounter
3.	Recommend and interpret common diagnostic and screening tests
4.	Enter and discuss orders/prescriptions
5.	Document a clinical encounter in the patient record
6.	Provide an oral presentation of a clinical encounter
7.	Form clinical questions and retrieve evidence to advance patient care
8.	Give or receive a patient handover to transition care responsibly
9.	Collaborate as a member of an interprofessional team
10.	Recognize a patient requiring urgent or emergent care and initiate evaluation and management
11.	Obtain informed consent for tests and/or procedures
12.	Perform general procedures of a physician
13.	Identify system failures and contribute to a culture of safety and improvement

EPAs, at the level of UME, consist of foundational clinical skill sets needed on the first day of residency, and are constructed so residents can more easily transition from student to resident. See Table 5 for a list of UME EPAs. Entrustment remains a critical component of the undergraduate EPAs and the concept of entrustment is similar to what has been previously discussed. Englander et al. (2016) believed that using similar frameworks along the UME-GME continuum would help align learners' development of progressive skills (Englander et al., 2016). The real success of EPAs, milestones, or competency initiatives is dependent on the ability of the field to operationalize outcomes across the entire continuum. Curricula should be thoughtfully designed so that learner knowledge, skills, and attitudes are appropriately scaffolded and integrated, and concepts are repeatedly presented at increasing levels of complexity (spiral curriculum). Learner expectations should be explicitly outlined at each step and learners should receive targeted feedback designed to help them progress along a developmental continuum (Carraccio et al., 2016; Chen, McNamara, Teherani, ten Cate, O'Sullivan, 2016; Chen, van der Broek, & ten Cate, 2015; Englander & Carraccio, 2014).

Table 5. Examples of UME Milestones (Adapted from Englander et al—Core Entrustable Activities)

EPA	Critical Competency	Pre Entrustable	Entrustable
Gather history and perform physical exam	Gather essential information about patients through history taking, physical exam, lab and imaging data, and other tests	Gather too list or too much information Unable to identify salient details Uses basic pathophysiology knowledge without being able to link to prior experience Incorrectly performs physical exam Misses key physical exam findings Does not alter exam to meet needs of patient Does not incorporate secondary data	Links current experience to past encounters Clinical information can be filtered and a prioritized differential diagnosis created Performs basic physical exam appropriately Can alter exam to meet needs of patient Uses secondary sources

Assessment of entrustment at the UME level, however, remains challenging given the fluid nature of the clinical teams that students encounter on clerkship rotations, and the brief period of time spent on each clerkship (Holmboe, Ginsburg, & Bernabeo, 2011). Medical schools will need to focus on defining a clear-cut process that addresses the following questions:

1. What are the best assessment methods?
2. How will data from multiple assessment methods be aggregated?
3. Who ultimately determines entrustment?
4. What is the role of basic/foundation sciences in this process?
5. Given the current structure of the clerkship years, with students rotating amongst various clerkship rotations and on various teams within a clerkship rotation, who will be in a position to evaluate the student?

Despite all the discussion around competency frameworks, EPAs, and milestones, medical educators are still challenged in determining the outcomes of training in specific, measureable terms that can assist a learner in charting a course to expertise. The outcomes of training should be meaningful for the learner and to the faculty member, and should be a point of discussion about direction of future learning plans. Carraccio et al. (2016), noted that assessment strategies must be closely aligned or mapped to the construct (EPA, milestone, or competencies) being assessed, multiple assessors should be used to bring varying perspectives of the learner, and developmental feedback to the learner should be targeted to specific skills or knowledge.

Even if assessment strategies are closely mapped to EPAs or competencies, the next challenges lie in first identifying the content needed in the curricula to support achievement of these competencies and then planning when and how that content should be taught to most benefit the learner. Unfortunately, learners cannot master the competencies in a UME program through a single course or discipline. Instead mastery of content relies on appropriately building and integrating knowledge and skills from many disciplines gradually throughout their medical school careers and beyond. As such, the integrated curriculum model is a logical partner for approaching CBME at the UME level, particularly in the context of backward design.

The Integrated Medical Curriculum in Support of CBME

Defining the Integrated Medical Curriculum

One of the challenges of the integrated curriculum in UME has been reaching a common understanding of exactly what constitutes 'integration.' In the context of UME, curricular integration traditionally seeks to remove the structural barriers between the basic and clinical sciences (Brauer & Ferguson, 2015). However, definitions and interpretations of integration widely vary. For the purposes of this chapter, the proposed definition by Brauer and Ferguson (2015) will be used: "a fully synchronous, trans-disciplinary delivery of information between the foundational sciences and the applied sciences throughout all years of a medical school curriculum" (Brauer & Ferguson, 2015, p. 318). In this definition, the term 'foundational sciences,' adopted from Bandiera, Boucher, Neville, Kuper, and Hodges (2013), incorporates not only the traditional basic sciences, such as anatomy and biochemistry, but also behavioral sciences, population health, and social sciences. In the same vein, 'applied sciences' parallels the traditional clinical sciences (Bandiera, Boucher, Neville, Kuper, & Hodges, 2013). Brauer and Ferguson's definition stresses the collaboration of both realms in deliberately structuring and delivering the curriculum as a whole over the entire four years. Models of implementing such integrated curricula will be addressed later in the chapter. The major limitation to this definition is the ongoing separation of two groups of 'sciences' rather than one, integrated whole. In addition, there is a lack of acknowledgement of the role of the arts and humanities in medical education. This dichotomous model has steered UME over the last 100 years.

Integration Through the Lens of Flexner

In his seminal report, Flexner (1910) emphasized the importance of including not only clinical skills, but also 'laboratory sciences' in the medical school curriculum: "In general, the four-year curriculum falls into two fairly equal sections: the first two years are devoted mainly to laboratory sciences, - anatomy, physiology, pharmacology, pathology; the last two to clinical work in medicine, surgery, and obstetrics" (Flexner, 1910, p. 57). This structure is often referred to as the 'two plus two' model and continues to this day to be the underpinning of medical school curricula.

Nevertheless, even in this early report, Flexner recognized the value of many disciplines in the learning and practice of medicine, "How far the earlier years should be at all conscious of the latter is a mooted question" (Flexner, 1910, p. 57) and that "No one [science] is sharply demarcated…medical education is a technical or professional discipline; it calls for the possession of certain portions of many sciences arranged and organized with a distinct practical purpose in view" (Flexner, 1910, p. 58). In this, Flexner maintains that in the context of medical education, the sciences are too intertwined to operate in silos and should collaborate no matter where their respective content is covered in the curriculum. Flexner's primary focus, however, remains on the two realms of the basic and clinical sciences.

Surrounding the 100-year anniversary of Flexner's report, the field of medicine has been seriously reflecting on the current structure of undergraduate medical education with calls to retire the 'two plus two' model and investigate alternative ways of approaching UME. In a commentary on Flexner's original report, Boelen (2002) argued the recommendations created 100 years ago were meant to formalize medical education, not be the ultimate model to follow without question (Boelen, 2002). He continues by saying the scope of Flexner's model needs to be expanded to accommodate the needs of modern medicine and that medical schools can emulate Flexner's critical approach in thinking about medical education reform (Boelen, 2002).

Shortly after Boelen's commentary, several reports were released by various foundations and professional bodies analyzing the current structure of UME including from The Commonwealth Fund Task Force on Academic Health Centers (2002), The Blue Ridge Academic Health Group (2003), the Committee on the Roles of Academic Health Centers in the 21st Century (2003), and the AAMC (2004). All coming to the same conclusion as well that modern medical education needs to critically reflect on current issues in science and medicine. In their review, Cooke, Irby, Sullivan, and Ludmerer (2006) summarized the major changes to the academic and clinical medicine environments in the 100 years since Flexner's seminal report. Among these changes, they posit the most impactful included: 1) the emphasis on research over clinical care and teaching; 2) the shift of research away from patients to a focus on lab-based research; and 3) the demands of profit-based models of care on physician priorities (Cooke, Irby, Sullivan, & Ludmerer, 2006). Ultimately, they believe Flexner would be among those in support of the reform:

No one would cheer more loudly for a change in medical education than Abraham Flexner. He recognized that medical education had to reconfigure itself in response to changing scientific, social, and economic circumstances in order to flourish from one generation to the next. The flexibility and freedom to change — indeed, the mandate to do so — were part of Flexner's essential message. He would undoubtedly support the fundamental restructuring of medical education needed today. Indeed, we suspect he would find it long overdue. (Cooke, Irby, Sullivan, & Ludmerer, 2006, p.1343)

Medical schools have started to address the call for curriculum restructuring by Boelen and these organizations through the inclusion of social sciences and humanities content within their curricula. Bandaranayake (2011) identified behavioral science and medical ethics as the two primary disciplines that medical schools have added in expanding the scope of the curriculum (Bandaranayake, 2011). The primary drawback of adding these disciplines is that they are mostly taught separately from the rest of the curriculum. As a result, both students and traditional basic science and clinical faculty have difficulty seeing the value of including such content in medical school curricula. Despite these challenges, he still believes integration of these topics into existing courses is the most effective approach for increasing learners' and teachers' appreciation of such content (Bandaranayake, 2011). Recognizing the value of multiple disciplines in medical education is indeed progress, but once again, the estrangement of disciplines continues rather than the creation of one, integrated whole.

It is clear that the profession of medicine is in support of medical education reform, but identifying the need for change and implementing that change are two very different things. As outlined earlier in this chapter, training at the GME level has successfully approached reform through the use of milestones and competencies. Developing a similar framework and plan for all medical schools to follow in reforming curricula at the UME level has remained a challenge. This is where partnering competencies and EPAs with the integrated curricular model may offer one potential solution.

Integration Models

Although integrated curricula have been discussed in the general education literature since the 1940s (Mcgroth & Washburne, 1949), it is really only in the last two decades that integration models have appeared in medical education. Bandaranayake (2011) nicely summarizes Dressel's (1958) three approaches to integration in the context of general education:

1. Those that develop interrelationships among existing courses;
2. Those that reorganise content into more general courses; and
3. Those that arrange content around vital problems relevant to students or society (Bandaranayke, 2011, p. 39).

The models proposed in the medical education literature incorporate and mirror these three overarching tenets. Table 6 provides a brief overview of each, including a definition, example, and the original citation in which the model was published. For further detail on these models, see Brauer and Ferguson's 2015 AMEE guide as well as Chapters 3 and 4 of Bandaranayke's "The Integrated Medical Curriculum" (2011), which provide excellent summaries and additional examples of how these models have been used at various medical schools.

Table 6. Models of Integration

Model	Definition	Example	Originating Citation
Horizontal Integration	"Integration across disciplines…within a finite period of time" (Brauer & Ferguson, 2015, p. 314).	An organ system course, such as a the cardiovascular system, that combines multiple disciplines, such as anatomy, biochemistry, and microbiology, into a single course.	Benor, 1982
Vertical Integration	"Integration across time, attempting to improve education by disrupting the traditional barrier between the basic and clinical sciences" (Brauer & Ferguson, 2015, p. 314).	Usually in the context of the traditional 'two plus two' model, vertical integration pairs clinical content with basic science content in the first two years and the basic sciences are revisited again in the clinical context in the third and fourth years.	Benor, 1982
Z Model	A form of vertical integration that emphasizes basic science with a little clinical content at the beginning of medical school with graduate increases in clinical content as the student progresses.	In the M1 year, the majority of course content focuses on basic science topics, but students have clinical visits once per week to promote early exposure to clinical experiences.	Wijnen-Meijer, Cate, Rademakers, Van Der Schaaf, and Borleffs, 2009
Spiral Integration	Combination of both horizontal and vertical integration where "the basic and clinical sciences are continually integrated" throughout the UME curriculum (Brauer & Ferguson, 2015, p. 317).	In Harden's original article, he uses the example of students progressing from the normal to abnormal with equal integration of basic science and clinical content throughout all years. Other themes, or threads, are also present throughout, such as preventative medicine and ethics.	Harden, Davis, and Crosby, 1997

Challenges of the Integrated Curriculum

There are a number of considerations medical schools should take into account when investigating the development of an integrated curriculum. Bandaranayake (2011) reviewed the major advantages and disadvantages of integrated curricula to both the student and teacher. For students, integration increases their retention of knowledge, encourages creative thinking, and reduces redundancy of content (Bandaranayake, 2011). Several case studies over the last 20 years have demonstrated the positive effect of integrated curricula on student learning and retention (Brooks, Panizzi Woodley, Jackson, & Hoesley, 2015; Dahle, Brynhildsen, Behrbohm Fallsberg, Rundquist, & Hammar, 2002; Dyrbye, Starr, Thompson, & Lindor, 2011; Schmidt et al., 1996; Woods et al., 2006). Schmidt et al. (1996) found that students trained in a new integrated curriculum were able to more accurately diagnose clinical conditions than students trained in a traditional curriculum (Schmidt et al., 1996). In their study, investigators in Sweden found that students who were trained in a problem-based, integrated curriculum were able to better link and apply basic science and clinical science (Dahle et al., 2002). Woods et al. (2006) also found that students who learned the anatomy and physiology behind four clinical conditions were able to better recall relevant clinical information after one week compared with students who were only given non-related epidemiological information, such as prevalence and prognosis (Woods et al., 2006). More recently, the Mayo Medical School implemented a yearlong Advanced Doctoring course that integrated basic science, clinical, surgical, diagnostic and simulation into six content blocks. Though the authors did not formally assess student knowledge or retention, student course evaluations indicated that this organizational structure helped them better apply class concepts to clinical experiences. In addition, on their AAMC Graduation Questionnaire reporting on their medical school experience, 46.4% of students strongly agreed that basic science content was sufficiently integrated in the curriculum, compared to two years earlier where only 11.4% reported this (Dyrbye et al., 2011).

Finally, Brooks et al. (2015) documented improved student United States Medical Licensing Examination (USMLE) scores in anatomy and embryology after implementing a fully integrated, organ system-based curriculum during the first two years of medical school where anatomy, embryology, and radiology were carefully tied to organ system content (Brooks et al., 2015). Although these case studies are promising, there is still little published data demonstrating the long-term impact of integrated curriculum in UME; a challenge we will discuss in detail below.

In addition to students, integration also offers benefits for faculty. Increased communication and collaboration with colleagues, particularly those outside their field, is the major benefit of integration. Related to this, faculty can discuss solutions to common educational problems with fellow colleagues as well as share the teaching load, which is of utmost importance to busy clinical faculty (Bandaranayake, 2011).

Although there are documented benefits of integration to both students and faculty, there are major limitations that could dissuade medical schools from pursuing integrated curricula. One of the major barriers is simply the time and effort required to develop, implement, and assess an integrated curriculum, particularly if it requires major curriculum reform (Goldman & Schroth, 2012; Muller, Jain, Loeser, & Irby, 2008). In their article, Malik and Malik (2011) outlined twelve tips for developing a successful integrated curriculum. Nearly all of their strategies involve careful planning, including training faculty on integration practices, choosing an appropriate integration approach or model, establishing working groups and timelines, determining the desired learning outcomes and content, and selecting assessment methods (Malik & Malik, 2011). These tips directly align with the tenets of competency-based education in terms of identifying educational outcomes and how to appropriately assess those outcomes.

Such careful planning also requires buy-in from a number of stakeholders including medical school administration as well as faculty to lead the integration process. Bandaranayke (2011) outlined the major challenges that faculty may encounter in implementing an integrated curriculum. These include: 1) forcing specialists to learn new content outside their traditional discipline area in order to develop integrated instructional sessions; 2) developing interdisciplinary relationships and working teams; and 3) developing material that is appropriate, timely, and interesting to medical students; and 4) sensing the need to protect their existing instructional time in the curriculum. To aid schools in overcoming the challenges of integration, Goldman and Schroth (2012) propose a three-level framework where integration is discussed, planned, and addressed at three distinct levels: the program level, the course level, and the session level (Goldman & Schroth, 2012).

The program level is most concerned with overarching school policies, such as the mission, goals, and objectives of the learning program. At the course level, integration should be addressed when developing course objectives and discussing content, sequencing of content, and assessment. Finally, at the session level, integration should drive session objectives and teaching strategies (Goldman & Schroth, 2012). The main goal of this approach is to use integration as the driver for all decisions at all levels, ultimately ensuring that all stakeholders are involved, including administration and faculty. For students, integrated curricula make it increasingly difficult to identify how much they should know on a particular topic in addition to not being as exposed to the various specialties during the course of their medical school careers (Bandaranayke, 2011).

By far, one of the most challenging aspects of the integrated curricula has been assessing its effectiveness. A narrative review conducted by Kulasegaram, Martimianakis, Myloploulos, Whitehead, and Woods (2013) analyzed literature on the integration of the basic and clinical sciences from 1982 – 2012. They found that although numerous studies describe methods of integration, assessment of student learning outcomes is scarce (Kulasegaram et al, 2013). Brauer and Ferguson (2015) also recognize the lack of studies in the literature analyzing the long-term effectiveness of integrated curricula. In their summary of the evaluation strategies published in the medical education literature, they discovered that reflection, multiple choice and/or short answer exams, exercises with standardized patients, and concept maps were the most commonly reported (Brauer & Ferguson, 2015). However, all of these were reported in a single study with no indication of how these methods faired over the long term. In Chapter 6 of his book, Bandaranayke (2011) also identified multiple-choice questions, free response questions, and clinical examinations as the major forms of assessing integrated knowledge. Above all, he stresses the importance of closely linking integrated material with integrated assessments:

If students are shown how the basic sciences they learn can be applied to clinical and community situations they are likely to encounter in the future...they should be presented with such situations in their examinations to assess their ability to apply basic science knowledge to new situations by interrelating the knowledge they gain from different disciplines. (Bandaranayke, 2011, p. 82)

No matter the model or assessment used, Bandaranayke (2011) contends that no single integration approach can be successful without encouraging the learner to pursue his or her own 'integrative activities.' In other words, faculty and the structure of the UME curricula must guide students in learning how to reflect and connect integrated content across the curriculum. Kulasegaram et al. (2013) also argue that approaching integration from a cognitive standpoint where the focus shifts to the learner may make the assessment and analysis of integration easier.

The best use of the basic sciences is as a tool for helping learners more effectively understand and organize clinical concepts. Integration should be understood as a cognitive function or operation that occurs within the learner as he or she links clinical concepts with basic science. (Kulasegaram et al., 2013, p. 1582)

Bandaranayke also believes that the success of integration is dependent on the ability of the facilitator to encourage integrative thinking and activities: "The skilled facilitator is one who encourages blurring of boundaries among disciplines, both horizontally and vertically, without establishing links among them himself" (Bandaranayke, 2011, p. 51). Kulasegaram et al. (2013) follow this same logic by concluding that it is the role of educators to review how the learning environment is helping or hindering the learner to 'cognitively integrate' knowledge (Kulasegaram et al., 2013). The conclusion is that there is no one universal method for implementing and assessing an integrated curriculum. As one of the tenets of CBME is identifying the desired learning outcomes and assessing whether students have achieved competence in these outcomes, these issues present additional challenges for medical educators.

Issues with Competency-Based Medical Education

As presented above, many challenges face medical educators in the current environment. With the advent of CBME in UME, outcomes (performance expectations) need to be clearly identified and communicated to the learner. Medical educators need to design curricula that aligns with the outcomes they desire students to achieve and be able to explicitly communicate the linkage between curricula and outcomes to the learner and other faculty. Integration of the basic/foundational science with clinical science will also pose a significant challenge for medical educators. All of this takes a substantial amount of time, effort, and collaboration to plan and execute. As the field moves forward, these challenges to designing strong curricula in UME will only increase. Backward design is instructional design model that may help medical educators conceptualize educational outcomes and curricula in a manner that clearly specifies outcomes and provides learners adequate training to achieve those outcomes.

SOLUTIONS AND RECOMMENDATIONS

Using the Backward Design Instructional Design Model for CBME

Backward Design is an instructional design method first proposed by Wiggins and McTighe (2005) and used primarily in K-12 to design curricula and assessment methods that link to national standards (Wiggins & McTighe, 2005). This model is unique in many respects. Instructional designers start with defining the outcomes, rather than starting with a needs assessment or teaching/content strategies. In many cases, these outcomes reflect national standards. Three basic principles form the core components of the Backward Design model: 'Identify Desired Results', 'Determine Acceptable Evidence', and 'Plan Learning Experiences and Instruction.' In addition, the Backward Design model encourages instructional designers to focus on defining content that includes "enduring knowledge," "important to know or do," and "worth being familiar with" concepts which help form the core of topics for integration. Figure 2 provide a visual illustration of this model applied to UME.

Identify Desired Results

Wiggins and McTighe (2005) recommend instructional designers spend significant time identifying the desired learning outcomes, based on national standards, before deciding on teaching strategies or content. In the case of medical education, entrustment on the UME EPAs represents national standards that medical students should achieve prior to graduation from medical school, and the desired result is entrustment to perform a specific EPA without direct supervision. Medical education leadership will need to define EPAs so that students and faculty have clarity about requirements for pre-entrustment/entrustment decisions for each of the 13 EPAs. In addition, significant time and effort will need to be given to investigating software systems that can collect and aggregate large amounts of data on student performance across multiple courses and years. A process for collecting this data will also need to be established to aid the faculty committee in determining whether each student has reached entrustment for each EPA. Although direct observation and multisource feedback are recommended assessment methods, medical schools will need to experiment with the implementation process so these tools are used in a manner that produce deliberate and targeted feedback to learners to improve performance. The

Figure 2. Backward Design: An Instructional Design Framework for UME

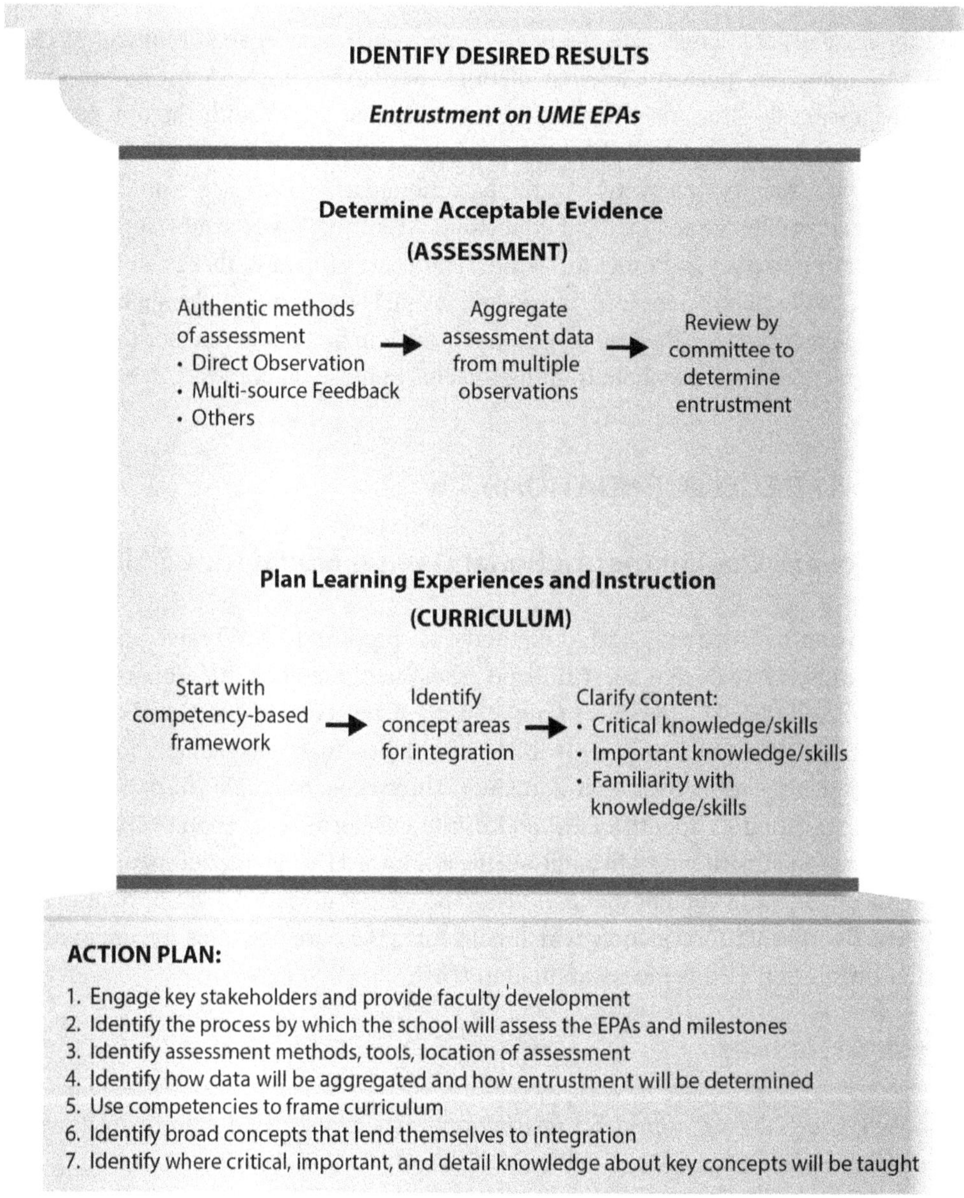

implementation process will vary between schools and should include stakeholders from administration, medical education, faculty, students and others involved in entrustment decisions.

At first glance, the EPAs and competencies appear to be straightforward outcomes of UME. EPAs should be thought of as the overarching outcome for UME while competencies and milestones provide a more granular and specific snapshot of student performance. Of course, a medical student should be able to: "Gather a history and perform a physical exam" or "Recommend and interpret common diagnostic and screening tests" (Englander et al., 2016). But, how does one measure that? How does one determine an acceptable level of performance? How does the instructional designer incorporate all the complexity inherent in an EPA to determine an outcome measure? How do faculty determine entrustment? Backward Design principles, along with review of best practices in the literature, may offer some solutions. The implementation and assessment of EPAs and entrustment is in its infancy and much remains to be learned about best practices for this.

Identify Desired Evidence

The second step in this model discusses identifying the evidence that faculty use to determine whether a student is entrusted to carry out the EPA without direct supervision. Here it is necessary to turn to the literature to determine best practices for assessment and entrustment of the EPAs. Holmboe (2015) recommends the use of authentic assessment methods, such as direct observation of the student performing the EPA or, in the case of some EPAs, multisource feedback from peers and others regarding whether the student adequately performs the EPA. "...Thus, the role and importance of direct observation and mentored deliberate practice in the development of expertise is and always has been central in medical education" (Holmboe, 2015). Recommendations also include multiple observations of student performance over time with the data from each of these observations being aggregated to form a clear picture of student performance. This aggregate data produces a summative assessment of student performance of a particular EPA (Carraccio et al., 2016; et al., 2016; Holmboe, 2015; ten Cate, 2005).. Multiple observations over time on a single student are challenging, particularly given the structure of clerkships with multiple rotations and multiple evaluators. More scholarship in this area is desperately needed as these national standards roll out. For now, it is safe to say that direct observation and multi-source feedback are two key assessment methods recommended by experts.

Assessment tools should also be mapped to the particular clerkship and milestones where students are being directly observed on that particular task. This requires instructional designers to think carefully about where to best observe student performance of EPAs within the clerkship. An example of this mapping in GME is described by Warm et al. (2014) who carefully identified milestones for internal medicine rotations and mapped assessment tools to specific rotations to measure those outcomes (Warm et al., 2016). Once the assessment data is collected on a particular resident, a group of expert faculty reviews that data to determine entrustment. As noted previously, entrustment, or the ability of the faculty to trust the learner to demonstrate the EPA without direct supervision, is a summative assessment. Milestones ("pre-entrustable vs. entrustable") provide formative assessment to the learner throughout training. Milestones help the learner identify where they are in relation to expectations and what skills they still need to refine.

Plan Learning Experience and Instruction

This stage of the Backward Design model is especially important for planning and implementing an integrated curriculum, which is a perfect partner to CBME. Outside of the medical education literature, combining the integrated curriculum model and competency-based education has already been conceptualized and applied in the K-12 environment. In her book "Creating Standards-Based Integrated Curriculum," Drake (2007) outlines several strategies for tackling the design of a competency-based, integrated curriculum through the use of backward design. One example from Drake that illustrates integration in K-12 is the development of an integrated unit on fables for fourth grade students to fulfill the standards set by the Ontario Grade 4 curriculum standards. The unit combines skills in English, math, social studies, arts, and physical education and has students work through a number of tasks related to fables such as reading and interpreting the stories (language arts) and creating drawings of the story (arts). The unit is assessed with a variety of methods including teacher observation, peer assessment, writing reflections, and creating objects (Drake, 2007). Though this example focuses on integrating disciplines taught in K-12, her techniques and strategies may provide a model for developing a structured, integrated curriculum based on existing standards in UME. Of particular interest is Chapter 8 of Drake (2007) on designing and implementing a curriculum process model, originally developed by national educational consultant, Tessie Torres-Dickson. The model includes four phases, which are easily translatable to medical education:

1. **Phase 1:** Obtaining Buy-in and Conducting Professional Development includes meeting with administrators and curriculum planners to gather support for and provide educational workshops for instructors on standards-based curriculum.
2. **Phase 2:** Planning the Curriculum Using Backward Design entails developing planning teams or units and tasking them with using standards to plan how content will be taught and assessed throughout the entire program of study.
3. **Phase 3:** Implementing the Curriculum including documenting how content is taught, assessed, and aligned with the standards.
4. **Phase 4:** Ongoing Assessment & Revision of the Curriculum based on emerging teaching or assessing strategies, changes to standards, and educator professional development (Drake, 2007).

These general phases are represented and broken down even further in the Malick and Malick (2011) article, which will also be of value to medical educators in planning and implementing an integrated curriculum. For UME curricula, using the EPAs and competencies to identify desired results can help curriculum developers then map out how topics will be integrated and taught both vertically and horizontally across the curriculum. Given the complexity of the curriculum in UME, it will be important for medical educators to determine what is "enduring knowledge" (key knowledge and skills necessary for practice), "important to know or do (prerequisite knowledge necessary for successful practice), and "worth being familiar with" (those concepts that enrich and provide key details for broader concept formation) (Drake, 2007).

FUTURE RESEARCH DIRECTIONS

The shift to competency-based education in UME is still in its infancy and little is known about creating an educational program that successfully delivers and assesses a competency-based, integrated curriculum in meaningful ways. There is much to do. Future research directions should focus on identifying best practices for creating and sustaining competency-based integrated curriculum in UME. Specific research areas should target the use of direct observation and multi-source feedback in the clerkship years to provide the student with direct feedback on performance. What are the best tools? Can some tools already used in the GME environment be customized to the UME environment? What are best practices for aggregating data, determining entrustment, and providing students feedback to improve their performance? Many more questions can be generated about the curricular, assessment, and infrastructure changes that will need to happen for EPAs, milestones, and competencies to become firmly rooted in UME.

CONCLUSION

A transformational shift is occurring in UME that will change the way medical schools structure curriculum, assess students, and determine educational infrastructure. For schools starting down the path of implementing EPAs and milestones, a review of strategies outlined by Drake (2007) will help medical educators develop an action plan. It is critical that administrators, curriculum designers, basic science and clinical faculty, residents, and others be involved in the design and development of the new curriculum. Identifying key people with sufficient knowledge, skills, and experience to lead these curricular change initiatives will be crucial. Using backward design as an instructional design model offers a unique approach to developing competency-based, integrated education with the 13 EPAs serving as the overarching outcomes for UME. Identifying authentic assessment methods and tools, implementing those tools, aggregating data, and providing deliberate and focused feedback to students will be a key task of successful implementation and will provide evidence of a student's entrustment of these core clinical skills.

Designing curriculum that focuses on integrating basic/foundational and clinical sciences should be in direct and transparent alignment with UME EPAs, competencies, and milestones. If assessment truly drives learning, then curriculum should be built and assessed using the desired outcomes. As it stands, medical educators often build curriculum based on their expertise and try to retrofit assessment methods. The challenge for medical educators will be to shift their frame of reference to truly consider outcomes first and curricular content second.

REFERENCES

Accreditation Council for Graduate Medical Education. (2016). *ACGME common program requirements*. Retrieved from http://www.acgme.org/What-We-Do/Accreditation/Common-Program-Requirements

Albanese, M. A., Mejicano, G., Mullan, P., Kokotailo, P., & Gruppen, L. (2008). Defining characteristics of educational competencies. *Medical Education*, *42*(3), 248–255. doi:10.1111/j.1365-2923.2007.02996.x PMID:18275412

Association of American Medical Colleges. (2004). *Educating doctors to provide high quality medical care: A vision for medical education in the United States*. Washington, DC: Association of American Medical Colleges. Retrieved from https://members.aamc.org/eweb/upload/Educating%20Doctors%20to%20Provide%20July%202004.pdf

Association of American Medical Colleges. (2014). *Core entrustable professional activities for entering residency*. Washington, DC: Association of American Medical Colleges. Retrieved from http://www.aamc.org/cepaer

Australian Medical Council Limited. (2010). *Competence-based medical education AMC consultation paper*. Retrieved from http://www.amc.org.au/publications/policy

Bandaranayake, R. C. (2011). *The integrated medical curriculum*. Radcliffe Publishing.

Bandiera, G., Boucher, A., Neville, A., Kuper, A., & Hodges, B. (2013). Integration and timing of basic and clinical sciences education. *Medical Teacher*, *35*(5), 381–387. doi:10.3109/0142159X.2013.769674 PMID:23444888

Batalden, P., Leach, D., Swing, S., Dreyfus, H., & Dreyfus, S. (2002). General competencies and accreditation in graduate medical education. *Health Affairs (Project Hope), 21*(5), 103–111. doi:10.1377/hlthaff.21.5.103 PMID:12224871

Benor, D. E. (1982). Interdisciplinary integration in medical education: Theory and method. *Medical Education, 16*(6), 355–361. doi:10.1111/j.1365-2923.1982.tb00950.x PMID:7176983

Boelen, C. (2002). A new paradigm for medical schools a century after Flexner's report. *Bulletin of the World Health Organization, 80*(7), 592-593. doi:S0042-96862002000700013

Brauer, D. G., & Ferguson, K. J. (2015). The integrated curriculum in medical education: AMEE guide no. 96. *Medical Teacher, 37*(4), 312–322. doi:10.3109/0142159X.2014.970998 PMID:25319403

Brooks, W. S., Woodley, K. T., Jackson, J. R., & Hoesley, C. J. (2015). Integration of gross anatomy in an organ system-based medical curriculum: Strategies and challenges. *Anatomical Sciences Education, 8*(3), 266–274. doi:10.1002/ase.1483 PMID:25132664

Carraccio, C., Englander, R., Van Melle, E., Ten Cate, O., Lockyer, J., Chan, M. K., & Snell, L. S et al.. (2016). Advancing competency-based medical education: A charter for clinician-educators. *Academic Medicine, 91*(5), 645–649. doi:10.1097/ACM.0000000000001048 PMID:26675189

Carraccio, C., Wolfsthal, S. D., Englander, R., Ferentz, K., & Martin, C. (2002). Shifting paradigms: From Flexner to competencies. *Academic Medicine, 77*(5), 361–367. doi:10.1097/00001888-200205000-00003 PMID:12010689

Carraccio, C. L., & Englander, R. (2013). From Flexner to competencies: Reflections on a decade and the journey ahead. *Academic Medicine, 88*(8), 1067–1073. doi:10.1097/ACM.0b013e318299396f PMID:23807096

Chen, H. C., McNamara, M., Teherani, A., Cate, O. T., & OSullivan, P. (2016). Developing entrustable professional activities for entry into clerkship. *Academic Medicine, 91*(2), 247–255. doi:10.1097/ACM.0000000000000988 PMID:26556295

Chen, H. C., van den Broek, W. E., & ten Cate, O. (2015). The case for use of entrustable professional activities in undergraduate medical education. *Academic Medicine, 90*(4), 431–436. doi:10.1097/ACM.0000000000000586 PMID:25470310

Committee on the Roles of Academic Health Centers in the 21st Century, & Kohn, L. (2003). *Academic health centers: Leading change in the 21st century.* Washington, DC: The National Academies Press.

Cooke, M., Irby, D. M., Sullivan, W., & Ludmerer, K. M. (2006). American medical education 100 years after the Flexner report. *The New England Journal of Medicine, 355*(13), 1339-1344. doi:355/13/1339

Covey, S. R. (1989). *The seven habits of highly effective people: Restoring the character ethic.* New York, NY: Fireside Books – Simon & Schuster.

Dahle, L. O., Brynhildsen, J., Behrbohm Fallsberg, M., Rundquist, I., & Hammar, M. (2002). Pros and cons of vertical integration between clinical medicine and basic science within a problem-based undergraduate medical curriculum: Examples and experiences from Linkoping, Sweden. *Medical Teacher, 24*(3), 280–285. doi:10.1080/01421590220134097 PMID:12098414

Drake, S. M. (2007). *Creating standards-based integrated curriculum: Aligning curriculum, content, assessment, and instruction*. Thousand Oaks, CA: Corwin Press, a SAGE Publications Company.

Dressel, P. L. (1958). The meaning and significance of integration. In N. B. Henry (Ed.), *The Integration of Educational Experiences* (pp. 3–25). Chicago, IL: University of Chicago Press.

Dreyfus, S. E. (2004). The five-stage model of adult skill acquisition. *Bulletin of Science, Technology & Society*, *24*(3), 177–181. doi:10.1177/0270467604264992

Dyrbye, L. N., Starr, S. R., Thompson, G. B., & Lindor, K. D. (2011). A model for integration of formal knowledge and clinical experience: The advanced doctoring course at Mayo Medical School. *Academic Medicine*, *86*(9), 1130–1136. doi:10.1097/ACM.0b013e31822519d4 PMID:21785316

Englander, R., Cameron, T., Ballard, A. J., Dodge, J., Bull, J., & Aschenbrener, C. A. (2013). Toward a common taxonomy of competency domains for the health professions and competencies for physicians. *Academic Medicine*, *88*(8), 1088–1094. doi:10.1097/ACM.0b013e31829a3b2b PMID:23807109

Englander, R., & Carraccio, C. (2014). From theory to practice: Making entrustable professional activities come to life in the context of milestones. *Academic Medicine*, *89*(10), 1321–1323. doi:10.1097/ACM.0000000000000324 PMID:24892405

Englander, R., Flynn, T., Call, S., Carraccio, C., Cleary, L., Fulton, T. B., & Aschenbrener, C. A. et al. (2016). Toward defining the foundation of the MD degree: Core entrustable professional activities for entering residency. *Academic Medicine*, *91*(10), 1352–1358; Advance online publication. doi:10.1097/ACM.0000000000001204 PMID:27097053

Flexner, A. (1910). *Medical education in the United States and Canada*. Retrieved from http://archive.carnegiefoundation.org/publications/medical-education-united-states-and-canada-bulletin-number-four-flexner-report-0

Frank, J. R., & Danoff, D. (2007). The CanMEDS initiative: Implementing an outcomes-based framework of physician competencies. *Medical Teacher*, *29*(7), 642–647. doi:10.1080/01421590701746983 PMID:18236250

Frank, J. R., Mungroo, R., Ahmad, Y., Wang, M., De Rossi, S., & Horsley, T. (2010a). Toward a definition of competency-based education in medicine: A systematic review of published definitions. *Medical Teacher*, *32*(8), 631–637. doi:10.3109/0142159X.2010.500898 PMID:20662573

Frank, J. R., Snell, L. S., Cate, O. T., Holmboe, E. S., Carraccio, C., Swing, S. R., & Harris, K. A. et al. (2010b). Competency-based medical education: Theory to practice. *Medical Teacher*, *32*(8), 638–645. doi:10.3109/0142159X.2010.501190 PMID:20662574

Goldman, E., & Schroth, W. S. (2012). Perspective: Deconstructing integration: A framework for the rational application of integration as a guiding curricular strategy. *Academic Medicine*, *87*(6), 729–734. doi:10.1097/ACM.0b013e318253cad4 PMID:22534596

Harden, R. M. (1999). AMEE guide no. 14: Outcome-based education: Part 1-an introduction to outcome-based education. *Medical Teacher*, *21*(1), 7–14. doi:10.1080/01421599979969

Harden, R. M. (2000). The integration ladder: A tool for curriculum planning and evaluation. *Medical Education, 34*(7), 551-557. doi:med697

Harden, R. M., Davis, M. H., & Crosby, J. R. (1997). The new Dundee medical curriculum: A whole that is greater than the sum of the parts. *Medical Education, 31*(4), 264–271. doi:10.1111/j.1365-2923.1997.tb02923.x PMID:9488841

Hauer, K. E., Ten Cate, O., Boscardin, C., Irby, D. M., Iobst, W., & O'Sullivan, P. S. (2014). Understanding trust as an essential element of trainee supervision and learning in the workplace. *Advances in Health Sciences Education: Theory and Practice, 19*(3), 435–456. doi:10.1007/s10459-013-9474-4 PMID:23892689

Holmboe, E., Ginsburg, S., & Bernabeo, E. (2011). The rotational approach to medical education: Time to confront our assumptions? *Medical Education, 45*(1), 69–80. doi:10.1111/j.1365-2923.2010.03847.x PMID:21155870

Holmboe, E. S. (2015). Realizing the promise of competency-based medical education. *Academic Medicine, 90*(4), 411–413. doi:10.1097/ACM.0000000000000515 PMID:25295967

Kulasegaram, K. M., Martimianakis, M. A., Mylopoulos, M., Whitehead, C. R., & Woods, N. N. (2013). Cognition before curriculum: Rethinking the integration of basic science and clinical learning. *Academic Medicine, 88*(10), 1578–1585. doi:10.1097/ACM.0b013e3182a45def PMID:23969375

Liaison Committee on Medical Education. (2016). *Functions and structure of a medical school: Standards for accreditation of medical education programs leading to the MD degree*. Retrieved from http://lcme.org/publications/

Malik, A. S., & Malik, R. H. (2011). Twelve tips for developing an integrated curriculum. *Medical Teacher, 33*(2), 99–104. doi:10.3109/0142159X.2010.507711 PMID:20874013

Megroth, E., & Washburne, V. (1949). Integration in education. *The Journal of Educational Research, 43*(2), 81–92. doi:10.1080/00220671.1949.10881753

Muller, J. H., Jain, S., Loeser, H., & Irby, D. M. (2008). Lessons learned about integrating a medical school curriculum: Perceptions of students, faculty and curriculum leaders. *Medical Education, 42*(8), 778–785. doi:10.1111/j.1365-2923.2008.03110.x PMID:18627445

Nasca, T. J., Philibert, I., Brigham, T., & Flynn, T. C. (2012). The next GME accreditation systemrationale and benefits. *The New England Journal of Medicine, 366*(11), 1051–1056. doi:10.1056/NEJMsr1200117 PMID:22356262

Royal College of General Practitioners. (2016). *The RCGP curriculum: Core curriculum statement*. Retrieved from http://www.rcgp.org.uk/training-exams/gp-curriculum-overview/document-version.aspx

Schmidt, H. G., Machiels-Bongaerts, M., Hermans, H., ten Cate, T. J., Venekamp, R., & Boshuizen, H. P. (1996). The development of diagnostic competence: Comparison of a problem-based, an integrated, and a conventional medical curriculum. *Academic Medicine, 71*(6), 658–664. doi:10.1097/00001888-199606000-00021 PMID:9125924

Simpson, J. G., Furnace, J., Crosby, J., Cumming, A. D., Evans, P. A., Friedman Ben David, M., & MacPherson, S. G. et al. (2002). The Scottish doctorlearning outcomes for the medical undergraduate in Scotland: A foundation for competent and reflective practitioners. *Medical Teacher*, *24*(2), 136–143. doi:10.1080/01421590220120713 PMID:12098432

Swing, S. R. (2007). The ACGME outcome project: Retrospective and prospective. *Medical Teacher*, *29*(7), 648–654. doi:10.1080/01421590701392903 PMID:18236251

Swing, S. R., Beeson, M. S., Carraccio, C., Coburn, M., Iobst, W., Selden, N. R., & Vydareny, K. et al. (2013). Educational milestone development in the first 7 specialties to enter the next accreditation system. *Journal of Graduate Medical Education*, *5*(1), 98–106. doi:10.4300/JGME-05-01-33 PMID:24404235

ten Cate, O. (2005). Entrustability of professional activities and competency-based training. *Medical Education, 39*(12), 1176-1177. doi:MED2341

ten Cate, O., & Scheele, F. (2007). Competency-based postgraduate training: Can we bridge the gap between theory and clinical practice? *Academic Medicine*, *82*(6), 542–547. doi:10.1097/ACM.0b013e31805559c7 PMID:17525536

The Blue Ridge Academic Health Group. (2003). *Reforming medical education: Urgent priority for the academic health center in the new century*. Retrieved from http://www.whsc.emory.edu/blueridge/publications/reports.html

The Commonwealth Fund Task Force on Academic Health Centers. (2002). *Training tomorrow's doctors: The medical education mission of academic health centers*. The Commonwealth Fund. Retrieved from http://www.commonwealthfund.org/publications/fund-reports/2002/apr/training-tomorrows-doctors--the-medical-education-mission-of-academic-health-centers

Warm, E. J., Mathis, B. R., Held, J. D., Pai, S., Tolentino, J., Ashbrook, L., & Mueller, C. et al. (2014). Entrustment and mapping of observable practice activities for resident assessment. *Journal of General Internal Medicine*, *29*(8), 1177–1182. doi:10.1007/s11606-014-2801-5 PMID:24557518

Wiggins, G. P., & McTighe, J. (2005). *Understanding by design*. Alexandria, VA: Assoc. for Supervision and Curriculum Development.

Wijnen-Meijer, M., Cate, O. T., Rademakers, J. J., Van Der Schaaf, M., & Borleffs, J. C. (2009). The influence of a vertically integrated curriculum on the transition to postgraduate training. *Medical Teacher*, *31*(11), e528–e532. doi:10.3109/01421590902842417 PMID:19909031

Woods, N. N., Neville, A. J., Levinson, A. J., Howey, E. H., Oczkowski, W. J., & Norman, G. R. (2006). The value of basic science in clinical diagnosis. *Academic Medicine, 81*(10 Suppl), S124-7. doi:00001888-200610001-00031

KEY TERMS AND DEFINITIONS

Backward Design: An instructional design model developed by Wiggins & McTighe (2005) proposing that instructors start with desired learner outcomes and work backward to design appropriate assessment tools and curricular content.

Competencies: A broad set of knowledge, skills, and attitudes that learners should master by the end of a program of study.

Competency-Based Education: An approach to designing and assessing curricula based on a set of national standards or competencies.

Curriculum Integration: The seamless delivery and assessment of all core content (basic science, clinical science, social science, and humanities) throughout all years of the undergraduate medical education program with no division between disciplines.

Entrustable Professional Activities (EPAs): A set of core professional knowledge, skills, and attitudes initially proposed by ten Cate and Scheele (2007) that graduating medical students should possess at the time of entering residency.

Milestones: Originating in graduate medical education, a series of developmental benchmarks for each sub-competency resulting in more accurate assessment of educational outcomes and resident performance.

Subcompetencies: A more narrowly defined set of knowledge, skills, and attitudes that reside within a competency.

Chapter 4
Designing Simulated Learning Environments and Facilitating Authentic Learning Experiences in Medical Education

Xun Ge
University of Oklahoma, USA

Kun Huang
Mississippi State University, USA

Qian Wang
University of Oklahoma, USA

Victor Law
University of New Mexico, USA

Dominique C. Thomas
Cameron University, USA

ABSTRACT

The purpose of this chapter is to provide some practical guidance and theoretical basis on designing simulated learning environments to researchers and instructional designers, medical educators, instructional design students, and others who are committed to improving learning and instruction in medical education. This chapter will benefit those who are interested in designing simulated learning environments and facilitating simulated learning experiences in instructional settings. The chapter first defines various types of simulations and their cognitive functions in support of students' authentic learning experiences. Following this, the chapter highlights critical components for designing simulated learning environments, including identifying learning objectives, developing problem scenarios, and facilitating students' learning experiences. It is hoped that this chapter will be a useful tool and resource for medical educators, researchers and instructional designers, and graduate students who are pursuing an advanced degree in instructional design and technology.

DOI: 10.4018/978-1-5225-2098-6.ch004

Copyright © 2017, IGI Global. Copying or distributing in print or electronic forms without written permission of IGI Global is prohibited.

INTRODUCTION

Simulations have been regarded as the most prominent innovation taking place in medical education over the past decade (Passiment, Sacks, & Huang, 2011). They have been used as a pedagogical method for training in both medical schools and teaching hospitals. As many as 91% of emergency residency programs use simulations to train their residents (Okuda, et al., 2008). According to the American Board of Anesthesiology (2016), simulator-based education is required for Maintenance of Certification in Anesthesia. It is clear that simulations have become "a central thread in the fabric of medical education" (McGaghie, Issenberg, Petrusa, & Scalese, 2010, p.51).

Simulations are defined as a model that represents a certain phenomenon or activity that allows learners to acquire knowledge by interacting with the model (Alessi & Trollip, 2001). The definition is further contextualized in medical education by being referred to as a method "to replace or amplify real patient experiences with scenarios designed to replicate real health encounters" (Passiment, Sacks, & Huang, 2011, p.35). In today's medical field, where there are increasing concerns about patient safety and quality of care as well as increasing outpatient treatment, simulations have become a means to bridge classroom instruction and actual clinical environments (Okuda et al., 2009).

Simulations offer advantages that may not be readily available in real patient encounters or through other media or instructional methods. First, simulations can emulate and reproduce patient physiology and physiological responses, even those of rare conditions that may not be available in real-life encounters, and allow learners to engage in repeated trials and errors (Issenberg, McGaghie, Petrusa, Gordon, & Scalese, 2005). Second, during repetitive practice, learners are also able to receive immediate and directed feedback through debriefing and discussion, especially for errors they make, while such teaching rarely takes place in reality due to legal concerns (Okuda et al., 2009). Third, simulations afford opportunities to train and assess competencies holistically in multiple domains, which facilitates transfer of learning to clinical settings. Fourth, many problems in medical education are complex and ill-structured, and simulations can help students build mental models and represent problems (Feltovich, Spiro, Coulson, & Feltovich, 1996). Through a carefully designed simulated learning environments, learners are able to acquire important teamwork and communication skills, in addition to basic science and clinical knowledge and skills. Fifth, simulations can present patient cases in a time efficient manner, which enables a focused learning experience (Alessi & Trollip, 2001). Lastly, simulations often gives trainers the flexibility to adjust levels of difficulty, which leads learners progressively through the trajectory of target competencies (Issenberg et al., 2005).

With the aforementioned advantages and the effectiveness of simulation-based medical education (e.g., Issenberg et al., 2005; McGaghie, Issenberg, Cohen, Barsuk, & Wayne, 2011; Okuda et al., 2009), there is an increasing motivation for medical educators to incorporate simulations in instruction. However, designing and delivering a simulated learning environment presents challenges to many medical educators and instructional designers. Part of the challenges comes from the complexity of designing learning environments, and part of the challenge is due to the lack of experiences in facilitating students' learning experiences that fully take advantage of simulations. As Okuda et al. (2009) stated, "simulators do not replace good educators" (p. 339); rather, instructors should play an essential role in facilitating, guiding and motivating learners (McGaghie et al., 2010). Indeed, the lack of faculty training in skillful use of simulations and debriefing has been identified as some of the major barriers to the effective use of simulation in medical education (Okuda et al., 2008; Okuda et al., 2009).

PURPOSE

Grounded in sociocultural learning theories and instructional design principles (e.g., Brown, Collins, & Duguid, 1989; Hannafin et al., 1999; Schank, Berman, & Macpherson 1999; van Merriënboer, 2007), the purpose of this chapter is to provide a practical guide on the design of simulated learning enivornments, and the facilitation of authentic learning experiences in medical education. Important aspects for instructional designers and educators in the medical field to consider when designing and implementing simulated learning environments are highlighted in this chapter. The authors start with a description and classification of various types of simulations and their cognitive functions in support of learning. Next, the authors focus on critical components in designing simulated learning environments and best practices for integrating simulations in instruction, including identifying learning objectives, developing problems or scenarios, and facilitating learning experience. Each of the facilitation components will be discussed at lengths, with in-depth discussion of key concepts followed with specific examples in the context of medical field to illustrate the concepts presented.

TYPES AND CHARACTERISTICS OF SIMULATIONS

There are various ways to categorize simulations in medical fields (e.g., Cumin & Merry, 2007; Durham & Alden, 2008; Gaba, 2004). Based on the concept of fidelity, simulations can be categorized as computer-based simulations or human-patient simulators. Fidelity is defined as "the degree of similarity between the training situation and the operational situation which is simulated" (Hayes & Singer, 1989, p.50). The first type, *computer-based simulation,* can be considered low in fidelity as it does not fully represent physical characteristics of patients. There are several types of computer-based simulations: *physical*, *iterative*, *procedural*, and *situational* simulations (Alessi & Trollip, 2001). Physical simulations provide knowledge about a real-world system, iterative simulations illustrate concepts about a particular process, procedural simulations illustrate a sequence of actions, and situational simulations focus on informing learners on how to do something in a real-world system. The second type of simulation is *human patient simulators* (a.k.a. high-fidelity mannequin simulators) which have high physical and functional fidelity and allow learners to physically interact with and receive real-time feedback (Okuda et al., 2009). The following section further elaborates the categories and subcategories with examples.

Computer-Based Simulations

Physical Simulations

In medical education, physical simulations are often used to illustrate a concept or object (Alessi & Trollip, 2001). Learners have an opportunity to interact with and manipulate the simulated object to gain a better knowledge of the system. Anatomical simulations belong to the category of physical simulations. One of the examples is a 3D heart simulation (http://thevirtualheart.org). Learners can interact with the simulation, manipulating the object, observing the structure, size and shape of the heart, and analyzing the muscle functions of a human heart. Physical simulations are particularly useful in studying objects or phenomena that are impossible to get a good perspective of, such as the live human heart or cells. *Neurophysiology Virtual Lab* (http://www.hhmi.org/biointeractive/neurophysiology-virtual-lab) is another example of physical simulations. In this simulation, learners can identify the neurons based on the morphology and the response to stimuli. It enables learners to use a micronmanuoulator and an electrode to probe for a cell. If learners find a cell, the screen will update itself. Learners can keep probing with the electrode until they find a cell.

Iterative Simulations

Iterative simulations aim to demonstrate interactive relationships among concepts. The difference between the physical simulations and iterative simulations is that iterative simulations are intended to demonstrate a process and highlight important aspects of a phenomenon or a system. Learners gain an understanding of a process by manipulating variables and observing how the change of one variable affects other variables in a system. Iterative simulations are often used in medical education to illustrate processes that are not directly or easily visible, such as the complexities of cancer and its causes.

ITS-SMR Micro-World (Figure 1) is an iterative simulation the authors designed to demonstrate the concept of blood glucose levels. This simulation is intended to help students better understand how blood glucose levels fluctuate through the change of variables such as food intake, physical activity, and medication consumption. The simulation separates the variables into three distinct categories. Each category contains a selectable list of variables. Notably, each list organizes variables by name (e.g., Bread), serving size (e.g.,1 slice), and duration (e.g., 2 hours) where applicable. Once the learner manipulates a variable in the simulation, the learner is provided with a description of the simulated character's blood glucose levels, a description of which variable was selected, a description of how much blood glucose levels have changed (e.g., +15 mg/dl), and a graph that illustrates a visual change in blood glucose levels. Figure 1 illustrates the manipulation of the *Whole Grain Bread* variable. The manipulation of this variable has resulted in a severe spike in blood glucose levels and has resulted in the character having high blood sugar or Hyperglycemia. This signifies that the learner should reconsider her choices made and select another variable to better regulate blood glucose levels. Processes like this can be difficult for learners to grasp and hard to observe in real life; therefore, iterative simulations allow students to better conceptualize the interrelationships of complex concepts.

Procedural Simulations

The purpose of procedural simulations it to engage learners in a sequence of actions or procedure to accomplish a particular goal (Alessi & Trollip, 2001). In order to perform a procedure, students are required to interact with or manipulate objects that constitute the procedure. Different from physical simulations, procedural simulations emphasize how to do things, such as extracting a wisdom tooth.

The simulation titled *Wisdom Tooth Extraction* (http://www.surgerysquad.com/surgeries/virtual-wisdom-tooth-extraction/), is an example of procedural simulation. This simulation provides an authentic clinical context that allows learners to go over the procedures of extracting a wisdom tooth. Students learn critical procedures without putting patients at risk (Good, 2003; Medina, Raccadio & Schwid, 2000). In addition, the simulation allows each procedure to be paused at any time for a close examination of a particular aspect of the procedure. Procedural simulations put emphasis on the correct sequences for completing a task. In procedural simulations, learners are encouraged to try incorrect procedures and observe the consequences as an important part of learning process (Alessi & Trollip, 2001; Kelsey

Figure 1. ITS-SMR Micro-World --An example of iterative simulation

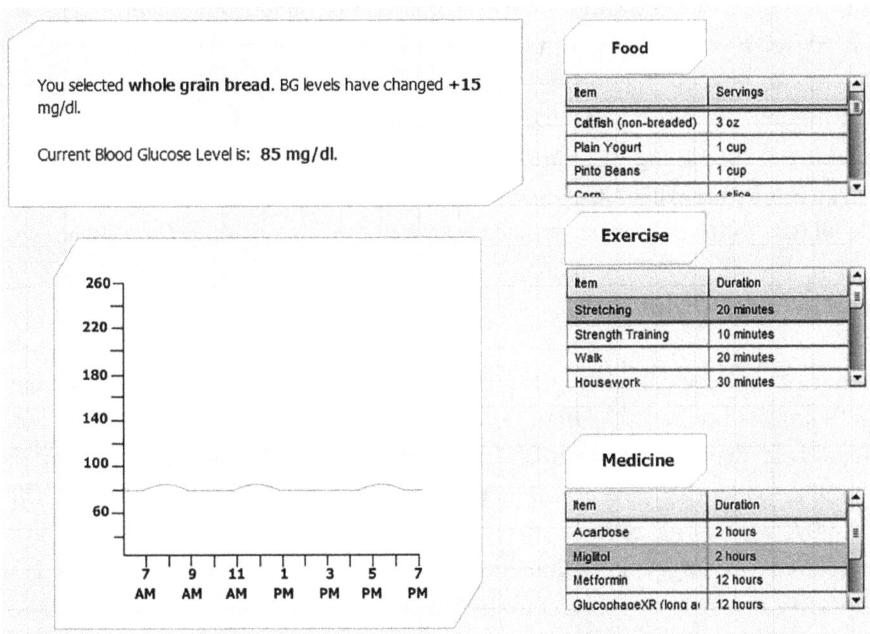

& Claus, 2016; Salas et al., 2005). Through repeated practice, learners gain not only proficiency but also confidence (Abrahamson, Denson & Wolf, 1969; Bremner, Aduddell, Bennett & VanGeest, 2006; Paver-Erzen & Cimerman, 2007; Rogers et al., 2000).

Situational Simulations

Situational simulations are simulations that deal with "the behaviors and attitudes of people or organizations in different situations, rather than with skilled performance" (Alessi & Trollip, 2001, p. 224). In medical education, situational simulations often present learners with a patient who needs some sort of help, which requires learners to take a course of action by interacting with the simulated environment, such as checking symptoms, forming a diagnosis based on symptoms, and developing a treatment plan. This type of simulations is often used to train and assess clinical skills such as decision-making, critical thinking, and application; furthermore, situational simulations provide an ideal way to train soft skills such as communication and teamwork (Cherry, Williams, George & Ali, 2007; Feingold, Calaluce, & Kallen, 2004).

DESIGNING FOR AND FACILITATING SIMULATED LEARNING EXPERIENCES

While simulations have many benefits in medical education, creating a simulated experience for successful learning is not an easy task. Grounded in instructional design theories (e.g., Ge, Huang, Zhang & Bowers, 2013; Morrison et al., 2007; Smith & Ragan, 2005) as well as research about simulation-based learning (e.g., Aebersold & Tschannen, 2013; Issenberg, 2005), the authors identify and describe three essential components for designing and implementing a simulated learning environment: (1) identifying learning objectives, (2) developing simulation scenarios, and (3) facilitating learning experience (Figure 2). *Learning objectives* provide a roadmap for instructional activities (Smith & Ragan, 2005; Morrison et al., 2007). *Scenarios* provide "enabling contexts" (Hannafin et al., 1999, p. 123) that guide students in identifying problems that needs to be addressed (Hannafin et al., 1999; Jonassen, 1999). *Facilitation* refers to external means or strategies to help learners move from their current state to the goal state of knowledge and skills (Gagné, Wager, Golas & Keller, 2005; Morrison et al., 2007; Smith & Ragan, 2005). In the remainder of this section, the authors discuss each of the three essential components with examples.

Identifying Learning Objectives

When a decision is made to design or implement simulation-based medical education, the first question to consider is, "*Where do we start?*" Often, a need to incorporate simulations into a curriculum often suggests that there is an existing or anticipated performance gap that requires intervention. Therefore, a good starting point is to identify the learning objectives that will close the gap (Jeffries, 2005; Morrison, Ross & Kemp, 2007; Salas et al, 2005).

Learning objectives are target skills that educators would like students to achieve. It is common for medical educators to come up with goals related to medical knowledge or psychomotor skills. However, it is important to keep in mind the capability of simulations to address multiple domains of competence. In addition to clinical knowledge and skills, the authors suggest that medical educators explicitly incorporate *soft* skills such as communication and teamwork skills in their list of learning objectives. For example, the learning objectives for a nursing simulation may include: apply knowledge and skills to make clinical decisions, communicate accurately and effectively, exhibit caring behaviors, and function well as team members. Some objectives are in the affective domain, with the intention to affect the change of individual's attitude or beliefs, for example, when communicating with a patient, a nurse should choose to communicate honestly, openly, and without judgment.

Figure 2. Overview of the three components for designing and implementing simulation-based learning

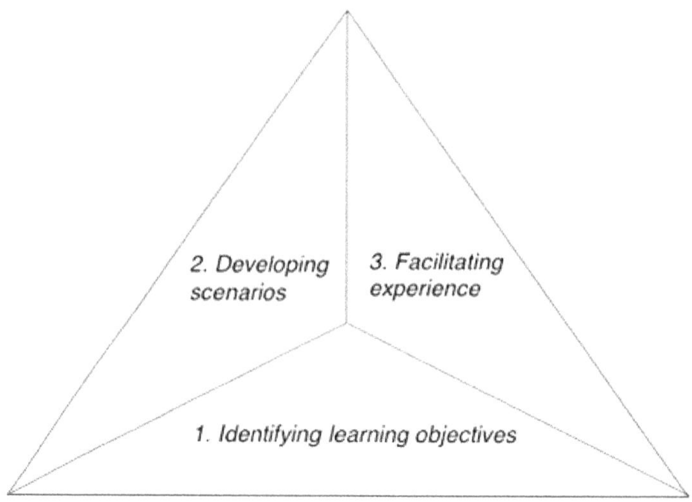

The AAMC survey (Passiment, Sacks, & Huang, 2011) provides a handy framework to consider different types learning objectives in the medical education context. Their list consists of medical knowledge, patient care, interpersonal communication skills, professionalism, practice-based learning/improvement, system-based practice, psychomotor tasks, leadership, team training, and critical thinking/decision making. Schank, Berman, and Macpherson (1999) proposed that each learning objective address two categories of knowledge: process knowledge, and content knowledge. *Content knowledge* refers to information required to accomplish a task while *process knowledge* refers to the knowledge of application. *Content knowledge* involves facts, concepts, rules and principles, whereas *process knowledge* involves application of *content knowledge* to solve problems and higher-order thinking skills, such as reasoning, interpretation, inference, deduction, analysis, synthesis, and evaluation. For example, an objective for content knowledge is "The learner will be able to describe relationships between a substrate, a Cytochrome P450 enzyme, and an inducer/inhibitor;" and an objective for process knowledge is, Given the description of a symptom(s) by a patient who has taken drugs, the learner will be able to explain possible cause(s) of the symptom(s) related to drug and enzyme interaction.

As seen from the examples above, learning objectives are intended to clarify desired learning outcomes and provide a basis for selecting instructional content and activities (Cannon-Bowers, 2008; Gagné et al., 2005; Morrison et al., 2007; Smith & Ragan, 2005). Appropriately identified learning objectives can inform the instructor about the levels of complexity and the types of simulation scenarios necessary for achieving the goals and objectives (Beaubien & Baker, 2004; Salas et al., 2005). Setting learning objectives in accordance with course content or curricular standards is one of the most important steps in designing a simulation (Hung, 2006). The ultimate purpose for implementing simulations is to create an authentic learning environment to construct process and content knowledge (van Merriënboer, 2007; van Merriënboer & Kirschner, 2001). Therefore, the learning objectives formulated need to include both content and process knowledge objectives in order for students to integrate and apply them simultaneously. A worksheet (see Appendix A) has been developed to facilitate the process of developing learning objectives. The worksheet is a step-by-step guide to help instructors generate a complete set of learning objectives.

Developing Authentic Scenarios for Simulated Experiences

When the learning objectives are clear, the next step is to develop simulated scenarios that lead to the achievement of the objectives. In integrating simulations in medical education, educators often encounter two types of situations regarding scenarios for a simulation: they either need to design their own scenarios, or modify existing ones. This section focuses on some important elements that can provide guidance in both situations. These components, a mission, an authentic storyline, and the role of the characters or players (Schank et al, 1999), are essential for creating a meaningful simulation environment. The authors will first outline the essential components, followed by a brief discussion on providing students with a sequence of well designed scenarios to facilitate transfer of learning.

A scenario is a patient case with a main storyline that holds specific tasks together, leading to desired learning outcomes (Alinier, 2010). Regardless of types of simulations, a good scenario orients learners to a problem that engages learners to transfer their classroom experience into a real-world environment (Cannon-Bowers, 2008; Hannafin, Land & Oliver, 1999; Jonassen, 2011; Schank et al, 1999). A good scenario has the following components: *a mission* for learners to accomplish, *an authentic storyline* that triggers learners' appropriate or inappropriate behaviors, and *a meaningful role* for learners to play in the storyline. In the scenario "Acute Pulmonary Edema" (Wald, Peet, Cripe, Kinloch, 2016, p. 2) below, the three components (i.e., mission, storyline, and roles) are illustrated.

You are an intern nurse on call tonight at a local hospital. The patient is a 66-year old man who was admitted to the hospital earlier this morning with biliary colic and is scheduled for a cholecystectomy the next day. While in the hospital, the patient develops progressive shortness of breath and severely elevates blood pressure resulting from acute pulmonary edema. Primary complaint is shortness of breath progressively worsening over the past 20 minutes. When asked, thee patient reports that he has had rightside upper abdominal pain for 2 days, associated nausea and that the pain worsened with eating. He was diagnosed with gallstones 2 years earlier.

According to Schank et al.'s (1999) Goal-based Scenario (GBS) theory, a good scenario should start with a *mission* so that learners are provided with an e*nabling context* for them to perform tasks and solve problems. The mission refers to an engaging task for learners to accomplish that replicates real-life applications of knowledge and skills. The mission presents objectives and a series of tasks for learners to carry out; therefore, it should be stimulating, exciting, motivating, and authentic. The mission must also allow learners to demonstrate both *process knowledge* and *content knowledge*, which challenges the learners as in authentic clinical settings (Barrows, 1994; Jonassen, 1999). In *Acute Pulmonary Edema*, the mission for learner is to save the life of a patient who has a hypertensive emergency. To accomplish the mission, learners need to have knowledge about hypertensive emergencies, and know how to initiate a diagnostic work up and management for a patient. Students engage in the tasks in this scenario, constructing knowledge, and practicing skills which leads to transfer to context outside of learning environments (Schank et al., 1999).

In a good scenario, learners also need to play a meaningful role. *The role* defines the learner's position in the simulation (Schank et al., 1999). The role learners play in a simulation needs to optimally enable them to practice targeted skills identified in the learning objectives. In *Acute Pulmonary Edema*, learners play the role of an intern nurse at a local hospital. This role is appropriate in the scenario which provides opportunities for nursing students to practice target knowledge and skills. On the other hand, learners are asked to play the role of the patient who wants to know how his medical condition develops, it may not be as meaningful for understanding the development of hypertension and applying diagnosis and patient management skills related to the condition. As noted, the role learners play needs to be meaningful.

Good scenarios also have an authentic storyline. *The storyline* creates the rationale for learners to accomplish the mission. Storylines should be as authentic as possible, creating the need for learners to accomplish the mission and motivating them (Jeffries, 2005; Schank et al., 1999) while addressing the learning objectives (Merrill, 2002). To be authentic, the story needs to contain sufficient rich contextual information that faithfully represents real-world situations, which helps learners link what they have learned in the classroom to real-world situations in order to facilitate transfer (Hung, 2006; Jonassen, 2011). In *Acute Pulmonary Edema*, the story begins as a patient complains about shortness of breath and progressively gets worse over the next 20 minutes, with blood pressure elevating severely. As an intern nurse on call, the learner has to assess the patient and initiate management for the patient.

In addition, the storyline needs to capture all the activities learners need to carry out in order to accomplish the mission; meanwhile, the storyline should be able to trigger learners' appropriate and inappropriate behaviors (Gordon, Wilkerson, Shaffer & Armstrong, 2001; Salas et al., 2005). Thus, the scenario should provide learners with enough opportunities to construct knowledge and practice skills,

Figure 3. An example of scenario structure

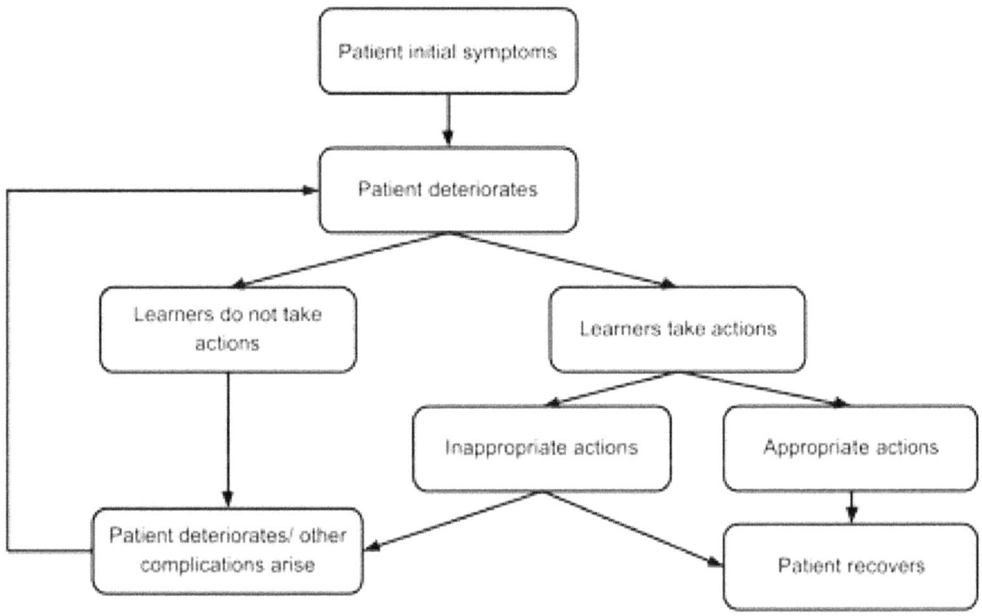

which leads to knowledge transfer (Schank et al., 1999). The storyline structure shown in Figure 3, which was adapted from Alinier (2009), illustrates all the activities and branching points based on appropriate or inappropriate actions as learners interact with simulator. The visual approach can be very helpful in developing storylines.

Simulation-based learning is often comprehensive and complex. It is often problematic to rely on one single scenario, because learners may use simple analogies and oversimplify the complex nature of clinical problems (Spiro, Coulson, Feltovich, & Anderson, 1988). Learners need to have the ability to restructure their knowledge in many ways to adapt to the situations (Spiro, Feltovich, Jacobson & Coulson, 1991). Providing learners with multiple scenarios that capture clinical variations is shown to be more useful than those with a narrow scope (Issenberg, 2005). Multiple scenarios can also be designed to achieve different learning objectives. For example, the first scenario of a human patient simulation can focus on clinical knowledge and skills. A subsequent scenario can incorporate additional components to address soft skills such as communication with patient's family. It is recommended that students learn from a sequence of well-designed scenarios that "crisscross the landscape" of target knowledge and skills, and build flexible cognitive structures (Spiro et al., 1991). In addition, it is beneficial to provide learners with multiple scenarios with increasing levels of difficulty (Issenberg, 2005).

Facilitating Learners' Simulated Experiences

Now that we have a good scenario, what are we going to do about it? A good scenario alone does not guarantee the acquisition of clinical competence. Learners must also be guided during the simulated experience to ensure the acquisition of appropriate procedures and skills (Issenberg & McGaghie, 2013). Particularly, *modeling* and *scaffolding* (Hannafin, Land & Oliver, 1999; Jonassen, 1999) are essential facilitation strategies to guide and engage learners in simulated learning environments. Often modeling and scaffolding strategies work hand in hand in the facilitation process.

Modeling refers to an expert demonstrating how a task is performed (Jonassen, 1999). The demonstration involves two aspects: demonstration of how to perform a task (i.e., behavior modeling), and articulation of the reasoning behind the demonstration (i.e., cognitive modeling) (Jonassen, 1999). Although behavior modeling is important to guide learners in understanding and completing a task, cognitive modeling is even more important to provide the reasoning behind tasks (Schön, 1983), because it makes the expert's internal thinking processes visible to learners (Collins, Brown & Holum, 1991). Compared with behavioral modeling that mainly focuses on procedural knowledge and relates to *content* learning objectives, cognitive modeling can better help learners to achieve *process* learning objectives. In a computer-based simulation learning environment, modeling can be provided by a pedagogical agent (i.e., a simulated character playing a role in the scenario, often a domain expert), whereas in a human-patient simulation environment, modeling is usually provided by the instructor or expert.

Scaffolding is a systematic approach to providing support to learners (Jonassen, 1999). It is a temporary assistance provided by an expert or a more capable peer for a learner to carry out and accomplish a task, which the learner would otherwise be unable to perform without the assistance (Lajoie, 2005). Scaffolding is adjustable as learners progress and their performance increases; when learners reach certain level of competence, scaffolding should be intentionally withdrawn (Palincsar, 1986; Wood, Bruner & Ross, 1976). Hannafin et al. (1999) categorized scaffolding into four types: conceptual, metacognitive, procedural and strategic. Conceptual scaffolding helps learners to understand concepts and directs their attention to areas of misconceptions, which guides learners to reason through complex problems. Metacognitive scaffolding provides support by engaging learners in reflections of their learning process, such as how to think, how to learn, how to plan and how to strategize the use of their learning resources and activities. Procedural scaffolding provides guidance on how to use available resources and tools. This type of scaffolding is often in the forms of directions for navigation, or orientation to features and functions of a technological system. Strategic scaffolding provides guidance on various approaches to solving complex and ill-structured problems, such as analysis, planning, and strategic and tactical decision-making. In computer-based simulations, scaffolding is often provided in the form of questions or cues prompted by a pedagogical agent who interacts with learners, through screen features such as menus, tabs and buttons.

In the remainder of this section, the authors illustrate how modeling and scaffolding strategies are applied in two settings: (1) the design of computer-based simulation environments, and (2) the facilitation of learning in human-patient simulation environments. For each setting, the authors use specific examples to demonstrate how modeling and scaffolding are actualized in the setting.

Modeling and Scaffolding in a Computer-Based Simulation Environment

In this section, the authors use two examples, *Pharmacokinetics Lab* and *Virtual Clinic*, to illustrate modeling and scaffolding strategies in computer-based simulation environments. *Pharmacokinetics Lab* (Figure 4) is a computer-based simulation the authors developed to teach students concepts and decision-making related to drug interactions in real life situations. Learners are guided through four different scenarios of possible drug interactions. The four scenarios are presented with increasing complexity. In each scenario, learners are prompted to consider the symptom(s) of patient as well as other sources of information in order to make a diagnosis.

Both *behavior* and *cognitive* modeling were applied in the simulation, along with scaffolding mechanisms. An expert nurse who acts as a pedagogical agent is always available in the simulation to guide the learner in the problem-solving task and decision-making process (see Figure 4). Behavior modeling is executed through the menu tabs, which prompt the learner to follow the steps by checking the patient's symptoms, examining the drugs the patient has taken, analyzing the different types of drugs, and then making decisions on diagnosis. Prompting learners to follow the steps is not only a behavior modeling process, but also a scaffolding process, where the simulated role of the expert verbally instructs and guides the learner to proceed from one step to the next, providing procedural scaffolding in completing the problem-solving task in identifying the causes for the effect failure of the drug. At the same time, question prompts, as procedural and metacognitive scaffolds, are provided at each of the problem-solving stages, such as examining the patient's symptoms, to engage the learner in considering the symptoms of the patient as well as the other possible information to make a diagnosis.

Cognitive modeling is provided at the end of each simulation scenario when learners has completed his/her problem-solving task and reaches a decision. At this point, the simulation provides the expert nurse's reasoning of the solutions so that the learners have a chance to learn the new knowledge by comparing and contrasting their solutions with the expert nurse's solution. In the problem-solving process, the learners have access to a "diagnosis notepad", which provides the tool for learners not only to take notes, but also to journal their reflections and decision-making process. The notepad feature can be considered as a metacognitive scaffolding tool, which supports learners with note-taking for decision-making, comparing notes with the expert's thinking and self-reflection. In addition, learners are prompted by the expert to reflect on the diagnosis process, identifying knowledge gap and skills needed to solve the problem. Some of the questions demonstrate the expert nurse's strategies in approaching the problem, as shown in the expert's script in Figure 4, "So let's ask the patient whether he took another drug in the

Figure 4. Modeling and scaffolding in the Pharmacokinetics Lab

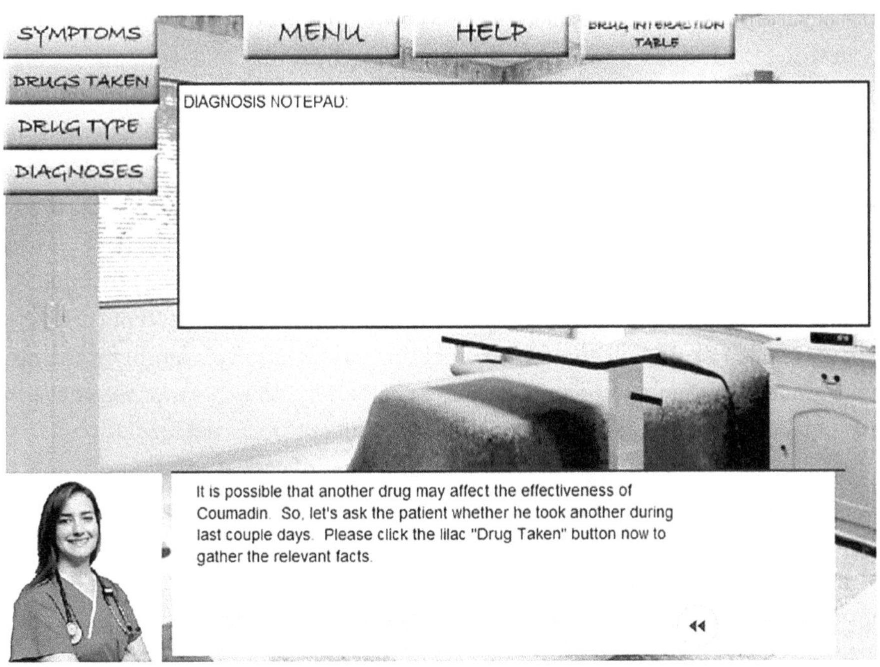

last couple of days." In this case, the expert's prompts also serves as a strategic scaffolding. Therefore, the expert's question prompts not only serves as a metacognitive scaffold, but also strategic scaffold in this computer-based simulation. Moreover, this simulation includes navigation buttons, such as Menu, Help, and Drug Interaction Table, which provide a procedural scaffolding.

Virtual Clinic (Figure 5) is a simulation that teaches nursing students ethical principles and decision-making skills in handling ethical dilemmas. Through a series of three scenarios featuring a variety of ethical dilemmas, learners gain an understanding of ethics principles and their application to authentic situations. Similar to *Pharmacokinetics Lab*, in this simulation, *cognitive* modeling is demonstrated through an expert nurse in the sharing of her thinking and decision-making processes when faced with an ethical dilemma. For example, in the second scenario after learners make a decision about a dilemma, the expert nurse shares with learners how she would approach the situation. *Behavior* modeling as well as *procedural* and *strategic* scaffolding is demonstrated in the expert nurse's prompts about tasks to perform, sharing of her perspectives and strategies, and provision of informative feedback. Further, built-in tabs at the top of the screen provide another means of procedural scaffolding. *Conceptual* scaffolding was provided through clickable buttons that show descriptions of ethical principles as well as confirmative or correct feedback after learners select an applicable code of ethics to a given dilemma. Lastly, scaffolding was not held constant in this simulation; it decreases as learners gain competence through solving similar problems. For instance, in the first scenario, the expert nurse walks learners through the entire process of handling an ethical dilemma and provides immediate guidance and feedback. In the second case, learners are left to figure out the issue on their own, and the expert nurse does not provide scaffolding and feedback until after learners have reached a decision. At that point, the expert nurse also provides *metacognitive* scaffolding by prompting learners to articulate the reasoning behind their decisions.

Facilitating Learning in a Human-Patient Simulation Environment

In a human-patient simulation environment, modeling is typically provided by humans, that is, an instructor or expert. In the aforementioned scenario *Acute Pulmonary Edema*, an expert would demonstrate the procedures by performing the steps to learners if they have difficulty in auscultating lungs. In this case, the expert demonstration is regarded as behavior modeling. In this modeling process, the expert performs cognitive modeling by articulating his/her reasoning, directing learners' attention to key patterns, and recommending resources and information. Other examples of modeling include experts' sharing of their past experience that is relevant to the current simulation, which provides learners with modeled behaviors and cognitive processes to follow.

Conceptual scaffolding can be in the form of a quick reference guide. For example, in a cardiac arrest simulation for nursing students, a quick reference sheet that shows different cardiac arrest rhythms and their key features can provide important conceptual information to facilitate the simulated learning experience. Conceptual scaffolding can also be provided by an expert, or instructor, in the form of feedback. In the cardiac arrest simulation example, if students perform defibrillation to a non-shockable rhythm, the instructor can then provide feedback and further clarify important concepts related to the task. The instructor's feedback, together with the physiological feedback by the simulator can be an effective strategy to identify and correct misconceptions.

Procedural scaffolding can be provided by a visual guide posted on a wall. As simulation continues, learners can quickly refer to the visual guide to see what to perform next. Obviously, the instructor is a main resource to provide procedural scaffolding. When students show signs of hesitation or uncertainty,

Figure 5. Modeling and scaffolding in the Virtual Clinic

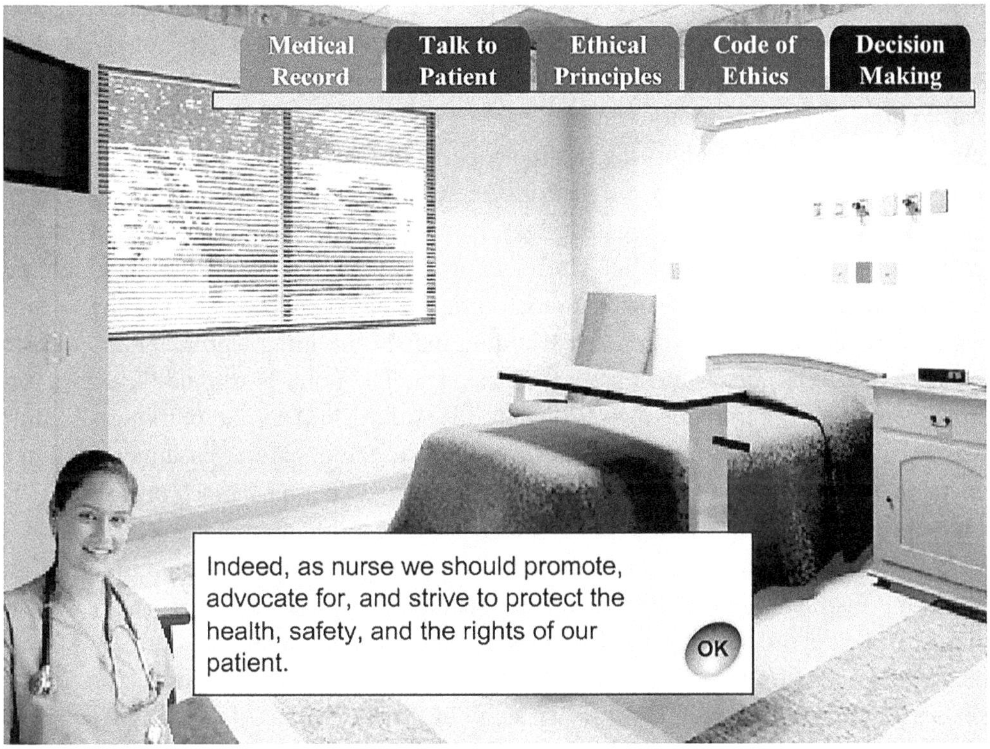

the instructor can prompt them with questions or direct them to pay attention to a certain aspect of the simulation.

Feedback has been utilized as a common scaffolding strategy to support conceptual understanding and metacognition (Buykx et al., 2012; Cannon-Bowers, 2008; Cannon-Bowers, burns, Salas & Pruitt, 1998), as demonstrated through cognitive apprenticeship (Collins, Brown & Holum, 1991). Feedback is helpful with learners' conceptual understanding in content areas and general cognitive skills (Bandura, 1991; Shute, 2008). Feedback also serves as a metacognitive scaffold to prompt students answer the three questions: *where am I going*? *how am I doing*? and *what should I do next*? (Hattie & Timperly, 2007).

In a human-patient simulation environment, metacognitive scaffolding is often manifested through debriefing, which is a brief meeting held after a task has been completed, when learners are prompted by an expert or an instructor to reflect on their learning experience, roles and responsibilities, and evaluate their cognitive and metacognitive processes. The expert may also ask learners to reflect on the roles and responsibilities they have taken, what they have learned, and what are some errors that can be avoided. In addition, debriefing also serves as a formative evaluation of learner' performance, during which learners are provided with tailored feedback and prompted to reflect on the effectiveness of their simulated experience (Ahmed et al., 2012; Akaike et al., 2012; Alinier, 2010; Cannon-Bowers, 2008; Fanning & Gaba, 2007; Jeffries, 2005; Motola et al., 2013; Sales et al., 2005).

Ahmed et al. (2012) indicate that effective debriefing requires an appropriate approach, a constructive and engaging environment, which allows learners to reflect, analyze, diagnose and apply knowledge to real clinical practice. In order to help learners maximize the benefits of debriefing in simulations, we have developed a worksheet (see Appendix B) based on Ahmed et al.'s (2012) recommendations to help students with their debriefing session. This worksheet identifies important questions for learners to reflect upon, including *what happened in the simulation*, *how the group acted*, and *how the learners felt*. This worksheet can be adaptively used for various cases, situations, and types of simulations.

When designing scaffolding for a simulated learning environment, it is important that the concept of scaffolding is understood. The authors discuss the concept of scaffolding earlier, and the authors would like to bring up the following issues again for consideration. First, it is important to understand that the instructor provide scaffolding only when necessary, not on students' first sign of uncertainty. Providing help when needed based on an individual's prior knowledge and needs is a fundamental principle of scaffolding (Wood et al., 1976). It helps learners to grapple with uncertainties, as long as the situation is not beyond learners' capability. Second, scaffolding means providing learners with questions, hints, cues, instead of providing direct information or guidance. The point is to guide learners through the critical thinking process, not focusing merely on the end results. Third, as part of the scaffolding process, it is necessary to remove scaffolds when needed. Similar to the computer-based simulation example, *Virtual Clinic*, in the beginning of the scenario when learners do not have much prior experience, more scaffolding is provided. When learners' competence increases, the instructor may withdraw scaffolds gradually. In the example cardiac arrest simulation for nursing students, it is recommended that in the first scenario, the instructor provide different reference materials, then he or she pause a simulator in order to demonstrate the process and provide guidance and feedback. Later, as students' knowledge and skills increase, the instructor may remove reference materials and withhold feedback until later debriefing, which is a key metacognitive scaffolding strategy in simulation-based medical education.

CONCLUSION

Simulations have promising affordances and possibilities for medical education to enrich students' real-world learning experience. They not only provide learners with real-world learning experiences, but also facilitate transfer of knowledge and skills. Most importantly, it creates a learning environment to enhance learners' motivation and self-regulation while controlling for the patient safety. In this chapter, the authors have illustrated different types of simulations for different learning purposes and specific contexts, including computer-based and human-patient simulators. The authors have also distinguished the affordances offered by both computer-based simulations and human-simulators, which would help instructional designers and medical education professors to make informed decisions regarding which type of simulators to use, when to use them and how to use them. Furthermore, it is demonstrated with some examples of authentic cases how to design effective simulated learning environments to facilitate learners' real-world learning experiences. The discussion of the support and facilitation focuses on the following aspects of instructional strategies and skillsets: how to develop learning objectives, how to write problem scenarios, and how to design simulated learning environments, and how to facilitate simulated learning experience, by providing provide instructional support aiming at modeling scaffolding, and coaching to learners. It is hoped that this chapter can be used as a useful tool for instructional designers, medical educators, and graduate students working on instructional design and technology.

Due to the limitation of space, the authors have not been able to discuss assessment, which is another important aspect in instructional design and delivery. However, the authors would like to mention in passing the importance of conducting valid and reliable assessment through objective-referenced assessments, that is, developing assessment items that are aligned with learning objectives that have been identified (Morrison et al., 2007; Smith & Ragan, 2005). Alternative assessment approaches need to be considered when it comes to testing students' performance in real-life contexts, including using a simulation for assessing learners' understanding and performance in authentic contexts (Gagné et al., 2005; Okuda et al., 2009). Since debriefing has already been considered as a scaffolding strategy used in the facilitation process in a human-patient simulation environment, it can also be used as an assessment tool to identify misconceptions, diagnose learners' difficult areas, and provide information about what remediation is needed and how to improve instruction for future instructional modules.

REFERENCES

Abrahamson, S., Denson, J. S., & Wolf, R. M. (1969). Effectiveness of a simulator in training anesthesiology residents. *Journal of Medical Education*, *44*, 515–519. PMID:5789592

Aebersold, M., & Tschannen, D. (2013). Simulation in nursing practice: The impact on patient care. *Online Journal of Issues in Nursing*, *18*(2). doi:10.3912/OJIN.Vol18No02Man06 PMID:23758424

Ahmed, M., Sevdalis, N., Paige, J., Paragi-Gururaja, R., Nestel, D., & Arora, S. (2012). Identifying best practice guidelines for debrie ng in surgery: A tri-continental study. *American Journal of Surgery*, *203*(4), 523–529. doi:10.1016/j.amjsurg.2011.09.024 PMID:22450027

Akaike, M., Fukutomi, M., Nagamune, M., Fujimoto, A., Tsuji, A., Ishida, K., & Iwata, T. (2012). Simulation-based medical education in clinical skills laboratory. *The Journal of Medical Investigation*, *59*(1-2), 28–35. doi:10.2152/jmi.59.28 PMID:22449990

Alessi, S. M., & Trollip, S. R. (2001). *Multimedia for learning: Methods and development* (3rd ed.). Boston, MA: Allyn & Bacon.

Alinier, G. (2010). Developing high-fidelity health care simulation scenarios: A guide for educators and professionals. *Simulation & Gaming*, *42*(1), 9–26. doi:10.1177/1046878109355683

American Board of Anesthesiology. (2016). Retrieved from http://www.theaba.org/MOCA/About-MOCA-2-0

Bandura, A. (1991). Social cognitive theory of self-regulation. *Organizational Behavior and Human Decision Processes*, *50*(2), 248–287. doi:10.1016/0749-5978(91)90022-L

Barrows, H. S. (1996). Problem-based learning in medicine and beyond: A brief overview. *New Directions for Teaching and Learning*, *68*, 3–12. doi:10.1002/tl.37219966804

Beaubien, J. M., & Baker, D. P. (2004). The use of simulation for training teamwork skills in health care: How low can you go? *Quality & Safety in Health Care*, *13*(Supplement 1), i51–i56. doi:10.1136/qshc.2004.009845 PMID:15465956

Bremner, M., Aduddell, K., Bennett, D., & VanGeest, J. (2006). The use of human patient simulators: Best practices with novice nursing students. *Nurse Educator*, *31*(4), 170–174. doi:10.1097/00006223-200607000-00011 PMID:16855487

Brown, J. S., Collins, A., & Duguid, P. (1989). Situated cognition and the culture of learning. *Education Researcher*, *18*(1), 32–42. doi:10.3102/0013189X018001032

Buykx, P., Cooper, S., Kinsman, L., Endacott, R., Scholes, J., McConnell-Henry, T., & Cant, R. (2012). Patient deterioration simulation experiences: Impact on teaching and learning. *Collegian (Royal College of Nursing, Australia)*, *19*(3), 125–129. doi:10.1016/j.colegn.2012.03.011 PMID:23101346

Cannon-Bowers, J. A. (2008). Recent advances in scenario-based training for medical education. *Current Opinion in Anaesthesiology*, *21*(6), 784–789. doi:10.1097/ACO.0b013e3283184435 PMID:18997530

Cannon-Bowers, J. A., Burns, J. J., Salas, E., & Pruitt, J. S. (1998). Advanced technology in decision-making training. In J. A. Cannon-Bowers & E. Salas (Eds.), *Making decisions under stress: Implications for individual and team training* (pp. 365–374). Washington, DC: APA Press. doi:10.1037/10278-014

Cherry, E., & Fenton, F. (2007). *The virtual heart*. Retrieved from http://thevirtualheart.org

Cherry, R. A., Williams, J., George, J., & Ali, J. (2007). The effectiveness of a human patient simulator in the ATLS shock skills station. *The Journal of Surgical Research*, *139*(2), 229–235. doi:10.1016/j.jss.2006.08.010 PMID:17161432

Collins, A., Brown, J. S., & Holum, A. (1991). Cognitive apprenticeship: Making thinking visible. *American Educator*, *15*(3), 6–17.

Cumin, D., & Merry, A. F. (2007). Simulators for use in anaesthesia. *Anaesthesia*, *62*(2), 151–162. doi:10.1111/j.1365-2044.2006.04902.x PMID:17223808

Durham, C. F., & Alden, K. R. (2008). Enhancing patient safety in nursing education through patient simulation. In R. G. Hughes (Ed.), *Patient safety and quality: An evidence-based handbook for nurses* (pp. 221–260). Rockville, MD: Agency for Healthcare Research and Quality.

Fanning, R. M., & Gaba, D. M. (2007). The role of debriefing in simulation-based learning. *Simulation in Healthcare*, *2*(2), 115–125. doi:10.1097/SIH.0b013e3180315539 PMID:19088616

Feingold, C. E., Calaluce, M., & Kallen, M. A. (2004). Computerized patient model and simulated clinical experience: Evaluation with baccalaureate nursing students. *The Journal of Nursing Education*, *43*(4), 156–163. PMID:15098909

Feltovich, P. J., Spiro, R. J., Coulson, R. L., & Feltovich, J. (1996). Collaboration within and among minds: Mastering complexity, individually, and in groups. In T. Koschmann (Ed.), *CSCL: Theory and practice of an emerging paradigm* (pp. 25–44). Mahwah, NJ: Erlbaum.

Gaba, D. M. (2004). The future vision of simulation in health care. *Quality & Safety in Health Care*, *13*(suppl_1), i2–i10. doi:10.1136/qshc.2004.009878 PMID:15465951

Gagné, R. M., Wager, W. W., Golas, K., & Keller, J. M. (2005). *Principles of Instructional Design* (5th ed.). Boston, MA: Cengage Learning.

Ge, X., Huang, D., Zhang, H., & Bowers, B. (2013). Three-dimension design for mobile learning: Pedagogical, design, and technological considerations and implications. In Z. L. Berge & L. Y. Muilenburg (Eds.), *Handbook of mobile learning* (pp. 329–345). New York, NY: Routledge.

Good, M. L. (2003). Patient simulation for training basic and advanced clinical skills. *Medical Education, 37*(s1), 14–21. doi:10.1046/j.1365-2923.37.s1.6.x PMID:14641634

Gordon, J. A., Wilkerson, W. M., Shaffer, D. W., & Armstrong, E. G. (2001). Practicing medicine without risk: Students and educators response to high-fidelity patient simulation. *Academic Medicine, 76*(5), 469–472. doi:10.1097/00001888-200105000-00019 PMID:11346525

Hannafin, M. J., Land, S., & Oliver, K. (1999). Open learning environments: Foundations and models. In C. Reigeluth (Ed.), *Instructional design theories and models: A new paradigm of instructional theory* (pp. 115–140). Mahwah, NJ: Erlbaum.

Hattie, J., & Timperley, H. (2007). The power of feedback. *Review of Educational Research, 77*(1), 81–112. doi:10.3102/003465430298487

Hayes, R., & Singer, M. J. (1989). *Simulation fidelity in training system design: Bridging the gap between reality and training*. New York, NY: Springer-Verlag. doi:10.1007/978-1-4612-3564-4

Howard Hughes Medical Institute. (2016). *Neurophysiology virtual lab*. Retrieved from http://www.hhmi.org/biointeractive/neurophysiology-virtual-lab

Huang, K., Ge, X., & Bowers, B. (2006). *The Virtual Clinic: Simulated ethical decision making in nursing education*. Paper presented at the annual convention of Association of Educational Communications and Technology, Dallas, TX.

Hung, W. (2006). The 3C3R model: A conceptual framework for designing problems in PBL. *The Interdisciplinary Journal of Problem-Based Learning, 1*(1), 55–77. doi:10.7771/1541-5015.1006

Issenberg, S. B., & McGaghie, W. C. (2013). Looking to the future. In W. C. McGaghie (Ed.), *International best practices for evaluation in the health professions* (pp. 341–359). London: Radcliffe Publishing.

Issenberg, S. B., McGaghie, W. C., Petrusa, E. R., Gordon, D. L., & Scalese, R. J. (2005). Features and uses of high-fidelity medical simulations that lead to effective learning: A BEME systematic review. *Medical Teacher, 27*(1), 10–28. doi:10.1080/01421590500046924 PMID:16147767

Jeffries, P. R. (2005). A framework for designing, implementing, and evaluating: Simulations used as teaching strategies in nursing. *Nursing Education Perspectives, 26*(2), 96–103. PMID:15921126

Jonassen, D. H. (1999). Designing constructivist learning environments. In C. M. Reigeluth (Ed.), *Instructional design theories and models: A new paradigm of instructional technology* (Vol. 2, pp. 215–239). Mahwah, NJ: Lawrence Erlbaum Associates.

Jonassen, D. H. (2011). *Learning to solve problems: A handbook for designing problem-solving learning environments*. New York, NY: Routledge.

Kelsey, N. C., & Claus, S. (2016). Embedded, in situ simulation improves ability to rescue. *Clinical Simulation in Nursing, 12*(11), 522–527. doi:10.1016/j.ecns.2016.07.009

Lajoie, S. (2005). Extending the scaffolding metaphor. *Instructional Science, 33*(5), 541–557. doi:10.1007/s11251-005-1279-2

McGaghie, W. C., Issenberg, S. B., Cohen, E. R., Barsuk, J. H., & Wayne, D. B. (2011). Does simulation-based medical education with deliberate practice yield better results than traditional clinical education? A meta-analytic comparative review of evidence. *Academic Medicine*, *86*(6), 706–711. doi:10.1097/ACM.0b013e318217e119 PMID:21512370

McGaghie, W. C., Issenberg, S. B., Petrusa, E. R., & Scalese, R. J. (2010). A critical review of simulation-based medical education research: 20032009. *Medical Education*, *44*(1), 50–63. doi:10.1111/j.1365-2923.2009.03547.x PMID:20078756

Medina, L., Racadio, J., & Schwid, H. (2000). Computers in radiology. *Pediatric Radiology*, *30*(5), 299–305. doi:10.1007/s002470050744 PMID:10836590

Merrill, M. D. (2002). First principles of instructional design. *Educational Technology Research and Development*, *50*(3), 43–59. doi:10.1007/BF02505024

Morrison, G., Ross, S., & Kemp, J. (2007). *Designing effective instruction*. Hoboken, NJ: Jonh Wiley & Sons.

Motola, I., Devine, L. A., Chung, H. S., Sullivan, J. E., & Issenberg, S. B. (2013). Simulation in healthcare education: A best evidence practical guide. *Medical Teacher*, *35*(10), 1511–1530. doi:10.3109/0142159X.2013.818632 PMID:23941678

Okuda, Y., Bond, W., Bonfante, G., McLaughlin, S., Spillane, L., Wang, E., & Gorden, J. A. et al. (2008). National growth in simulation training within emergency medicine residency programs, 2003–2008. *Academic Emergency Medicine*, *15*(11), 1113–1116. doi:10.1111/j.1553-2712.2008.00195.x PMID:18717652

Okuda, Y., Bryson, E. O., DeMaria, S., Jacobson, L., Quinones, J., Shen, B., & Levine, A. I. (2009). The utility of simulation in medical education: what is the evidence?. *Mount Sinai Journal of Medicine: A Journal of Translational and Personalized Medicine, 76*(4), 330-343.

Ottestad, E., Boulet, J., & Lighthall, G. (2007). Evaluating the management of septic shock using patient simulation. *Critical Care Medicine*, *35*(3), 769–775. doi:10.1097/01.CCM.0000256849.75799.20 PMID:17235260

Palincsar, A. S. (1986). The role of dialogue in providing scaffolded instruction. *Educational Psychologist*, *21*(1-2), 73–98. doi:10.1080/00461520.1986.9653025

Passiment, M., Sacks, H., & Huang, G. (2011). *Medical simulation in medical education: Results of an AAMC Survey*. Washington, DC: Association of American Medical Colleges.

Paver-Erzen, V., & Cimerman, M. (2007) The value of clinical simulation-based training. In T. Jarm, P. Kramar, & A. Zupanic (Eds.), *11th Mediterranean Conference on Medical and Biomedical Engineering and Computing 2007* (pp. 327-328). Berlin, Germany: Springer. doi:10.1007/978-3-540-73044-6_82

Rogers, P. L., Jacob, H., Thomas, E. A., Harwell, M., Willenkin, R. L., & Pinsky, M. R. (2000). Medical students can learn the basic application, analytic, evaluative, and psychomotor skills of critical care medicine. *Critical Care Medicine*, *28*(2), 550–554. doi:10.1097/00003246-200002000-00043 PMID:10708198

Salas, E., Wilson, K. A., Burke, C. S., & Priest, H. A. (2005). Using simulation-based training to improve patient safety: What does it take? *Joint Commission Journal on Quality and Patient Safety*, *31*(7), 363–371. doi:10.1016/S1553-7250(05)31049-X PMID:16130979

Schank, R. C., Berman, T. R., & Macpherson, K. A. (1999). Learning by doing. In C. M. Reigeluth (Ed.), *Instructional design theories and models: A new paradigm of instructional technology* (Vol. 2, pp. 161–182). Mahwah, NJ: Lawrence Erlbaum Associates.

Schon, D. A. (1983). *The reflective practitioner: How professionals think in action*. New York: Basic Books.

Shute, V. J. (2008). Focus on formative feedback. *Review of Educational Research*, *78*(1), 153–189. doi:10.3102/0034654307313795

Smith, P. L., & Ragan, T. J.(2005). *Instructional design* (3rd ed.). Hoboken, NJ: John Wiley & Sons, Inc.

Spiro, R., Feltovich, P., Jacobson, M., & Coulson, R. (1991). Knowledge representation, content specification, and the development of skill in situation-specific knowledge assembly: Some constructivist issues as they relate to cognitive flexibility theory and hypertext. *Educational Technology*, *31*(9), 22–25.

Spiro, R. J., Coulson, R. L., Feltovich, P. J., & Anderson, D. K. (1988). *Cognitive flexibility theory: Advanced knowledge acquisition in ill- structured domains. In 10th Annual Conference of the Cognitive Science Society* (pp. 375–383). Hillsdale, NJ: Erlbaum.

Squad, S. (2016). *Wisdom tooth extraction*. Retrieved form http://www.surgerysquad.com/surgeries/virtual-wisdom-tooth-extraction/

van Merrienboer, J. J. G. (2007). Alternate models of instructional design: Holistic design approaches and complex learning. In R. A. Reiser & J. Dempsey (Eds.), *Trends and issues in instructional design and technology* (2nd ed., pp. 72–81). Upper Saddle River, NJ: Merrill/Prentice Hall.

van Merrienboer, J. J. G., & Kirschner, P. A. (2001). Three worlds of instructional design: State of the art and future directions. *Instructional Science*, *29*(4/5), 429–441. doi:10.1023/A:1011904127543

Wald, D., Peet, A., Cripe, J., & Kinloch, M. (2016). *A simulated night on call experience for graduating medical students*. MedEdPORTAL Publications. Retrieved from https://doi.org/10.15766/mep_2374-8265.10483

Wood, D. J., Bruner, J. S., & Ross, G. (1976). The role of tutoring in problem solving. *Journal of Child Psychology and Psychiatry, and Allied Disciplines*, *17*(2), 89–100. doi:10.1111/j.1469-7610.1976.tb00381.x PMID:932126

ADDITIONAL READING

Al-Elq, A. H. (2010). Simulation-based medical teaching and learning. *Journal of Family and Community Medicine*, *17*(1), 35. doi:10.4103/1319-1683.68787 PMID:22022669

Alinier, G., Hunt, B., Gordon, R., & Harwood, C. (2006). Effectiveness of intermediate-fidelity simulation training technology in undergraduate nursing education. *Journal of Advanced Nursing*, *54*(3), 359–369. doi:10.1111/j.1365-2648.2006.03810.x PMID:16629920

Barnes, S., Golden, B., & Price, S. (2013). Applications of agent-based modeling and simulation to healthcare operations management. In B. T. Denton (Ed.), *Handbook of healthcare operations management* (pp. 45–74). New York, NY: Springer. doi:10.1007/978-1-4614-5885-2_3

Belland, B. R. (2014). Scaffolding: Definition, current debates, and future directions. In J. M. Spector, M. D. Merrill, J. Elen, & M. J. Bishop (Eds.), *Handbook of research on educational communications and technology* (4th ed., pp. 505–518). New York, NY: Springer. doi:10.1007/978-1-4614-3185-5_39

Bowles, K. (2000). The relationship of critical-thinking skills and the clinical-judgment skills of baccalaureate nursing students. *The Journal of Nursing Education*, *39*, 373–376. PMID:11103976

Cant, R., & Cooper, S. (2010). Simulation-based learning in nurse education: Systematic review. *Journal of Advanced Nursing*, *66*(1), 3–15. doi:10.1111/j.1365-2648.2009.05240.x PMID:20423432

Cooper, J. B., & Taqueti, V. (2004). A brief history of the development of mannequin simulators for clinical education and training. *Quality & Safety in Health Care*, *13*(suppl 1), i11–i18. doi:10.1136/qshc.2004.009886 PMID:15465949

Dieckmann, P., Gaba, D., & Rall, M. (2007). Deepening the theoretical foundations of patient simulation as social practice. *Simulation in Healthcare*, *2*(3), 183–193. doi:10.1097/SIH.0b013e3180f637f5 PMID:19088622

Dieckmann, P., & Rall, M. (2008). Designing a scenario as a simulated clinical experience: The TupASS scenario script. In R. R. Kyle & W. B. Murray (Eds.), *Clinical simulation: Operations, engineering and management* (pp. 541–550). San Diego, CA: Academic Press. doi:10.1016/B978-012372531-8.50096-0

Ge, X., & Land, S. M. (2003). Scaffolding students problem-solving processes in an ill-structured task using question prompts and peer interactions. *Educational Technology Research and Development*, *51*(1), 21–38. doi:10.1007/BF02504515

Gopher, D., Weil, M., & Bareket, T. (1994). Transfer of skill from a computer game trainer to flight. *Human Factors*, *36*(3), 387–405.

Gordon, J. A. (2000). The human patient simulator: Acceptance and efficacy as a teaching tool for students. *Academic Medicine*, *75*(5), 522. doi:10.1097/00001888-200005000-00043 PMID:10824795

Gordon, M. S. (1974). Cardiology patient simulator: Development of an animated manikin to teach cardiovascular disease. *The American Journal of Cardiology*, *34*(3), 350–355. doi:10.1016/0002-9149(74)90038-1 PMID:4136577

Greeno, J. G. (1989). Situations, mental models, and generative knowledge. In D. Klahr & K. Kotovsky (Eds.), *Complex information processing: The impact of Herbert A. Simon* (pp. 285–318). Hillsdale, NJ: Erlbaum.

Huffman, J. L., McNeil, G., Bismilla, G., & Lai, A. (2016). Essentials of scenario building for simulation-based education. In V. J. Grant & A. Cheng (Eds.), *Comprehensive healthcare simulation: Pediatrics* (pp. 19–29). Switzerland: Springer International Publishing. doi:10.1007/978-3-319-24187-6_2

Hung, W. (2009). The 9-step problem design process for problem-based learning: Application of the 3C3R model. *Educational Research Review*, *4*(2), 118–141. doi:10.1016/j.edurev.2008.12.001

Issenberg, B., Gordon, M. S., Gordon, D. L., Safford, R. E., & Hart, I. R. (2001). Simulation and new learning technologies. *Medical Teacher*, *23*(1), 16–23. doi:10.1080/01421590020007324 PMID:11260734

Kardong-Edgren, S. E., Starkweather, A. R., & Ward, L. D. (2008). The integration of simulation into a clinical foundations of nursing course: Student and faculty perspectives. *International Journal of Nursing Education Scholarship*, *5*(1), 1–16. doi:10.2202/1548-923X.1603 PMID:18673294

Khan, K., Pattison, T., & Sherwood, M. (2011). Simulation in medical education. *Medical Teacher*, *33*(1), 1–3. doi:10.3109/0142159X.2010.519412 PMID:21182376

Kim, J., Park, J. H., & Shin, S. (2016). Effectiveness of simulation-based nursing education depending on fidelity: A meta-analysis. *BMC Medical Education*, *16*(1), 152. doi:10.1186/s12909-016-0672-7 PMID:27215280

Kolb, D. (1984). *Experiential learning as the science of learning and development*. Englewood Cliffs, NJ: Prentice Hall.

Langdale, L. A., Schaad, D., Wipf, J., Marshall, S., Vontver, L., & Scott, C. S. (2003). Preparing graduates for the first year of residency: Are medical schools meeting the need? *Academic Medicine*, *78*(1), 39–44. doi:10.1097/00001888-200301000-00009 PMID:12525408

Lapkin, S., Levett-Jones, T., Bellchambers, H., & Fernandez, R. (2010). Effectiveness of patient simulation manikins in teaching clinical reasoning skills to undergraduate nursing students: A systematic review. *Clinical Simulation in Nursing*, *6*(6), 207–222. doi:10.1016/j.ecns.2010.05.005 PMID:27820553

Lateef, F. (2010). Simulation-based learning: Just like the real thing. *Journal of Emergencies, Trauma, and Shock*, *3*(4), 348–352. doi:10.4103/0974-2700.70743 PMID:21063557

Lave, J., & Wenger, E. (1991). *Situated learning: Legitimate peripheral participation*. New York: Cambridge University Press. doi:10.1017/CBO9780511815355

LeBlanc, V. R., MacDonald, R. D., McArthur, B., King, K., & Lepine, T. (2005). Paramedic performance in calculating drug dosages following stressful scenarios in a human patient simulator. *Prehospital Emergency Care*, *9*(4), 439–444. doi:10.1080/10903120500255255 PMID:16263679

Levine, A. I. DeMaria. Jr. S., Schwartz, A. D., & Sim, A. J. (2013). The comprehensive textbook of healthcare simulation. New York, NY: Springer.

Loudon, D., Taylor, A., & Macdonald, A. (2014). The use of qualitative design methods in the design, development and evaluation of virtual technologies for healthcare: Stroke case study. In M. Ma, L. C. Jain, & P. Anderson (Eds.), *Virtual, augmented reality and serious games for healthcare 1* (Vol. 1, pp. 371–390). Berlin, Germany: Springer. doi:10.1007/978-3-642-54816-1_19

Ma, M., Jain, L. C., & Anderson, P. (2014). Future Trends of Virtual, Augmented Reality, and Games for Health. In M. Ma, L. C. Jain, & P. Anderson (Eds.), *Virtual, augmented reality and serious games for healthcare 1* (Vol. 1, pp. 1–6). Berlin, Germany: Springer. doi:10.1007/978-3-642-54816-1_1

Ma, M., Jain, L. C., & Anderson, P. (Eds.). (2014). *Virtual, augmented reality and serious games for healthcare 1* (Vol. 1). Berlin: Springer. doi:10.1007/978-3-642-54816-1

Maran, N. J., & Glavin, R. J. (2003). Low- to high-fidelity simulation - a continuum of medical education? *Medical Education*, *37*(suppl 1), 22–28. doi:10.1046/j.1365-2923.37.s1.9.x PMID:14641635

McGaghie, W. C., Issenberg, S. B., Barsuk, J. H., & Wayne, D. B. (2014). A critical review of simulation-based mastery learning with translational outcomes. *Medical Education*, *48*(4), 375–385. doi:10.1111/medu.12391 PMID:24606621

McPherson, K., Headrick, L., & Moss, F. (2001). Working and learning together: Good quality care depends on it, but how can we achieve it? *Quality in Health Care*, *10*, 46–53. doi:10.1136/qhc.0100046 PMID:11700379

Murphy, J. G., Cremonini, F., Kane, G. C., & Dunn, W. (2007). Is simulation based medicine training the future of clinical medicine? *European Review for Medical and Pharmacological Sciences*, *11*(1), 1–8. PMID:17405343

Nehring, W. M., Ellis, W. E., & Lashley, F. R. (2001). Human Patient Simulators in Nursing Education: An Overview. *Simulation & Gaming*, *32*(2), 194–204. doi:10.1177/104687810103200207

Puntambekar, S., & Hubscher, R. (2005). Tools for scaffolding students in a complex learning environment: What have we gained and what have we missed? *Educational Psychologist*, *40*(1), 1–12. doi:10.1207/s15326985ep4001_1

Qayumi, K., Pachev, G., Zheng, B., Ziv, A., Koval, V., Badiei, S., & Cheng, A. (2014). Status of simulation in health care education: An international survey. *Advances in Medical Education and Practice*, *5*, 457–467. doi:10.2147/AMEP.S65451 PMID:25489254

Reigeluth, C. M. (1999). The elaboration theory: Guidance for scope and sequence decisions. In C. M. Reigeluth (Ed.), *Instructional-design theories and models: A new paradigm of instructional theory* (Vol. 2, pp. 425–453). Mahway, NJ: Lawrence Erlbaum Associates.

Rhodes, M. L., & Curran, C. (2005). Use of the human patient simulator to teach clinical judgment skills in a baccalaureate nursing program. *Computers, Informatics, Nursing*, *23*(5), 256–262. doi:10.1097/00024665-200509000-00009 PMID:16166827

Schank, R., Fano, A., Bell, B., & Jona, M. (1993/1994). The Design of Goal-Based Scenarios. *Journal of the Learning Sciences*, *3*(4), 305–345. doi:10.1207/s15327809jls0304_2

Schön, D. A. (1983). *The reflective practitioner: how professionals think in action*. New York: Basic Books.

Seropian, M. A., Brown, K., Gavilanes, J. S., & Driggers, B. (2004). Simulation: Not just a Manikin. *The Journal of Nursing Education*, *43*(4), 164–169. PMID:15098910

Shinnick, M. A., Woo, M., Horwich, T. B., & Steadman, R. (2011). Debriefing: The most important component in simulation? *Clinical Simulation in Nursing*, *7*(3), 105–111. doi:10.1016/j.ecns.2010.11.005

Tseng, S. C., & Tsai, C. C. (2007). On-line peer assessment and the role of the peer feedback: A study of high school computer course. *Computers & Education*, *49*(4), 1161–1174. doi:10.1016/j.compedu.2006.01.007

Weller, J. M. (2004). Simulation in undergraduate medical education: Bridging the gap between theory and practice. *Medical Education*, *38*(1), 32–38. doi:10.1111/j.1365-2923.2004.01739.x PMID:14962024

Ziv, A., Small, S. D., & Wolpe, P. R. (2000). Patient safety and simulation-based medical education. *Medical Teacher*, *22*(5), 489–495. doi:10.1080/01421590050110777 PMID:21271963

KEY DEFINITIONS AND TERMS

Computer-Based Simulation: A model or representation of a real world object, situation, or system that is delivered through a single computer or multiple computer network for the purpose of recreating a real world environment for study in a classroom setting.

Human-Patient Simulator: A model or natural physical representation of a human subject (mannequin) that returns real world output of behaviors or vital functions for the purpose of practical experience and instantaneous feedback in patient interaction and assessment.

Designing: The process of the development of instruction and authentic instructional environments through a planned approach that considers each facet of a system to be represented and includes identifying objectives, problem scenarios, and facilitation of learning experiences in the final product.

Facilitation: The process of applying reasoned instructional strategies that model, scaffold, support, and offer immediate feedback for learners in developing theory and practical skills in a clinical setting.

Modeling: A facilitation strategy where demonstration is integrated into instruction for the purpose of guiding learners in their development of behavioral processes or cognitive expectations and problem solving in a clinical setting.

Scaffolding: A facilitation strategy where learning support specific to the individual learner is integrated into real-time instruction for the purpose of guiding learners in their development of behavioral processes or cognitive expectations in problem solving in a clinical setting.

Debriefing: A metacognitive scaffolding strategy for the purpose of formative evaluation where feedback specific to individual learners is presented and learners are asked to reflect on their performance in a clinical experience.

Simulation-Based Medical Education: A teaching and learning design approach that integrates real world representations of systems and situated scenarios within instructional experiences that presents opportunity for medical students to obtain practical experience through these representations in demonstrating knowledge and skills for real world application.

APPENDIX A

Identifying Learning Objectives

Purpose: This worksheet is developed to assist you in identifying the learning objectives for creating simulated learning experience. Fill in this form as completely as possible to generate a complete set of learning objectives for each scenario that you would like to run.

Table 1.

Identified performance gaps/learning needs	
The purpose(s) of simulation	
Person needs to be trained	
Tasks need to be trained	
Expected learning outcomes	
Learning Objectives ● Process ● Content	
Assessment strategies	

APPENDIX B

Debriefing

Purpose: This worksheet is to help you to benefit the most from the debriefing session. You insights and your feedback are critical to the team and the development of reasoning skills through reflective learning processes.

Table 2.

Learning Objectives:	• •
Critical Events & Rationales:	• •
Group Considerations	• How effective was management of the situation? o What went well? Why? o What could be improved? • Was communication clear and effective before team deployment? During the event? • Were roles and responsibilities of all the team members clear? • If the team were going to do this again, how would you like to handle it differently? • Were there errors made that can be avoided? How?
Individual Considerations	• What learning objectives were you able to achieve? • What learning objectives were you not able to achieve and why? • How did you feel throughout the simulated experience? • What are the main take-aways? • Additional thoughts and comments?

Chapter 5

Medical Simulation as an Instructional Tool in Health Education:

A Worked Example for Clinical Training

Anna Lerant
University of Mississippi Medical Center, USA

Jeffrey D. Orledge
University of Mississippi Medical Center, USA

Oliver Jason Bates
University of Maryland Medical Center, USA

Robin (Rob) W. Rockhold
University of Mississippi Medical Center, USA

Michael G. Holder
University of Mississippi Medical Center, USA

Richard Kyle
Independent Researcher, USA

Willie Bosseau Murray
Pennsylvania State University, USA

ABSTRACT

The purpose of this chapter is to provide a background and a worked example of using the Instructional Design System (ISD) as applied to a complex real life example. Specifically, the authors demonstrate the use of ADDIE (Analysis, Design, Development, Implementation, and Evaluation) for building the instruction curriculum of the skills of intubation. The majority of the planning time should be spent on the Needs Analysis and Design. The Learning Objectives, prepared during the Design phase, should be written as Objective Observable Behaviors, which can then serve as the assessments for Evaluation. The content includes two examples of the application of ADDIE: firstly a task that requires a large cognitive component and where simulators and mannequins are readily available. Secondly, a task that requires a high level of psychomotor skills where suitably realistic mannequins are not available, and virtual reality needs to be used as an additional educational modality.

DOI: 10.4018/978-1-5225-2098-6.ch005

Copyright © 2017, IGI Global. Copying or distributing in print or electronic forms without written permission of IGI Global is prohibited.

INTRODUCTION

Simulation has been recommended as a valuable addition to health care training (Kohn 2000). To gain the maximum value from simulation training, a rigorous educational underpinning is required. These principles are encapsulated in the concepts of ADDIE: Analysis, Design, Development, Implement, and Evaluation, which is an example of Instructional Systems Design (ISD) (Dick 2009, Causer 2014, Steinert 2012).

Building a curriculum starts with a thorough Analysis (diagnosis) of who the learners are, what are the learners' current conditions, what are the learners' goals for change for which they seek our help; Design training interventions and Develop (prescribe) the interventions most likely to succeed; Implement the intervention and Evaluate the results. The evaluation phase ties back to the analysis phase, i.e., the observable learning objectives which were written in the design phase become the points for evaluation. Revisit this spiral cycle of analysis, design, development, implementation and evaluation, and adjust as needed until the learners' results are good enough to assert that the training program has met established expectations.

The work is shown as an instructional example applied for teaching airway intubation. Figure 1 demonstrates the process of intubation.[1] Intubation is not only a skill that is required by many disciplines and professions, but also, like so many other interventional skills, is a risky (Cormack 1984, Knill 1993, Mallampati 1985) and time-consuming procedure to teach in the clinical setting. Therefore, intubation should be taught for the first time in simulation and not on real patients. The examples given will be applicable to a wide range of health care training programs responsible for intubation, and readily adaptable for training programs responsible for tasks with inherent patient risks.

The goal of this chapter is therefore to reveal the value of deliberately designed instruction by providing a worked example suitable for adaption to most clinical training needs.

Figure 1. The figure shows an intubation training mannequin with the laryngoscope already inserted into the airway. The endotracheal tube ("breathing tube") is shown outside the airway to demonstrate the curved pathway required for the insertion through the airway.

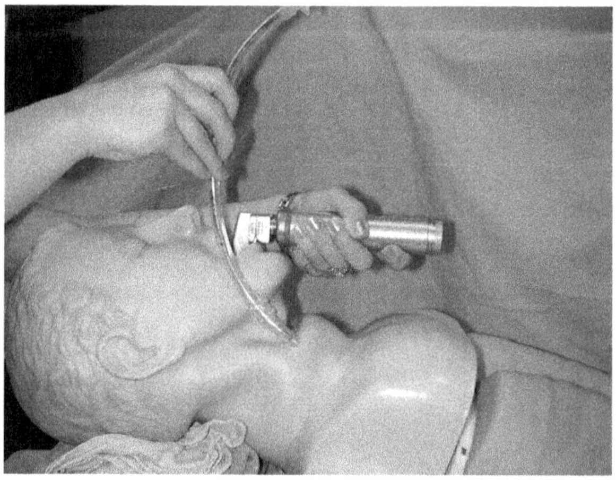

BACKGROUND

Intubation is a critical skill required by most acute care providers. It is taught in a simulation setting to a wide array of trainees from pre-hospital first-responders, to in-hospital care givers such as respiratory technicians as well as advanced practice nursing and medical personnel. It is critical to complete intubation in the least number of attempts, with the least trauma to the patient's mouth, airways and the adjacent tissues.

Observation of these acute care providers in both the clinical milieu and in simulation has shown that intubation skills have been declining. Multiple factors are involved, including fewer clinical hands-on hours, a wider audience required to learn intubation skills with fewer patients requiring intubation due to the widespread use of laryngeal mask airways (LMA), and more use of conscious sedation with minimally invasive surgery, where intubation is mostly not required. Also, the present intubation mannequins were designed primarily to look anatomically correct, rather than to teach the specific steps of the intubation process and reveal the consequences of poor execution. This chapter is designed to show how to make use of imperfect intubation simulators to demonstrate poor techniques and their consequences, as well as to teach good techniques, by applying Instructional System Design (ISD) principles.

The examples will enable the demonstration of how the deconstruction of an overall clinical task, e.g. intubation, produces a series of subtasks. Deliberate practice of each of the subtasks is performed using simple, cheap, part task trainers. The speed of execution of these subtasks is deliberately slowed for easier presentation of nuances. Initially, every part-task training session is performed slowly in "student time." The time expended during this training phase is focused upon the participants' explicit practice of just one or two new concepts and maneuvers. They continue practicing these maneuvers slowly until they have "mastered the moves" by demonstrating proficiency in these new subtasks.

Once the participants have grasped each subtask in the series of the tasks, and demonstrated each of them successfully in a "student-time", or "slow-time" session, the next phase will be a "patient time", or "real-time" scenario. They have to demonstrate the entire series of task at real-time speed. At this point, the overall clinical task can be performed successfully because the students have succeeded in a "crawl, walk, run" sequence with frequent evaluations after each subtask, thereby reinforcing the habit of self-evaluation.

Only after the student can successfully complete the overall clinical task in benign conditions, do the instructors add confounding complexities. For example, during intubation, a rapidly decreasing oxygen saturation might require the learner to make the decision to interrupt the intubation process to provide temporary mask ventilation.

The Problem: Difficulties of Teaching

For many years, clinical teaching has consisted of two almost independent portions: i.) the didactic portion, presenting facts and factoids to learners in a lecture, followed by ii.) the bedside hands-on apprenticeship. During didactic sessions, learners "succeeded" by memorizing the facts, and regurgitated those facts in a paper and pencil examination (and now their computerized equivalencies). There was also no measurement of any change in observable behavior, which should be the main goal of education. In the apprenticeship model, so typically employed in health care fields, an individual instructor shaped the trainee to fit each instructor's own preferred set of beliefs, ideas and behaviors. There is typically no formal design in such a clinical instructional process.

A further weakness in the clinical arena is that the instructors are quite willing to indicate their personal belief of a "good enough" performance: "This is an excellent trainee/resident/student!", but there are no observable behavior criteria, let alone objective measurements, in the clinical milieu. Many clinical instructors are expecting the simulation community to develop objective measures of success while using simulators with varying degrees of fidelity. It will not be possible to develop and validate measurements in an imperfect simulator, until the clinical instructors have succeeded in developing objective measures in the perfect fidelity of the human patient.

Intubation as an Instructional Example

Intubation was selected for this chapter as it is a complex procedure which can serve as an excellent demonstration for implementing ADDIE concepts, and enabling examples of utilizing ADDIE principles.

- High risk procedure.
- Intubation in the clinical arena is stressful.
- Too stressful to learn adequately in the clinical milieu.
- The simulation models are insufficient to teach and assess proficiency.
- The simulation models are only sufficient to teach certain steps of intubation.
- The simulation models can, and do, teach and ingrain bad habits, especially if not used carefully, e.g. as per ISD principles.
- Intubation requires much prior understanding, specifically of anatomy, to truly understand normal and abnormal actions.
- 99 out of 100 successful intubations still means: "fully unsuccessful for that one failed patient".
- Requires individual attention to trainees, i.e. coaching.
- Hands-on training in patients is improved with prior simulation.

Simulation as an Instructional Strategy

Simulation was selected for this chapter as it enables the demonstration of the ADDIE sequence:

- High risk procedure. It would be unethical to teach novices on live, anesthetized patients.
- Allows individual attention to trainees – coaching.
- Hands-on training "needs" simulation.
- Part task trainers are available to teach and test specific actions.
- Unrealistic aspects of part task trainers need to be addressed.

Anatomy as a Worked Example

For this book chapter the focus will be on anatomical aspects. Anatomy is poorly understood (Benumof 2006) by novices and by practitioners alike, because it is, and has been for many years, poorly taught in most health care teaching institutions. For instance, the structures that most clinicians call the "arytenoids" are actually the corniculate and cuneiform cartilages. The real arytenoids, which constitute the posterior anatomy of the vocal cords, are actually seldom seen during intubation, as the arytenoids are often hidden by the corniculate and cuneiform cartilages. This first worked example relates to placing the patient to be intubated in the correct "sniffing" (Adnet 2001) position, which involves both flexion and extension of the neck of the patient.

Teaching the correct direction of force to be applied to flip up the epiglottis is extremely difficult due to a lack of understanding of anatomy. Incorrect directions of force are often applied: i.) due to the lack of understanding of the anatomy of the vallecula (the angle between the tongue and the epiglottis), and ii.) the inability to predict flipping up the epiglottis, and iii.) lack of understanding the movements of the tip of the blade of the laryngoscope interacting with the anatomical structures (i.e., functional anatomy of the base of the tongue and epiglottis).

- Since the 1930s, prior teaching of intubation consisted of the instructor looking from the outside, with no idea of what the trainee was actually seeing inside the airway. The teacher could not see the tip of the blade of the laryngoscope, nor the anatomy encountered by the tip of the blade.
- Only recently has videolaryngoscopy, as shown in Figure 2, enabled the teacher to see what the trainee is seeing.
- We chose this "relationship of the epiglottis to the vallecula" as shown in Figure 3, to show how new technology can be disruptive ("change in long established habits") technology in teaching, in this case, beneficial disruption.
- We also specifically selected a topic where there is no physical simulator available to teach (or even show) the anatomy of the glosso-epiglottic ligament, as shown in Figure 4. Therefore teaching has to include "virtual reality" including pictures, videos and explanations.

Instructional Design

In the typical apprenticeship health care educational model, information is given to trainees, often in a haphazard and non-structured fashion, depending on the amount of time available in the clinical milieu. This is typically triggered by a randomly presenting patient where the trainee attempts a procedure,

Figure 2. The figure shows a videolaryngoscope with an endotracheal tube demonstrating similar curvatures. The videolaryngoscope has a camera near the tip of the blade, which provides improved vision of the vocal cords

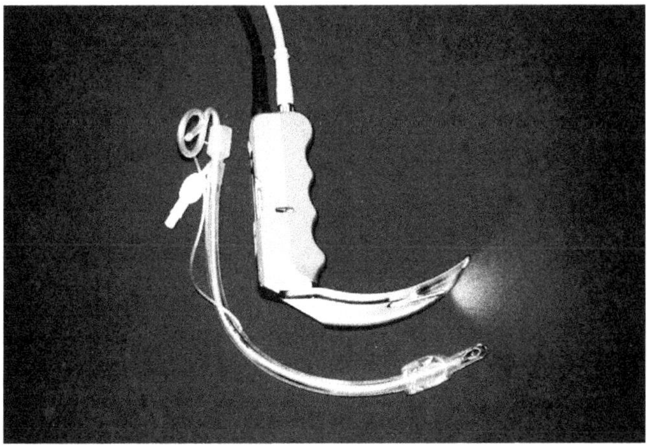

Figure 3. The figure shows the tip of the videolaryngoscope blade approaching the vallecula, which is the angle between the tongue and the epiglottis

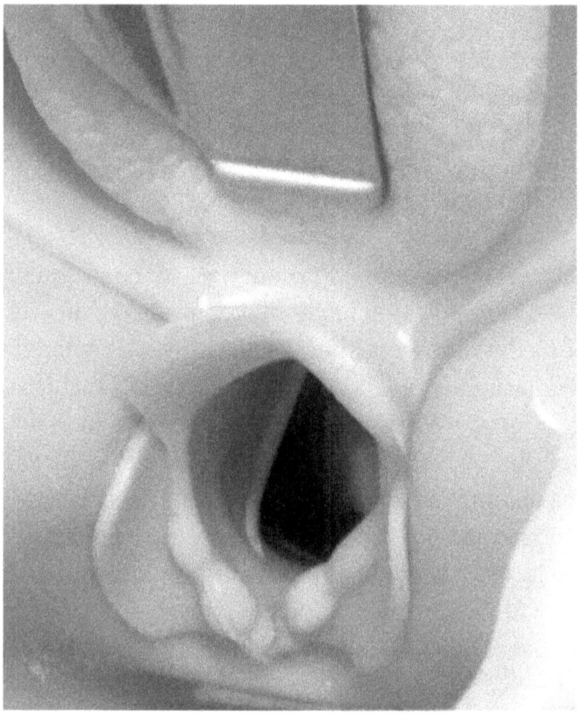

Figure 4. The figure shows the glosso-epiglottic ligament to the left of the tip of the blade of the videolaryngoscope

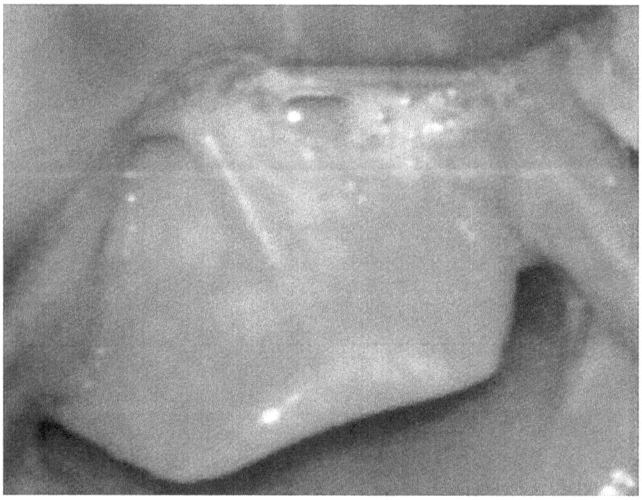

but due to time limitations, the instructor often takes over. There is no underlying educational theory underpinning such training.

In contrast, as a part of the application of ADDIE in this worked example, elements of educational theories are employed. The application of the *behaviorist* learning theory suggests that a stimulus/response system is employed along with a reward for accomplishing a task (think Pavlov's dog). Applying the *constructivist* theory a base is developed and then built upon. The same approaches should be used here. Start by teaching the individual steps slowly in simulation, and thereafter build the learner's ability to perform in real life.

An example of a teaching session devoid of any educational theory is the following: Medical students in their first week in medical school are sent to the simulation center. The beginner medical students have to manage a crisis event in real time (e.g. anaphylaxis.) There is much activity and much non-medical discussion: "I do not know what to do!" and "I do not know the dosage!" The students say afterwards that "I enjoyed the session!", but they do not say that they learned anything (nor were there really any formal Objectives, other than to use the brand new simulation center, and to let the trainees and trainers, have some "fun.")

This example clearly indicates that more formal approaches to education, such as ISD and ADDIE, are needed to properly establish the learner's needs, identify the appropriate level of objectives, develop a course that is specific to the students' knowledge, skills and abilities, as well as apply evaluation procedures to identify the impact on the learner, i.e., to change behaviors and improve clinical outcomes.

To successfully apply ISD models, one has to understand that ISD is a process. (Causer 2014, Steinert 2012) It provides a systematic approach to develop education. It is implemented through an understanding of the learner, development of specific objectives, the careful selection of learning theories and application of educational strategies, as well as applying evaluation techniques to improve future education. ADDIE is one example of an ISD model. (Almomen 2016, Dent 2016, Khalil 2016) ADDIE is also the most widely known and most widely applied. In the opinion of the authors, all other ISD models (Leppink 2015, Kolb 2012) are nothing more than derivatives of ADDIE. Implementation of ADDIE requires the use of an educational strategy such as simulation. Other educational strategies include a round table discussion, didactic lectures, blended learning, and table top exercises.

ADDIE is also an iterative process because analysis and evaluation are applied repeatedly throughout the entire process. As the design progresses, the question is repeatedly asked: "How can we make this better?" This question is repeated after the Development and Implementation.

Implementing ISD in general, and using the phases of ADDIE specifically, forces and encourages a step-wise approach, explicitly expecting learners to master each step before taking on the challenge of the next step. The eventual quality of graduates can be improved just by clearly describing explicit expectations for each step, and then providing students with clearly objective means to demonstrate their attainment of said expectations.

Before delving into details of a specific example, this section provides a high level discussion of each of the aspects of ADDIE, to enable the reader to follow the principles when applied to the two examples.

Analysis

ADDIE starts with the Analysis phase (also called "Needs Analysis".) This is one of the most important, but often neglected, sections of ADDIE. The majority of the preparation time should be spent on Analysis. A comprehensive analysis almost automatically "dictates" and shows the pathway to the

Table 1.

ADDIE Activities	Description of Activities	Examples of activities
Doing Analysis	The process of breaking down or "deconstructing" a complex topic into a series of subtasks to gain a better understanding of it	In simulation education, it allows us to understand our learners, simulation technologies, procedures, and performance
Doing Design	Ensures systematic development of the learning process, and creation of observable learning objectives	During design, objectives are written, learning theories, education strategies and evaluation techniques are selected
Doing Development	Building on objectives and performance expectations	Curriculum, evaluation tools, scenarios, presentations, etc. are all built during this phase
Doing Implementation	Conducting ("running") the course	A pilot course, leading to refinements, followed by the full course
Doing Evaluation	The systematic determination of merit, worth, and significance of a learning or training process by comparing criteria against a set of standards	Ensure that the stated goals of the learning process will actually meet learning objectives

method of instruction, i.e. the educational strategy to be selected. The analysis also DIRECTLY leads to the Learning Objectives (see the first section of Design.)

Analysis includes analysis of multiple items and issues. For instance:

- Who are the learners?
- A knowledge of the trainees, their prior experience, knowledge, skills, and attitudes is essential in the analysis phase.
- Multiple levels of trainees need to be addressed separately: novice students will need a different curriculum compared to experienced practitioners (for refresher and/or advanced courses.) There is a tendency to build a single "Simulation Experience", and all levels of trainees are "pushed through" the same curriculum.
- There are certain basic issues and principles (e.g. anatomy) that ALL trainees have to know. It is important to select what to teach to various levels of trainees, e.g. when working with medical students tell them the laryngoscope goes in the left hand, while more advanced practitioners will feel insulted if one told them: "Left hand, NOT right hand".
- What are the problems? What do the trainees "not get?" What does the instructor have to say over and over again?
- The problem needs to be deconstructed into a series of steps: each individual action needs to be analyzed and described
- Educational material and issues
- Trainers / instructors
- Available time (trainees, trainers, simulation/learning facility)
- Available equipment and resources
- What is typically done (incorrectly) when preparing a simulation session?
- Why it is incorrect? For example, thoughtless use of real patients as "teaching material" is not based on ISD theories

Analysis should be done on every aspect of the course. This includes learner analysis, procedural analysis (in this case the indications, contraindications, and steps to successfully intubate), analysis of education modalities and simulation tools, as well as technologies that will help meet the objectives and standards. Poor outcomes are also analyzed.

The central reason for poor design is because of a lack of understanding of the level of knowledge of the learner. The analysis of gaps in knowledge, skills and attitudes form the basis for the Learning Objectives as outlined in the next phase of Design.

Design

The first step of Design is to use the gaps and problems from the Analysis phase to describe what the trainees should be able to do better, i.e. what is the change in behavior that needs to occur after the training session. Writing the change in behavior in plain English helps the instructors to focus on the behavior, rather than on the construction and phrasing of the Learning Objectives. At a later stage, the "change in behaviors" can be formally written as formal educational objectives.

The next step of Design is to select an Educational Strategy that will help to engender the change in behavior. Simulation is an educational strategy which can be used in conjunction with other educational strategies such as round table discussions, didactic lectures, blended learning, table top exercises, etc.

Design also includes the selection of the education modalities, associated tools and technologies that will be used. Evaluation modalities are also considered during Design. Depending on the level of learner and their availability in the future, one may select one or multiple evaluation types: factual tests and quizzes, performance reviews, or actual training impact on performance, for example.

From a conceptual point of view, design is sitting around a table having a theoretical discussion:

- Identify examples of Design in general, and examples from specifically "intubation"
- Given a solid Analysis of needs and issues (and, as indicated before, most time should have been spent on the analysis), the Design becomes relatively clear
- The formal Design phase consists of a theoretical expansion of the needs: the Design formally transforms the needs to an implementable, hands-on teaching session
- The sequence of each element in relation to other elements needs to be planned (for instance, understand anatomy of the neck before practicing the flexion and extension of the neck)
- The amount of time available for the session will dictate how many of the elements of the needs could be addressed in a single session (and how many sessions will be needed in total for the list of needs and the whole curriculum)
- The group sizes and any rotations need to be addressed
- The Learning Objectives are designed as observable behaviors
- The Learning Objectives are used to Design the assessments that will be used in the evaluation phase.

After each step of ADDIE, the prior steps are revisited. For example, after the Design phase, the Design is scrutinized to ensure that it fulfills the requirements and gaps as outlined in the Analysis phase.

Development

Development includes building of all documents, presentations, and evaluation tools as well as scenarios, flow sheets and anything else that will support the course's teaching objectives. For simulation purposes, it also includes setting up the environment and equipment and assigning any supporting roles (rehearsing the script, training instructors and actors, as well as testing equipment.)

From a conceptual point of view, development is working in the Simulation Center doing a hands-on practical set-up, creating and testing of the training session as designed in the previous portion of ADDIE:

- The formal Development phase consists of a *Conceptual* expansion of the Analyzed Needs and Design. The *Practical* Development formally transforms the Needs and Design to an implementable, hands-on teaching session by selecting the identified items and equipment.
- The instructors will also trial (pilot) the time needed for each element.
- The sequence of each element in relation to other elements needs to be planned and tested in the Development phase: for example, teaching how to select the size and shape of the laryngoscope blade best matched to the given patient size precedes teaching how to insert the blade into the patient.

Analysis should be conducted on every aspect of the course. For instance, after the Development, the instructor checks back to see that the elements from the Needs Analysis are being fully covered, and all the design elements have been transformed into implementable actions. For instance, the technology and resources must support the selected strategy, and are also in line with the objectives and learners identified in the Analysis

Implementation

Many simulation centers tend to start with the Implementation step – they spend an inordinate amount of time on trying to put together ("Implement") a highly realistic simulation, and only then see what can be taught with such a session.

In contrast, Implementation should be the execution of all the prior planning. Each step and action in the Implementation has been carefully considered in the Design phase, and comprehensively outlined in the Development phase. Therefore, the Implementation phase should be relatively simple to implement.

Using a pilot group of trainees. presentations are given, patient scenarios and performance expectations are briefed, and the course is tested on a pilot group of trainees. After refinements, the course is hosted for the trainees.

Further points include checking the timing of each section, as well as ensuring sufficient time for Evaluation. As before, each prior phase of ADDIE should be revisited to check that every aspect of the course contributes to, and is consistent with, the Learning Objectives and required change in behavior.

Evaluation

Ideally, the observable, objective Learning Objectives become the measurements used for Evaluation of the learners. It is not just the learners who are evaluated. The instructors, the selection of strategies, theories, technologies, the implementation, etc. should all be evaluated and the results of those evaluations should be recycled into the next iteration of the training. Evaluation is what makes ISD a process, because the results and recycling of those results makes the effort ongoing.

The results of the Evaluation should be compared to the Analysis and Learning Objectives to determine if the assessment of the trainees encapsulates the changes in behaviors envisaged in the earlier phases. The purpose of the first sections of this chapter is to provide an overview of the concepts of ADDIE. The next section will be used to illustrate the detailed application of those principles to a real life educational problem. Two worked examples of preparing a simulation offering solidly based on Instructional System Design (ISD) theories are provided in the next sections.

MAIN FOCUS OF THE CHAPTER

The main focus of this chapter is to provide worked examples of a real life problem which involves multiple professions and disciplines at multiple levels of expertise and training, i.e. intubation of the airway. The authors indicate how the large subject of intubation is dissected ("deconstructed") into separate steps which need to be mastered before moving on to the next step.

The first seemingly simple step is the positioning of the patient prior to attempting the intubation. However, the anatomy of the cervical vertebrae and their movements are not simple, and cannot be adequately appreciated simply looking at an articulated skeleton. Failure to understand this functional anatomy leads to an increased incidence of failure to place the breathing tube expeditiously.

The second step addressed is placing the tip of the laryngoscope blade correctly in the vallecula. The available mannequins are inadequate to teach this step, and virtual images are required to help the trainees grasp the concept. The authors explain the thought process underlying the implementation of ADDIE for each example so that these examples can serve as generic templates to address multiple other educational needs.

First Worked Example of ADDIE: Anatomy of Positioning

The importance of a knowledge of anatomy to patient care is underappreciated (Benumof 2006) and poorly taught, hence poorly understood thereby leading to failures in the clinical milieu.

Doing Analysis: Anatomy of Positioning

The predominant reason for poor instruction is a lack of understanding of learners' incoming levels of comprehension and competence. This leads to misidentifying performance gaps and learning objectives and subsequently selecting the wrong learning theories and teaching strategies when designing the course. Hence, most of the instructional development time and effort should be devoted to the Analysis of needs phase.

To begin analysis, a course designer needs to identify major questions aimed at discovering the underlying problems in performance. Given the authors' example as identified in this chapter, the questions relating to the problems of anatomy are identified in Table 2.

Based on the authors' analysis, here are answers to the questions above as applicable to the example of anatomy of positioning.

Table 2.

Universal Questions to Address as a Part of the Analysis Phase of ADDIE	
1.	Who are the learners and what are the learners responsible for? What are their backgrounds and prior experiences?
2.	What do the learners "not get"? What do we (teachers) have to say over and over again, and yet the learners exhibit the incorrect behaviors? (They just do not do it correctly.) What is the gap between present behaviors and desired behaviors? How does the simulation instructor get information from the clinicians about what the trainees "do not get?"
3.	What domain(s) of knowledge (Knowledge, Skills, and/or Attitudes) is/are missing? What level of Knowledge (according to Bloom's Taxonomy) is missing?
4.	What specific skills need to be taught differently and/or remedied? Is the failure due to a lack of knowledge of the steps of the procedure, or due to lack of eye-hand coordination?
5.	Do the trainees believe that they need to change their behaviors? Do they want to change their behaviors? Do they have the attributes of adult learners?
6.	What teaching methods have been tried before, and did not work? What reading material, lectures, web based instruction and resources did the instructor try before?
7.	Who are the instructors and what are they responsible for?
8.	What resources are available to the instructor? (think widely: include time, teaching materials, etc.)

1. Who are the learners? What are the learners responsible for? What level of performance is expected of them?

The level of performance expected from the learners varies according to their background. During the early phases of training, the learners are not expected to be experts. Therefore, it is important to define what is "good enough" for them to progress to the next step.

Given a novice learner, there is minimal expectation that the trainee will have a grasp of anything. Use safe simulation to allow novices to demonstrate what they already know, while clearly showing what they still need to learn. This will help to focus on their gaps in knowledge and skills.

Given mid-level learners, background and prior formal training raises expectations above those of a novice. As the mid-level learners are expected to take on greater patient care responsibilities than the novice, they have an even greater need to explicitly demonstrate their current range of competence and determine which behaviors need improvement.

Given an experienced clinician, continuing competence can be demonstrated in simulation, while new concepts and equipment can be introduced and practiced.

2. What do the learners "not get"? What is the performance gap between present behaviors and desired behaviors?

Students need to:

a. Demonstrating an understanding of the anatomy and names of structures, specifically the anatomy and movements of the spine and cranium on the spine (movements of the atlanto-occipital joint).

b. Demonstrating an understanding of the anatomy of the cervical vertebrae with emphasis on functional movements, what is meant by "flexion of the neck" and "extension at the atlanto-occipital joint" (as shown in Figure 5.) This is the instruction given to trainees to obtain a "sniffing position." (Adnet 2001)
c. Differentiate between the sniffing position and "neck extension" ("sword swallowing") position as shown in Figure 6. Multiple times a trainee simply places a blanket under the shoulders, causing extreme extension of the neck, and incorrectly calling this the sniffing position.

Figure 5. The figure shows the model's head on several blankets, producing flexion of the neck. Note that the tragus of the ear is at the level of the sternum. The head is also extended on the neck due to extension at the atlanto-occipital joint. This "sniffing" position produces a relatively straight line through the mouth, the hypo-pharynx and the trachea

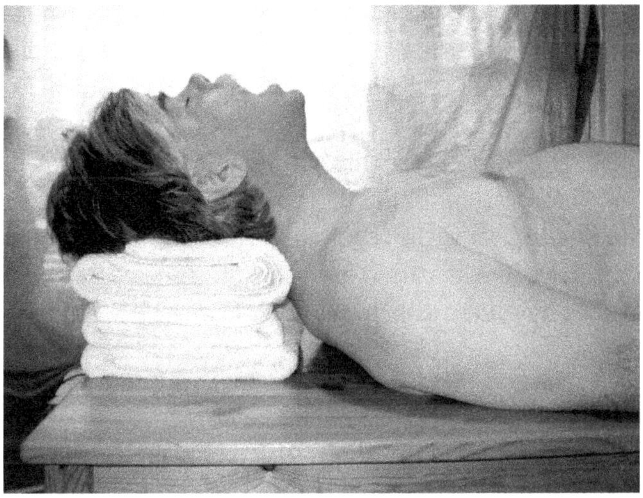

Figure 6. The figure shows the model with blankets under the shoulders, forcing the neck and head into an extremely hyperextended position. Note that the trachus of the ear is well below the level of the sternum

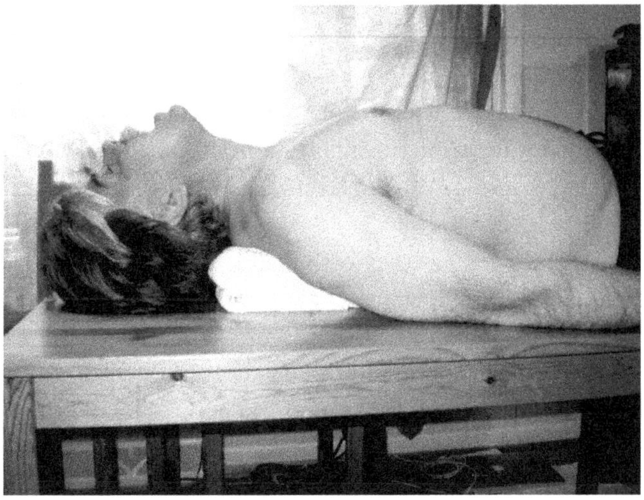

Instructors need to consider:

1. What does the instructor have to say over and over again, and still students exhibit the incorrect behaviors? Whatever the trainees just do not do correctly strongly suggests that the teaching methodology is in need of review and revision. For instance, the trainees do not seem to understand the changes in anatomy of the neck in the supine position caused by a 2-3 inch layer of obesity on the back of the patient: when supine, this "self padding" leads to severe neck extension, as well as extension at the atlanto-occipital joint. Trainees do not seem to take body habitus in consideration when positioning a patient for intubation.
2. How is the simulation instructor informed by the clinicians about what the trainees "do not get?"
3. This can be accomplished through surveys aimed at the correct steps in the procedures or observable practice of the learners prior to the simulated event.
    3. What domain(s) of knowledge (Knowledge, Skills, and/or Attitudes) is/are missing? It is important for the instructor to establish if the problems are due to a lack of Knowledge, due to a lack of Skills (including a lack of knowledge about the skills and/or the steps of the skills), or due to an incorrect Attitude: the trainee does not believe it is necessary to understand and implement position changes.
    4. What specific skills need to be taught differently and/or remedied? Is the failure due to a lack of knowledge of the steps of the procedure, or due to lack of eye-hand coordination? A discussion with the clinicians who reported the problems will help to elucidate these aspects.
    5. Do the trainees believe that they need to change their behaviors? Do they want to change their behaviors? Do they have the attributes of adult learners?

When the needs analysis indicates that the trainees believe their present skills are sufficient, it might be worthwhile to consider letting them experience the problem (e.g., with hyper-extension) in simulation. By experiencing a problem, the trainees realize what they do not know, which is one of the attributes of an "adult learner." For instance, they can be shown a simulated case, based on a real case of a morbidly obese patient on a flat X-ray table for cardiac catheterization under local anesthesia, now going into pulmonary edema and requiring urgent intubation, with no possibility to re-position the patient. The trainees will have great difficulty in intubating such a patient. The trainees can then be asked to suggest changes of the anatomical position which would make it easier to intubate. The trainees can then experience the improvement in their performance.

6. What teaching methods have been tried before, and did not work? Very often the answer to this question is "We tried either a lecture or an exhortation." The latter occurs while the trainee is trying to "get the tube in." But at that stage of high stress the learner is not listening or taking in anything. (Yerkes 1908)
7. Who are the instructors and what are they responsible for? The instructor should have the teaching knowledge, skills and attitude to be able to teach the anatomy. The teacher must be able to acknowledge that no one person can know everything, and there will be questions that a specific instructor cannot answer. This also provides an example to the trainee that it is acceptable to say: "I do not know, but I am willing to learn something new." This willingness to admit needing to learn is one of the first, and most crucial, steps towards becoming an adult learner. Teachers mod-

eling themselves as adult learners in front of their students is an excellent way to give the students permission to express their own need to learn.

8. What resources are available to the instructor? At this stage it is important to think widely, not only about the simulator that could be used, but also about the time available to the trainees as well as the instructors. Using didactic, factual teaching materials prior to the trainees coming to the simulation facility saves on the expensive time in the simulation center. To demonstrate all the issues that the trainees need to master necessitates a variety of teaching materials, as well as sufficient time to let the trainees work in small groups while experiencing effects of correct and incorrect anatomical positioning.
9. Correct and incorrect teaching points from the Analysis, related to the Sniffing Position

This section (sniffing position versus the sword swallowing position) demonstrates the results of an Analysis of Needs related to gaps in the understanding of anatomy that instructors have noticed. Better intubation training programs reveal, through the trainees' actions, the consequences (success or failure) of patient positioning, and instill correct application of their understanding of anatomy.

The training is mostly correctly presented: trainees are taught that the "sniffing" position consists of flexion of the lower cervical vertebrae and extension at the atlanto-occipital joint. Using an x-ray of the neck, as shown in Figure 7, in conjunction with a human model (Figure 5) helps to get the message across. However, the message is often incorrectly understood: most trainees remember this as "flexion of the neck, and extension of the head", others only seem to remember the "extension of the head" advice. The positioning of the head is therefore often sub-optimal.

McGill first described the position called "sniffing the early morning air." (McGill 1930). McGill described two anatomical components: cervical flexion and atlanto-occipital extension. (see Figure 5)

There are several classic training errors related to the flexion position: every trainee is able to recognize the correct answer from the choices in the multiple choice question (MCQ), and they can sometimes even re-state the remembered words. However, assessment of true understanding requires the trainee to demonstrate effective use of the concepts conveyed by the vocabulary.

Figure 7. The figure shows an x-ray of a model with blankets under the head to produce the correct "sniffing position." A normally curved breathing tube can readily be advanced down the trachea

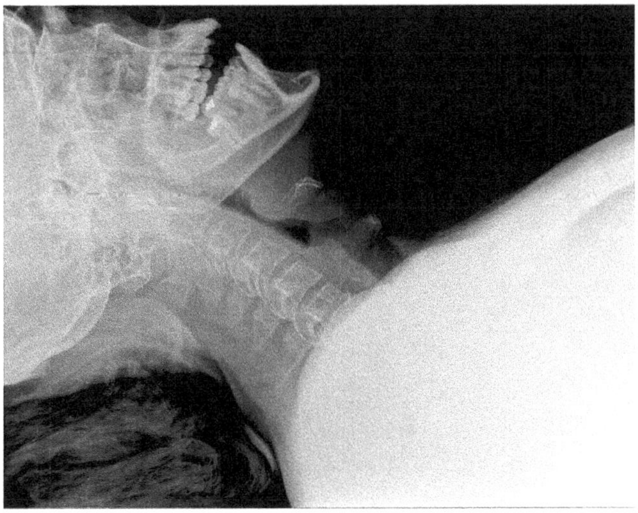

Without observable demonstration, there is:

- Neither true *"understanding" nor "application"* of the anatomy (in the sense of "higher levels of cognition" as described by Bloom (Bloom 1956)
- No valid assessment of their understanding

This lack of understanding is demonstrated by the following examples of trainees' classic actions that add to their patients' problems. For instance,

- They use a folded roll under the shoulders, forcing the neck and head into a severely extended position (Figure 8), compromising their ability to intubate, while they say that this is the sniffing position.
- They use a folded roll under the neck, again forcing the neck and head into a severely extended position, also calling this the "sniffing position".
- Another common scenario is that a morbidly obese patient is placed on the operating room table with a small pillow under the head because "everyone in our OR always gets a small pillow under the head". Due to the layer of obesity on the patient's upper back ("hump"), the head is still in a markedly extended position due to the patient's own internal pillow.
- The "ramp" position is a variation of the "sniffing" position. Several blankets are positioned such that the whole upper body is at a 30 degree angle. It has been described to make intubation in the morbidly obese patient easier, more successful, and give a better laryngoscopic view. The trainees diligently build up the ramp, but then they let the neck "hang" over the upper end of the ramp, again placing the head in a markedly extended position.

Figure 8. The figure shows an x-ray of a model with a roll under the shoulders forcing the neck into a severely extended position. The curved endotracheal tube will impinge on the anterior wall of the trachea and present an impediment to advancing the breathing tube down the trachea

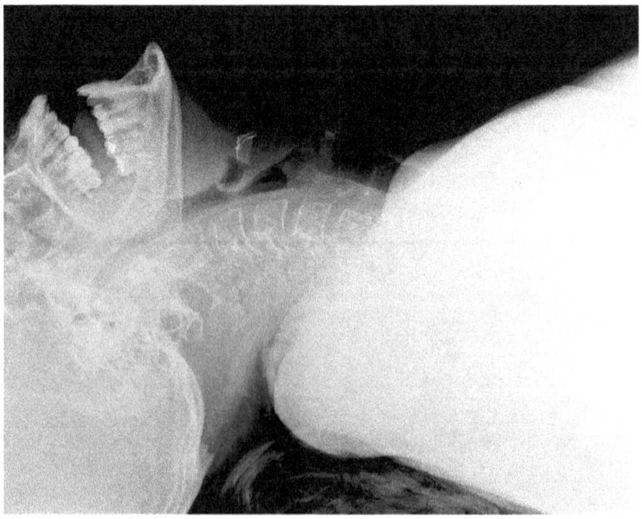

When students are seen to implement incorrect positioning, such mistakes indicate inadequate prior preparation, as well as the need for changing the students' current learning ways: for intubation, they just want to "get the tube in" and they do not want to be bothered with anything that delays this gratification. What they fail to understand is that it is all about the mind BEFORE the hand (as outlined in the new Bloom's 1995 cognitive errors in skills training.)(Anderson 2001) They must want to change their ways of performing the task, an attribute of an adult learner. To promote the desire to change behaviors, it is necessary to let the trainee experience the consequences of prior actions. In this case, poor anatomical positioning has the consequence of a difficult, or even failed intubation. This is followed by an opportunity to correctly position the mannequin which leads to an easy intubation. The trainee, in future cases, would be more likely to change behaviors, to continue to experience easy intubations.

Instructors' attempts to negate these errors have not had uniform success: To overcome this lack of understanding, various teaching methods and descriptions have been attempted. For instance:

- Instructors "demonstrate" the sniffing position to the trainees in the clinical milieu, just before the trainee is going to intubate. The stress on, and expectation for, the trainee is so much that learning does not occur. Loading all student training into the patient care environment does not work, as indicated by the common lack of understanding of the correct anatomical positions, as outlined above.
- A mental model has been published to try to generate understanding. The image is that of a winning athlete at the end of a 100 meter run "pushing out the chin to be the first to cross the line." Unfortunately, trainees remember the "winning" image as that of the athlete, after winning, throwing up the arms in the air, and looking towards the sky, which is a severely extended neck position.
- Some instructors have tried to use a contrasting image, to help the trainees understand when they are not in the correct position. The instructors verbally describe the "sword-swallowing position." In this position, an absolutely straight object, such as a sword, could pass through the mouth and straight down into the neck. This mental image might not be considered relevant to some trainees, possibly because the sword swallower places the sword into the esophagus, and the trainee is interested in the trachea.

Design: Anatomy of Positioning

The second step in the ADDIE process is that of Design. This can also be thought of as the planning of the learning session while sitting around a table. Included in the Design phase is the writing of the Learning Objectives. To be able to write the Learning Objectives, it is necessary to identify in which domain of knowledge the problem resides.

It is therefore necessary to classify each analyzed problem as a Knowledge, a Skill or an Attitude issue (Bloom1956), as each will require a different remedy. The knowledge problems will further have to be classified as to the level of knowledge that needs to be remedied. See Table 3 with Bloom's Taxonomy. One of the steps of Design is to write the Learning Objectives, which will be based on how far down the Bloom's Taxonomy the instructor has to go to fulfill the training needs of the trainee.

Table 3. provides a generic, universal description of Bloom's Taxonomy (Bloom 1956) followed by an application of the Bloom's Taxonomy for Anatomy of Positioning.

Table 4. describes the Bloom's Taxonomy as applicable to this section on anatomical aspects identified in the Needs Analysis.

Table 3. Description of Bloom's Taxonomy

GENERALIZABLE Description of Bloom's Taxonomy	
Bloom's Taxonomy	**The Trainee Will**
Knowledge (Head)	
Facts	Know the words and actions
Understanding	Appreciate how it all fits together; why it has to be done this way
Application	Be able to implement Understanding to manage the problem
Analysis	Identify, scrutinize and investigate the problem(s); break problem down into elements
Synthesis	Make several potential plans, i.e., "figure it out"
Comparison / Evaluation	Assess the various plans, and choose one, then evaluate the outcome of the selected plan compared to the desired outcome
Skills (Hands)	Be able to perform the task(s)
Attitudes (Heart)	Want to perform the tasks; Want to perform the tasks correctly and well

Table 4. Bloom's Taxonomy as it relates to patient positioning

Description of Bloom's Taxonomy Related to Positioning of the Patient Prior to Intubation	
Bloom's Taxonomy	**The Trainee Will Be Able To**
Knowledge	
Facts	List the anatomical names, the characteristics and movements of the neck, the orientations and maneuvers of the different approaches to sniffing and sword swallowing positioning
Understanding	Explain the differences in the approaches and conditions for using each position – e.g., why is it easier to intubate in the sniffing position
Application	Demonstrate proper arrangement of supporting towels and table height adjustment required for the different approaches
Analysis	Assess patient's anatomy and support equipment for suitability with the different approaches
Synthesis	Make several different action plans for implementing the different approaches with variations in anatomy
Comparison / Evaluation	Compare the relative merits of various approaches: decide on the one approach that is considered to be most beneficial for this patient; after completion of intubation, compare the actual outcome results with the expected results
Skills	Correctly orient and support patient's head and neck to obtain the sniffing position, as well as adjust table height as required for the different approaches
Attitudes	Accept that the presently used technique (by the trainee) is not the only way to provide the sniffing position – there might be other, or even better, techniques; Request placement of the patient in the optimal position for intubation; Communicate with the team members the need for the items used for orienting and supporting the patient's head and neck position as well as table height.

The least complex (simplest) level of Bloom's Taxonomy is the FACTS classification (see Table 3 and Table 4). The focus of Facts is for the trainees to have at least a minimal *knowledge base* to be able to perform the tasks. As simulation center time is expensive and limited, it is probably wise (efficient and economical) to have the trainees acquire this knowledge at their own pace, and using the learning modalities and learning styles most favored by each learner. A variety of learning modalities should therefore be available to the trainees.

The description of facts applicable to anatomy, as given in the table, is as follows: "know the materials, orientations and maneuvers of the different approaches to flexion and extension positioning." There are multiple methods better and more efficient than simulation to get the knowledge and facts across to the trainees. For instance:

- An important part of this exercise is to understand the anatomy of the neck. Homework to study such as anatomy references could be used, followed by a video of movements of the neck and head.
- A series of graphics can be used to demonstrate the extent of neck extension. The graphics can have pictures with various degrees of flexion and extension of the neck (e.g., looking down at the floor and up at the ceiling).
- A series of pictures and graphics can be used to demonstrate sufficient (correct) flexion of the neck and sufficient extension of the head at the atlanto-occipital joint.
- As mentioned before, it is also important to demonstrate the incorrect positions, e.g. insufficient flexion and extension, so that the trainee can recognize the errors.

The next level of Bloom's Taxonomy is the level of UNDERSTANDING. It is described in Table 4 as "describe the differences in the approaches and conditions for using each position (flexion and extension.)" The focus of Understanding is the *movement of the skeleton* (cervical vertebrae). There are two parts to Understanding: a theoretical understanding, and a hands-on understanding.

- The theoretical level of understanding can actually start prior to the simulation center experience – this saves valuable and expensive simulation time. For instance, this can be based on a series of pictures, x-rays and videos showing various degrees of head extension.
- As a part of the "homework" described above, the trainee has to demonstrate understanding by answering questions. For instance, estimate how many degrees of extension are represented in each of a series of pictures. Trainees also have to explicitly indicate if the extension is sufficient or not. A web-based program can be used to give feedback, provide a score, and document that the trainee did the prior learning exercises.
- Similarly, the trainees have to show understanding of the anatomy and relevant movements (specifically flexion) of the neck by answering questions based on another series of images and videos.
- An x-ray or MRI of the head and neck can be used to elucidate the very complex anatomy and movements of these structures
- The hands-on understanding involves the homework being reinforced in the simulation center: for instance, the trainees demonstrate flexion of the neck on a skeleton, and extension of the head at the atlanto-occipital joint – specifically to show too little, sufficient, and too much extension. The trainees can also demonstrate flexion and extension maneuvers on one another.

The next level of Bloom's Taxonomy is the level of APPLICATION. For the purposes of describing the process in this chapter, the levels of Understanding and Application are separated. However, in the practical implementation in the simulation center, Understanding and Application can flow seamlessly from one to the other. The focus of Application is the *resulting position* of the patient's head and neck.

- Demonstrate application of knowledge by a hands-on exercise: the trainee demonstrates to the instructor how to position a mannequin or another trainee. The trainee measures the height of the occiput from the bed, and also measures the degree of extension of the atlanto-occipital joint, by using a large protractor with degrees marked on it.
- The trainees can demonstrate on one another, to obtain more experience with a variety of anatomies.

The next level of Bloom's Taxonomy is the level of ANALYSIS. The focus of Analysis is *determining if the position is correct or not*, being able to describe why the position is correct or not, and finally, how to obtain a correct position in a patient with this anatomy.

- To train and demonstrate mastery of the Analysis step, the trainee can practice with a series of exercises of recognizing correct and incorrect positions in the simulation center.
- The trainee has to set-up the patient/mannequin as per the homework, both in correct and incorrect positions, and indicate (complete a questionnaire) why it is correct or incorrect.

The next level of Bloom's Taxonomy is the level of SYNTHESIS. Similar to Understanding and Application which flow into one another, Analysis and Synthesis typically flow into one another, and can be managed together. The focus of Synthesis is coming up with a *series of plans or steps* to remedy an incorrect position.

- A series of exercises of recognizing correct and improving incorrect positions in the simulation center should be performed.
- The trainee has to avoid changing a correct position, but demonstrate (or describe) a remedy for an incorrect position.

The highest level of Bloom's Taxonomy is the level of EVALUATION AND COMPARISON. The focus of Evaluation and comparison is *determining which is the best (optimal) plan of action.*

- Given a limited amount of extension of the head, the usual amount of flexion might be insufficient to place the head in a horizontal position needed for intubation.
- Given a patient with a potential neck injury, no neck movement is advised.
- In both these cases the trainee should come to the decision that the usual typical flexion position and intubation with a laryngoscope should not be attempted, but a different modality (e.g. flexible fiber-optic intubation) should be instituted.

As mentioned, ISD and ADDIE are repetitive, spiral processes. Now is the next time to go back to the Needs Analysis and determine if the needs are being covered. (Table 2)

As a part of the Design phase, Learning Objectives need to be created. Once the level of knowledge has been identified, the next step in Design is to write the Learning Objectives. Preferably, the Learning Objectives are written as *objective, observable behaviors*. One way to think about Learning Objectives is to say: "Show me ...." This forces the instructor to think about and write an observable behavior as a Learning Objective, i.e., something the trainee will be able to do.

For instance, after the training session, the trainee will be able to "*Show the Instructor how to*":

- Place supports for the patient's body, head and neck to obtain the correct orientation ("sniffing position")
- Adjust the table height as required for a typical intubation

Note that each of the levels of Knowledge in Bloom's Taxonomy in Table 4 has been written as an observable behavior, and each learning objective becomes a behavior to be assessed in the Evaluation phase of ADDIE. As a part of the design, failure modes and remedies are discussed. For instance, if the trainee fails to perform the task satisfactorily, the instructor determines at which of the Bloom's domains the failure seems to be. The instructor can then revisit that aspect of knowledge, skill or attitude and let the trainee practice at the appropriate level. Each Bloom's level also functions as a Learning Objective for the failure modes.

As noted, ADDIE is an iterative process. Therefore, the last item for Design is to circle back to the Analysis, and confirm that all the tasks addressed in the Analysis are actually in the Design, and also that all the items in the Analysis have been addressed.

Development: Anatomy of Positioning

As mentioned before, the planning that occurred in the Analysis and Design phases typically identify what needs to taught, what methods will be used to teach those skills, and how the skills will be evaluated. In the Development phase, the ideas generated in the Design phase are "brought to life" and tested prior to student participation.

In the Development phase, the instructor will produce all the relevant self-teaching materials (e.g. the videos and series of graphics mentioned in the Design phase), as well as collect all the hands-on skeletons, mannequins, OR tables, sheets and blankets for positioning the head and neck. The instructor will also evaluate and test the functionality of the teaching instruments, check that the timing for the exercise fits in the allotted time, etc.

Successful live theaters learned the hard way the value of spending the time and energy for technical rehearsals to reveal issues with equipment as well as dress rehearsals to reveal issues with participants. Successful simulation-based training programs borrow these same lessons learned, for the same reasons. The instructors walk through the whole session, from beginning to end, to check for a logical sequencing, completeness, and smooth functioning.

As mentioned before, the instructor needs to go back to Analysis and Design to ensure that all the issues are being covered.

Implementation: Anatomy of Positioning

In the implementation phase, the instructor will have a pilot group of trainees go through the exercise. This step should not be overlooked or skipped. This step will further test the educational offering and also provide feedback from the pilot trainees as to the efficacy and value the trainees attribute to the training.

For instance, the instructor will set up correct and incorrect head and neck positions. The trainees have to say whether it is good enough, thereby developing their clinical judgment. Such clinical judgement is refined ("honed") by making mistakes in simulation. For instance, the trainees can try to intubate mannequins which they have identified as "good enough" or "not good enough." They will fail to intubate in some "good enough" cases, and succeed in some "not good enough" cases. The purpose of the simulation exercise is to allow (enable) the trainees to make these mistakes in the simulation center, on a mannequin and under supervision, where immediate feedback can be given with re-training, and re-testing until meeting criteria.

The need for the trainee to adjust the bed height might be used as an assessment method for both the trainee and the facilitator. With the mannequin's head in an extreme extended position, the trainee has to have a line-of-sight which is horizontal. Either the bed height has to be adjusted higher, or the trainee has to go down on the knees to obtain the horizontal line of sight. The endo-tracheal tube will also be bent over the upper teeth in an attempt to reach the vocal cords. These position changes can be used to force the trainee to acknowledge that the position might not have been optimal, and lead to a change in behavior.

It has been noted multiple times in the clinical milieu that a trainee places a blanket under the shoulders, causing extreme extension, and calling this the sniffing position. The trainee does this after having observed such a practice by other clinicians. The trainee has to understand the fallacy of such a practice. Unless the trainee believes this to be an incorrect practice, the trainee will not alter any behavior, and the training exercise will have no effect. Hence the emphasis that is being placed on Understanding as well as objective assessment methods.

Learning from mistakes in simulation emphasizes that simulation is a *preparation* for clinical experience: it is NOT a replacement. Future studies will have to quantify the value of simulation and the amount of clinical transfer achievable.

The instructor will again go through Analysis, Design and Development, in the light of the feedback, and make changes as needed.

The instructor will perform the first formal teaching session, get feedback and make adjustments as before.

Evaluation: Anatomy of Positioning

In the Evaluation phase, the instructor will evaluate everything and everybody, including an evaluation of the instructors. The instructor will evaluate the success of the teaching and learning with observable, objective measures identified as Learning Objectives in the Design phase. For instance, measuring the height of the head above the bed is an indicator of neck flexion, and measuring the degrees of extension of the neck is a measure of the atlanto-occipital joint movement. Objective measurements also prevent the trainees from arguing with the instructor over what exactly "adequate" positioning is. Therefore, such objective measurements are preferable over the instructor saying: "In my opinion, this is adequate flexion."

The Evaluation needs to ensure that the trainees truly understand (and can demonstrate) the difference between the sniffing position and extension ("sword swallowing") position. Such true understanding can be tested by providing a different body habitus for the trainee to position. For instance, given an obese person with 2-3 inches (5-7 cm) of obesity on the posterior chest wall (simulated by blankets under the body (or chest) of a mannequin), the usual height ("small pillow") of the positioning the head will be insufficient, and the head will not be in the "sniffing" position. The trainee should recognize this incorrect position, analyze the problem, and synthesize a solution (i.e. place more folded blankets or sheets under the head.) The trainee should then evaluate the new position of the head, compared to the correct and incorrect positions encountered during the training.

The Evaluation should also include evaluating the instructors, the duration of the exercise, the applicability of the exercise to the trainees, the instructional materials, the mannequins, and the facility. This whole exercise will stand or fall by how well the Evaluation of the trainee is written by the instructors. Without a believable evaluation, there will not be any learning, defined as "a change in behaviors."

Second Worked Example of ADDIE: Teaching the Anatomical and Functional Relationships of the Epiglottis to the Vallecula

The anatomical and functional relationships of the epiglottis to the vallecula have specifically been chosen as an example of using ADDIE for several reasons (see below). This also demonstrates an instance where the lack of adequate simulation models may lead to erroneous instruction, resulting in poor habits and incomplete skills.

The glosso-epiglottic ligament, (Figure 4) which is situated in the vallecula. It is an important factor in prompt and atraumatic intubation, has been left out of most simulation intubation training programs. Its value is rarely discovered during subsequent teaching. Hence, correct understanding and use of the anatomical connections of the glosso-epiglottic ligament in the vallecula should be addressed in intubation training programs.

While there are physical simulation models demonstrating the epiglottis, there are no mannequins adequately demonstrating the existence or the *anatomy* of the glosso-epiglottic ligament (Figure 3). There are no models demonstrating the *movement* of the epiglottis when the tip of the laryngoscope blade encounters (and pulls on) the glosso-epiglottic ligament.

As there are no physical simulators exhibiting a glosso-epiglottic ligament, the training exercise as described in this chapter has to be built using mainly non-physical (e.g. graphics and Virtual Reality) materials. This enables the authors of this book chapter to demonstrate such "non-physical" materials under the ADDIE rubric.

A high fidelity mannequin with its "enclosed larynx", would also not be ideal as the sole teaching aid, as it would not be possible to observe the exact position of the tip of the laryngoscope blade, as is possible with the "open larynx" model (as shown in Figure 3) deliberately designed to reveal the airway, related structures, and their interactions during intubation manipulations.

Clinical experience with intubation, for most of the last century, has been based upon the use of a standard laryngoscope where only one person (instructor or trainee) can visualize the internal anatomy. The person not performing the intubation (instructor or trainee) has to guess what the other person is doing to the patient's airway during intubation. In the absence of a shared experience of what is actually happening to the patient while it is happening, what passes as formal expert-guided education, is in fact nothing more than *ad-hoc, consequence-based guessing* by teacher and student alike.

However, new technology, specifically the videolaryngoscope with a camera near the tip, makes it possible for the instructor and student to share in real time the unfolding events. Furthermore, recording and replaying of deliberately chosen examples of good and poor behaviors is possible for debriefing.

What are the normal steps of successful intubation?

The typical steps to successful intubation are outlined here to enable the reader to understand the concepts discussed in this section:

1. Using the right hand, open the mouth of the patient (various methods are available to accomplish this step)

2. Holding the laryngoscope in the left hand, insert the laryngoscope blade towards the right side of the mouth
3. Move the blade to sweep the tongue to the left (out of the way), while continuing to insert the blade and moving towards the midline of the airway
4. Identify the tip of the epiglottis
5. Position the blade tip towards the space between the epiglottis and the tongue, i.e., the vallecula (the space where the epiglottis and the tongue meet)
6. Move the tip of the laryngoscope blade into the vallecula
7. "Flip up" the epiglottis with the blade tip by pulling the laryngoscope handle 45 degrees upwards and towards the feet
8. Obtain an overall view of the glottic opening and vocal cords
9. With the right hand, insert the tip of the breathing tube through the vocal cords
10. Advance the breathing tube to the correct depth

Steps 6 and 7 are the steps we describe in this section. Note that in a typical description of intubation such as this, the glosso-epiglottic ligament is not mentioned at all, hence the need for application of ADDIE related to this subject.

Analysis: Vallecula Relationships

Analysis is the step of listing all the problems that the trainees have of "not getting it." It is the instructor's purpose to formally reveal how actions connect with consequences, hence the need for better instruction methods that help the instructor reveal those connections. Furthermore, this example shows how adding live video of the airway from the point of view of the intubation device being manipulated by the intubator reveals these connections to the trainee and instructor simultaneously.

This is an example of APPLIED ANATOMY. At this point in their academic progression, all the students can recognize and name the anatomical structure known as the epiglottis. However, the implications of knowing and understanding the movements of the epiglottis, and how it responds to forces by devices, is not that well known. Also, the existence of the glosso-epiglottic ligament (see Figure 4), and its role in hindering the movement of the tip of the blade to the midline, is not known to the majority of intubators who do not use videolaryngoscopy.

The next section takes the general statements above and applies the concepts in a more detailed list of a formal Needs Analysis, i.e. list the problems that intubators typically experience, and that should be remedied.

- The trainees do not manage to "flip up the epiglottis" correctly to reveal the glottic opening where they are to insert the breathing tube. Figure 9 shows adequate flip up clearly showing the vocal cords, while Figure 10 shows inadequate flip up – the vocal cords are not visible.
- The insertion of the tip of the laryngoscope blade might be too shallow, (see Figure 3 where the tip of the bade is not yet exactly in the vallecula) i.e. not deep enough, with the tip still on the tongue, and not positioned perfectly in the vallecula. There is then a tendency to lean back ("lever") the blade on the upper teeth to produce the "flip up."

- The insertion of the tip might be too deep, (Figure 11) thereby pushing the epiglottis into the glottic opening and blocking the view of the vocal cords, again with a tendency to lean back on the upper teeth to improve the view.
- The insertion of the tip might be too lateral, (see Figure 4) making the flip up much more difficult than it needs to be.
- The trainees get the blade tip hung up on the glosso-epiglottic ligament. (Figure 12)
- This ties back to the first point: if the trainee is in the midline, this ligament helps to flip up the epiglottis, whereas if the tip of the blade is too lateral, then epiglottis flip up is difficult.
- The trainees get the blade tip "hooked on" or "hung up" on the left or right side of the glosso-epiglottic ligament – the epiglottis is then tilted (Figure 12) to one side or the other, the epiglottis will also not "flip up" easily, and it is difficult to visualize the glottic opening.
- Many very experienced intubators have never even seen this ligament. Because they would typically insert the laryngoscope blade in the midline, they never noticed the glosso-epiglottic ligament, even in multiple decades of intubating with a standard laryngoscope. Only with the advent of the video-laryngoscope, and video recording of the intubation process, was this ligament noticed.
- Some trainees do not know or understand or apply their knowledge of the importance of the vallecula. Figure 13 shows a trainee where the tip of the laryngoscope blade is far to the left of the vallecula. The danger to the patient is that major complications may arise at this anatomical position. For instance, perforation of the wall of the pharynx. This trainee still manages to obtain a view of the glottic opening, even from this incorrect position. This specific trainee actually also manages to place the breathing tube through the vocal cords as shown in Figure 14. In prior years, with the instructor watching from the outside, this would have been accepted as an expeditious (33 second) and otherwise "successful" intubation. However, with the newer technology of videolaryngoscopy, the instructor is able to review the video and suggest remedial actions for this specific individual. Showing this video to other trainees also helps them to understand that "placing the breathing tube" is not the main objective. Performing a safe intubation is actually the goal.
- Many experienced intubators insert the laryngoscope in the midline "up to the hilt" and then withdraw the laryngoscope until the glottic opening comes into view. These experienced intubators have an "*intuitive feel*" for the anatomy of the upper airway: they have to insert the laryngoscope blade far enough posterior so that they deliberately enter the esophagus. However, if the tip of the blade is too far anterior, it might enter the glottic opening as shown in Figure 15. The laryngoscope blade is seen to impinge upon the vocal cords, potentially leading to swelling and airway obstruction.

Design: Vallecula Relationships

To demonstrate the anatomy and movements of the tip of the blade in relation to the glosso-epiglottic ligament, the Design phase will have to rely extensively on real life examples and videos (from novices through experts.): presently available physical simulator mannequins do not enable demonstration of many of these anatomical structures, movements and principles.

The first section from the Analysis phase included a lack of understanding exactly where the tip of the blade should be, how the enclosed larynx training contributes to this misunderstanding, and how it is critical to successful intubation to be precise in this placement. A part-task-trainer such as the open larynx (see Figure 3) can be used to let the trainee practice while directly observing how to place the tip

Figure 9. The figure shows adequate flip up of the epiglottis revealing clearly the vocal cords and glottic opening

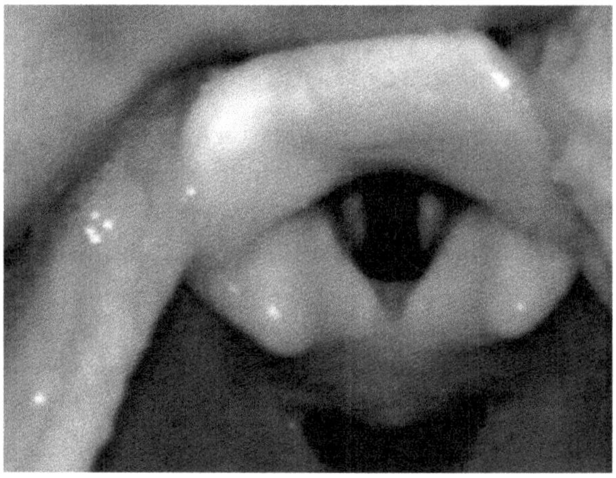

Figure 10. The figure shows inadequate flip up of the epiglottis and the vocal cords are not visible

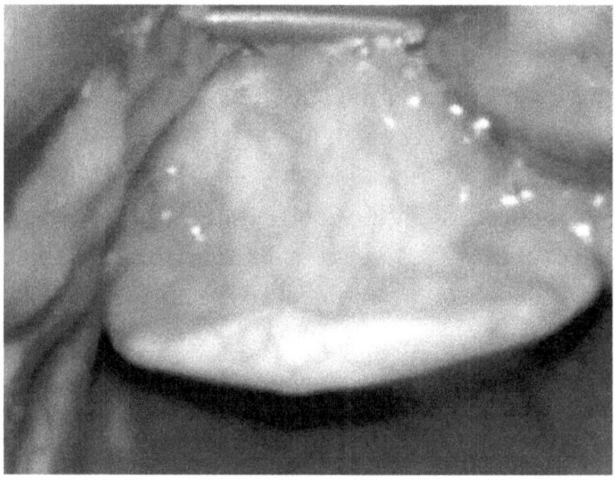

of the blade in the exact, correct position. This correct Knowledge and Understanding (from Bloom's taxonomy – see Table 3) can be reinforced with still pictures from human intubations using videolaryngoscopy. The Bloom's Analysis and Synthesis phases can be enhanced using a series of videos of successful and unsuccessful intubations where the video is frozen with the tip of the blade in the midline, but at various distances from the vallecula (e.g. too shallow or too deep.) The trainee has to predict if the "flip up" would be successful from this position or not. The Bloom's phase of Evaluation can then follow by continuing the video to reveal success or failure. By viewing multiple variants of human anatomy and multiple successful and unsuccessful placements, the trainees can add to their correct understanding through valid, risk-free "clinical experiences" prior to their first real clinical attempts.

The second section from the analysis phase was the Knowledge and Understanding (from Bloom's taxonomy) of the value of the glosso-epiglottic ligament in helping to flip up the epiglottis, and the problems of getting caught up with the ligament (a hindrance.) A series of still photographs can be used in an interactive fashion (as in the prior paragraph) to highlight the "help" and "hindrance" of the

Figure 11. The figure shows the tip of the blade of the laryngoscope has passed the vallecula, and is pushing down on the epiglottis, thereby obscuring the view of the glottic opening and the vocal cords

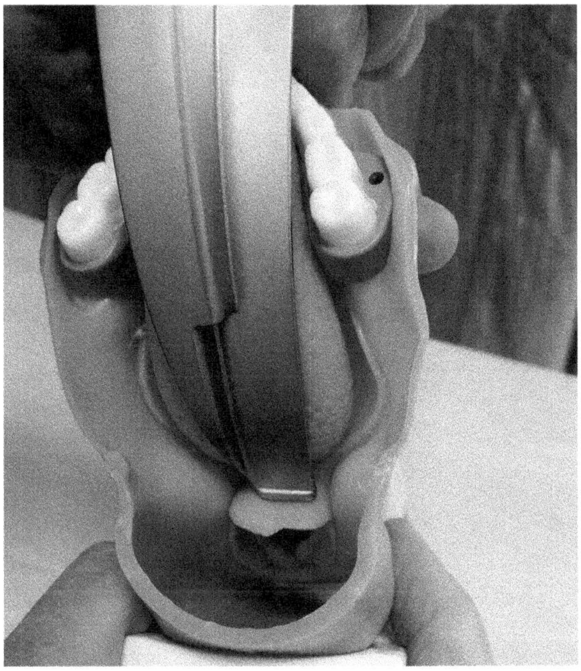

Figure 12. The figure shows the tip of the laryngoscope blade caught on the left side of the glosso-epiglottic ligament and, with movement of the tip of the blade towards the right, is causing the epiglottis to tilt, thereby obscuring the view of the vocal cords

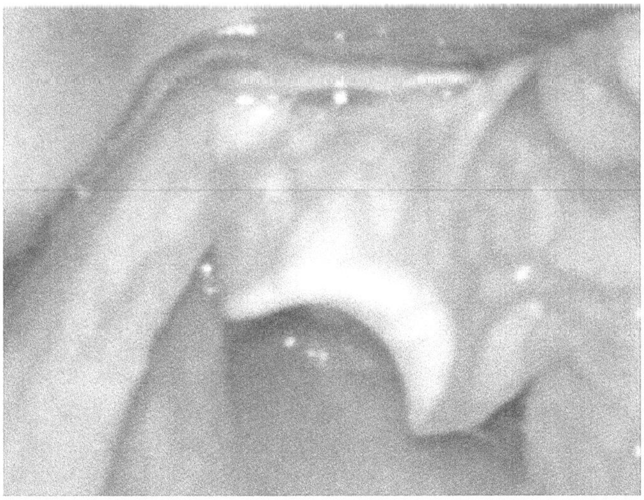

Figure 13. The figure shows a laryngoscopic view with the tip of the laryngoscope blade to the left of the glottic opening. The vallecula and other anatomic landmarks are not easily recognizable

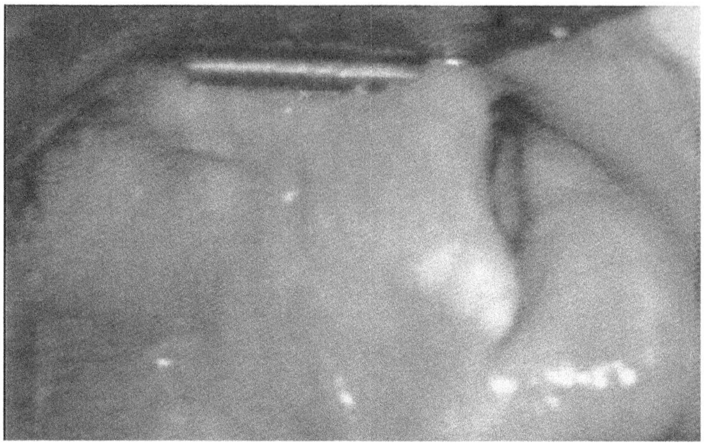

Figure 14. The figure shows an incorrect procedure (laryngoscope blade far to the left of the glottic opening), which still results in a successful intubation, as evidenced by the endotracheal tube seen passing through the vocal cords. This is an example of lack of application of the Understanding of anatomy

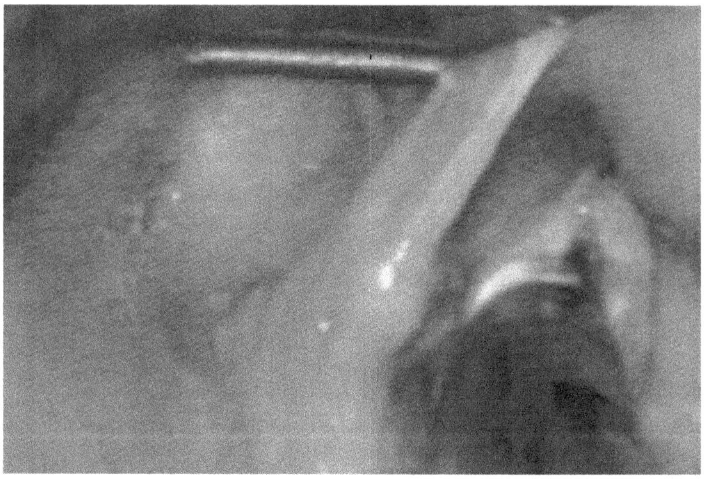

ligament. The Bloom's Analysis and Synthesis phases can be achieved using a series of videos of successful and unsuccessful intubations where the video is frozen with the tip of the blade in various lateral relationships to the vallecula. A position of the tip which is a short distance off the midline, with the epiglottis tilted at an angle (Figure 4) can still allow placement of the tube. However, placement of the tip that is too far lateral makes it quite difficult to "flip up" the epiglottis and prevents placement of the breathing tube in an expeditious and timely fashion. The Bloom's phase of Evaluation can then follow by continuing the video to demonstrate success or failure.

Figure 15. The figure shows an instance where the tip of the laryngoscope blade has passed the glottic opening and is now touching the vocal cords, with potential post-intubation edema, swelling and stridor

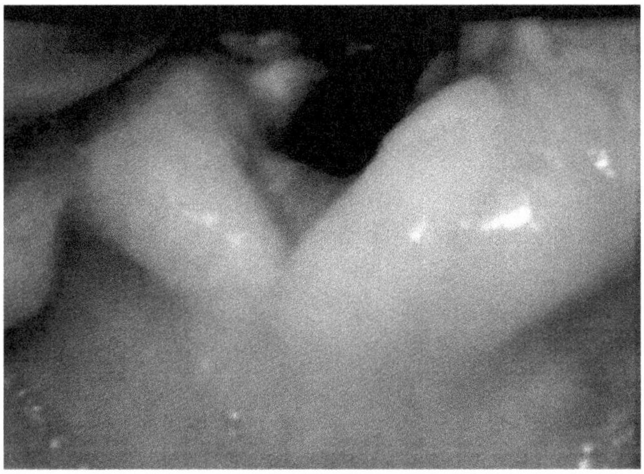

Development: Vallecula Relationships

The development of the teaching materials includes the use of the "open larynx" part task trainer (see Figure 3), as well as screen captures from videos of intubations in patients. For the purposes of demonstrating errors (too shallow and/or too deep) in the midline, a standard intubation head, as shown in Figure 1 could be used to generate video material. Using a videolaryngoscope, the trainee can also be asked to demonstrate the positions of too shallow and too deep, and experience how the "flip up" is adversely affected by incorrect positioning of the tip of the blade. The very stiff epiglottis in most presently available intubation mannequins, requiring quite a bit of force to manipulate, does not accurately respond to the typical blade tip "flip up" as experienced with the very flexible epiglottis in real patients.

Caught up laterally on the glosso-epiglottic ligament: (Figure 12) As mentioned, there are no physical simulators available today that include this anatomy, nor reproduce the movements of the epiglottis caused and prevented by this ligament. Therefore, the ligament training will have to be based mainly on photographic and video material from real patients.

In the Development phase of a formal curriculum, the photographic and video material is prepared for use by the instructor giving real time explanations. Once the instructor has determined the optimal format and extent of the explanations, the material can be further expanded with annotations (written and/or audio) for initial self-study (Implementation), and/or continued education by the trainees. This formal curriculum is in contrast to the trainee randomly picking through thousands of images and videos on the internet, where the lesson to be learned from the graphic is unclear, or mostly not even stated.

Implementation: Vallecula Relationships

As mentioned before, a significant part of this training can be completed by the students on their own prior to their instructor-directed simulation center experiences. The trainees will then have a solid basis for those lessons that are best learned through hands-on training. The trainees will be required to demonstrate correct and incorrect maneuvers on the open larynx, as well as on the intubation mannequin.

By using videolaryngoscopy while practicing on the intubation mannequin, the instructor will be able to observe the actions of the trainees in real time. As discussed in the Analysis, the trainees are given intubation sequences which can be "frozen" at a specific point for the trainee to analyze the position of the tip of the blade and then predict the likely success or failure when doing their next step.

Even with a mannequin, there is much stress experienced by the trainees during training, and they find it difficult to observe and absorb all the teaching points simultaneously. It has also been found to be useful to videotape the actions of the trainee while using the intubation mannequin for reviewing and debriefing purposes. By having the ability to replay and freeze the video, each separate teaching point can be addressed one at a time until the student performs "well enough" to progress to the next learning level.

Evaluation for Vallecula Relationships

As noted in the prior section, Evaluation includes "everything and everybody", rather than just evaluating the trainees. Considering evaluation of the change in behavior of the trainees, Evaluation of the placement of the tip of the laryngoscope blade is the main teaching point. The position of the tip of the blade can be phrased as objective measurements:

- The tip of the laryngoscope blade must be precisely positioned in the angle of the vallecula, defined as: the tip of the blade must not be no further than 3 mm (1/8th of an inch) either too shallow (proximal on the tongue), or too deep (pushing distally on the epiglottis).
- The tip of the laryngoscope blade must be exactly in the midline of the vallecula, defined as: the center of the tip of the blade must not be no further than 3 mm (1/8th of an inch) from the midline.

Having a video recording will be of value to make this determination. The size of the tip of the blade could be used as a known dimensional gauge appearing within the video camera image. The effect of being hung up on the lateral side of the glosso-epiglottic ligament can be evaluated by using videos from patients as in the prior section. The trainee has to predict if the flip-up would be successful given an image of the tip of the blade in a lateral relation to the ligament.

The instructor's responsibility is to keep trainees away from learning on patients until the trainees have been trained correctly as far as their simulators can take them. Ideally, the first time that any aspect of intubation is explained and experienced should not be in the clinical arena just before the patient is intubated. As mentioned, this intubation example was chosen to demonstrate ADDIE in an area where correct and complete simulators are not available. This demonstrates an important point: where the simulators are good enough, the instructor can confidently shift the risk of some of the training from patients to simulators. Where simulators are not good enough, the instructor's responsibility is to keep trainees away from practicing upon those incorrect features and thus instilling misunderstandings. Building instruction using the ADDIE principles will assist the instructors to fulfill this obligation.

CONCLUSION

ADDIE consists of a series of logical steps that can be used in the creation of a curriculum for a simulation session. While it might seem that the process is drawn out and labor intensive, it saves time in the long run due to the efficiency of learning.

By using this systematic way to "figure out" who the trainees are, and what they need, and addressing those needs during training, the measured outcomes can be expected to be improved. By having a plan for educational offerings based on ISD and ADDIE principles, many more changes in behaviors are expected to occur. Instituting ISD principles and using a process such as ADDIE will help trainees gain the most from their training sessions in simulation in preparation for their training in the clinical milieu.

REFERENCES

Adnet, F., Borron, S. W., Dumas, J. L., Lapostolle, F., Cupa, M., & Lapandry, C. (2001). Study of the "sniffing position" by magnetic resonance imaging. *The Journal of the American Society of Anesthesiologists*, *94*(1), 83–86. PMID:11135726

Almomen, R. K., Kaufman, D., Alotaibi, H., Al-Rowais, N. A., Albeik, M., & Albattal, S. M. (2016). Applying the ADDIE—Analysis, Design, Development, Implementation and Evaluation—Instructional Design Model to Continuing Professional Development for Primary Care Physicians in Saudi Arabia. *International Journal of Clinical Medicine*, *7*(08), 538–546. doi:10.4236/ijcm.2016.78059

Anderson, L. W., Krathwohl, D. R., & Bloom, B. S. (2001). *A taxonomy for learning, teaching, and assessing: A revision of Bloom's taxonomy of educational objectives*. Allyn & Bacon.

Benumof, J. L. (2006). Corniculate cartilages are wrongly labeled arytenoid cartilages. *The Journal of the American Society of Anesthesiologists*, *104*(2), 377–377. PMID:16436864

Bloom, B. S. (1956). *Taxonomy of educational objectives: The classification of educational goals. Cognitive domain*. New York: David McKay.

Causer, J., Barach, P., & Williams, A. M. (2014). Expertise in medicine: Using the expert performance approach to improve simulation training. *Medical Education*, *48*(2), 115–123. doi:10.1111/medu.12306 PMID:24528394

Cormack, R. S., & Lehane, J. (1984). Difficult tracheal intubation in obstetrics. *Anaesthesia*, *39*(11), 1105–1111. doi:10.1111/j.1365-2044.1984.tb08932.x PMID:6507827

Dent, J., & Harden, R. M. (2013). *A practical guide for medical teachers*. London: Elsevier Health Sciences.

Dick, W., Carey, L., & Carey, J. (2009) The Systemic Design of Instruction (8th ed.). Boston, MA: Pearson e-text.

Khalil, M. K., & Elkhider, I. A. (2016). Applying learning theories and instructional design models for effective instruction. *Advances in Physiology Education*, *40*(2), 147–156. doi:10.1152/advan.00138.2015 PMID:27068989

Knill, R. L. (1993). Difficult laryngoscopy made easy with a BURP. *Canadian Journal of Anaesthesia*, *40*(3), 279–282. doi:10.1007/BF03037041 PMID:8467551

Kohn, L. T., Corrigan, J. M., & Donaldson, M. S. (2002). *To err is human: building a safer health system*. Washington, DC: National Academy Press.

Kolb, A. Y., & Kolb, D. A. (2012). Experiential learning theory. In *Encyclopedia of the Sciences of Learning*. New York, NY: Springer.

Leppink, J., & van den Heuvel, A. (2015). The evolution of cognitive load theory and its application to medical education. *Perspectives on Medical Education, 4*(3), 119-127.

Magill, I. W. (1931). Technique in Endotracheal Anesthesia. *Anesthesia and Analgesia, 10*(4), 164–168.

Mallampati, S. R., Gatt, S. P., Gugino, L. D., Desai, S. P., Waraksa, B., Freiberger, D., & Liu, P. L. (1985). A clinical sign to predict difficult tracheal intubation; a prospective study. *Canadian Anaesthetists Society Journal, 32*(4), 429–434. doi:10.1007/BF03011357 PMID:4027773

Steinert, Y., Mann, K., Centeno, A., Dolmans, D., Spencer, J., Gelula, M., & Prideaux, D. (2006). A systematic review of faculty development initiatives designed to improve teaching effectiveness in medical education: BEME Guide No. 8. *Medical Teacher, 28*(6), 497–526. doi:10.1080/01421590600902976 PMID:17074699

Yerkes, R. M., & Dodson, J. D. (1908). The relation of strength of stimulus to rapidity of habit-formation. *The Journal of Comparative Neurology and Psychology, 18*(5), 459–482. doi:10.1002/cne.920180503

KEY TERMS AND DEFINITIONS

Atlanto-Occipital Extension: The highest cervical vertebra (C1) articulates with the base of the skull enabling extension (looking up at the sky).

Epiglottis: A flexible cartilage situated at the base of the tongue, just above the glottic opening, thereby preventing food from entering the trachea, but also preventing visualization of the vocal cords.

Intubation: The process of placing an endotracheal tube ("breathing tube") through the vocal cords and into the lungs to enable assisted ventilation.

Laryngoscope: A device placed in the upper airway that enables visualization of the glottic opening and vocal cords during intubation.

Sniffing Position: By placing the patient's head on a pillow, the lower cervical vertebrae are flexed, and the upper vertebrae are extended. The sniffing position improves the ability to perform intubation, and requires less force.

Vallecula: The area where the base of the tongue and the epiglottis come together. The tip of the blade of the laryngoscope is placed in this area to be able to flip up the epiglottis to visualize the vocal cords.

Videolaryngoscope: A laryngoscope with a digital camera near the tip of the blade improving the view of the vocal cords. A video screen enables an indirect view of the vocal cords visible to the trainee as well as to the instructor.

ENDNOTE

1 All human images are used with informed consent by the subject, or with ethical approval of the use of anonymized videolaryngoscopic images for teaching purposes.

Chapter 6
The Nurse Educator's Role in Designing Instruction and Instructional Strategies for Academic and Clinical Settings

Patricia J. Slagter van Tryon
East Carolina University, USA

ABSTRACT

Nursing education programs seeking to equip graduates with needed tools to integrate medical expertise with experience in the systematic design of instruction have the opportunity to better ensure positive learning outcomes in varied settings as graduates take on their new roles as nurse educators. The learning environment of the nurse educator is complex yet with skill in the reasoned approach to the design of instruction can progress into more knowable contexts for which to problem solve. Nurse educators possessing interdisciplinary skills in their field facilitated by expertise in instructional design will enhance their practice by developing and delivering precision instruction.

INTRODUCTION

Nurse educators are guided in their practice by the Core Competencies of Nurse Educators proposed by the National League for Nursing (NLN) (National League for Nursing, 2005). Within the core competencies, nurse educators are called to "Participate in Curriculum Design and Evaluation of Program Outcomes" (National League for Nursing, 2005). However, even the most exhaustive examination of university based Master's degree programs in Nursing Education will return little reference to coursework for learners in content or theory in the systematic design, development and evaluation of instruction. While many nurse educator programs include course work in curriculum development, it is important to note that curriculum development is not synonymous with instructional design.

The design of instruction is a systematic approach to the development of instruction and instructional materials focused on solving educational problems where a reasoned assessment of the need for

DOI: 10.4018/978-1-5225-2098-6.ch006

Copyright © 2017, IGI Global. Copying or distributing in print or electronic forms without written permission of IGI Global is prohibited.

the instruction is determined up front and the evaluation of the instruction is precisely aligned with the assessment of learning outcomes identified prior to the delivery of instruction. In addition, instructional design is deeply embedded within learning theory and as such, assessing the characteristics of the target learner audience becomes a key facet of the instructional design process such that instruction is relevant and immediately applicable (Dick, Carey & Carey, 2015). Curriculum development is content-based development outside of the learning environment and while high quality curriculum development will often be readily aligned with standards and inclusive of evaluation methods, curriculum development is not a systematic process in addressing the full scope of an educational problem at hand. To support nurse educators in their design efforts, this chapter aligns a brief yet concise guide for an integration of principles from the field of instructional design to scaffold the core competencies for nurse educators in the realm of curriculum development.

BACKGROUND

In considering that a consistently reported mission of Master's degree programs in Nursing Education is to prepare its graduates for the role of nurse educator in a highly dynamic academic setting as well as in complex clinical settings, it may be efficacious to move a step beyond the linear curriculum development model that many programs maintain as a core element in informing the nurse educator's practice. Further, and specific to the mission in nurse educator programs, precision in the design of instruction may serve to support confidence in addressing emergent technologies that require a skilled approach in practice, support effective communication in assessment, and help to develop highly efficient problem solving skills in a demanding interdependent work environment. Each of these areas offer support in leadership as nurses gain needed confidence in areas where they may be called upon to lead however potentially feel unprepared to do so (Ashton, 2012).

A deeper understanding of the instructional process and the environment for which the learning takes place mirrors the reasoned decision process nurses must engage in consistently and efficiently each day of their practice. Without focused skill building in a reasoned approach to the design and delivery of instruction, nursing education programs may fall short of their goal of equipping future nurse educators with the needed tools to integrate their medical expertise with experience in high quality design of instruction that might better ensure positive learning outcomes for their own learners in the varied settings in which they will teach.

In an assessment of the state of the practice by nurse educators in the instructional design process, Krouse (2015) noted that adherence to design principles is often lacking and in order to better prepare future nurse educators, programs in nursing education should not only be collaborating with instructional designers but should consider the challenge of designing instruction themselves. As more and more nurse educator programs are being offered online, nurses are looking to resources for both the design of instruction and successful practices for delivering instruction online once completed. Nurse educators are therefore faced with a twofold demand of their time and resources in first expanding the depth and breadth of their approach to the development of instruction for their courses and programs but also taking that new approach into the online learning environment. Oftentimes nurse educators have not been offered concentrated training in either realm even though consistently pressed upon to write this type of innovative and relevant curriculum for their programs (Egerton, McConnell, Corazzini, Kitzmiller, & Crook, 2010). These researchers further note that indeed demands for this quality instruction then to be delivered online is becoming the norm. Johnson (2008) noted that in addition to being asked to maintain curriculum aligned current standards, and thrust into new learning environment of the online learning world, few resources are even allocated toward making the transition.

The benefits of reasoned design and development of instruction abound. Intense focus on the design process maintains relevance for learners (see Driscoll, 2005), drives close alignment of learning objectives to assessment of learning (Mayer, 2011), works to ensure that the instruction proposed is specifically aligned with the educational need (see Smith, & Ragan, 2004), and results in reliable and precision process in decision points for achieving positive learning outcomes (see Hannafin, Hannafin, Land, & Oliver, 1997). A focused approach therefore such as collected in this current volume for medical professionals, supports real time and just in time content, theory, and strategies for designing effective instruction for the medical field specifically.

This chapter will focus on principles in instructional design that might be implemented in the instruction delivered in nursing education programs and that learners in these programs may immediately apply as they begin to design their own instruction in their new roles as nurse educators. In essence the work addresses constructs for the nurse educator to teach the process of instructional design to future nurse educators to offer support in their own development of instruction in the environments in which they will teach. While this chapter points to design strategies for instruction delivered in the online learning environment and through a learning management system, all principles and strategies proposed here are transferrable and appropriate for face-to-face and blended learning environments alike.

The Design Process in Assessing Need

The instructional design process begins as an educational problem arises. At this time it is necessary to critically examine the focus of the problem and the desired change expected as result of a proposed solution to the problem. This critical examination supports the design of instruction in ensuring alignment with desired outcomes in performance and takes place through determining goals, assessing need, and recognizing the learner and learning context for which the solution is to take place. Further, determining preliminary goals for successful educational outcomes is a priority in the design and development of quality instruction and a key component of the iterative process of the aforementioned assessment of need. In essence, this time is reserved for the nurse educator to envision the overall big picture of what is to be accomplished in instruction. As nurse educators begin in this way to solve educational problems in their varied work environments, they no doubt experience varied avenues from which a multitude of educational problems have arrived in their programs of instruction. For example, increasingly nurse educators have been faced with a need to deliver nursing education at a distance and as such have been called upon to prepare goals for successful transition from the face-to-face mode of teaching to the online mode of teaching in their practice regardless of prior experience. Potential needs for instruction in addressing educational problems can be presented in many forms and precise clarity in the need for instruction, through close examination of the indicators within the system, is a key facet of a successful instructional design process.

Rossett (1995) details the rationale in design for determining needs in educational problems and points to three avenues or initiators of impending need, 1) Performance Problems, 2) New Stuff, and 3) Mandates. For nurse educators in many cases a mandate is present in meeting nursing program requirements and curriculum is developed as a result of this mandate. Beyond curriculum and program mandates, need presented as "New Stuff" often carries with it an urgency to become up to date and proficient in a limited amount of time. The accelerated growth in technologies for example available to support healthcare professionals has had a staggering effect on need for training. Patient health portals and digital patient record systems alone have required countless hours of training for the healthcare professional. Need presented as "Performance Problems" in clinical or academic work environments are often recognized when student/staff evaluation scores are below a set benchmark. The ongoing analysis of performance in nursing care in clinical situations is one such area garnering resources as health care institutions' reviews are heavily reliant on patient reports of satisfaction with the institution overall. Regardless of the means by which an educational problem is presented, further examining and analyzing need is a priority in the design of high quality instruction in successfully solving educational problems. It is always possible that after closely examining the problem however that some other form of intervention is determined as opposed to instruction and it will be the detailed assessment of need that will initiate the decision making process here.

It is important that nurse educator programs, and the nursing instructors in charge of their delivery, consider all initiators of need for instruction that future nurse educators may face in their own academic or clinical learning environment. How does one begin to examine need more closely? It is important to seek out those individuals involved in the educational problem, such stakeholders as the administrators, educators, families, and student learners (Brown & Green, 2016). Time must be allocated to determine who holds any data and materials/resources to support examination efforts as well as planning for collecting those evidences in further determining need. In total, evidences can successfully be collected in the following ways as access permits:

- Interviewing.
- Observing performance.
- Examining prior records.
- Conducting group discussions.
- Surveying.

Each of the above will support identifying and analyzing the problem by collecting data and perceptions of those involved in the problem to be addressed (see Brown & Green, 2016). Clear articulation of the problem will lend itself to the organization of the instructional tasks that learners will move through in order to meet the goals set for instruction. Goals include articulation of the skills and competencies required of learners and tasks include the stages of development learners must advance through to meet the goals.

Assessing Tasks of Instruction

While often times little attention is given in curriculum development to the analysis of tasks in instruction, it is a valuable and revealing process that allows a critical eye on the precise skills and competencies expected of learners. Determining the skills needed to achieve the learning that results from the needs assessment supports the development of both the structure of the instructional materials as well as the development of learning objectives to address the specific learner skills and characteristics. A myriad of approaches exist in the literature to initiate the process of assessing and analyzing tasks in instruction and perhaps an approach such as the procedural analysis (see Dick, Carey, & Carey, 2015, Morrison, 2006, Shepard, 2000) where both cognitive and psychomotor skills can be mapped out in steps is most readily applicable here. For example, consider each step that would be required of a posted procedure for dressing a simple wound. The procedure may begin with washing hands, procuring materials for dressing, washing the wound, applying antiseptic, then bandaging the wound however this procedure may have additional decision points if the wound has not stopped bleeding, or if the wound is determined to need further medical attention. Visualizing the tasks required through flowcharts offers a view into the precise advancement through pre-defined procedures. The figure below (see Figure 1) represents the simple example of dressing a simple wound. The process of detailing tasks in this way is indeed time consuming however even minor efforts in this facet of the development of instruction will allow for identifying gaps in narratives in instruction for learners such that the content and skill requirements are clear and attainable for learners.

Figure 1. simple task flowchart

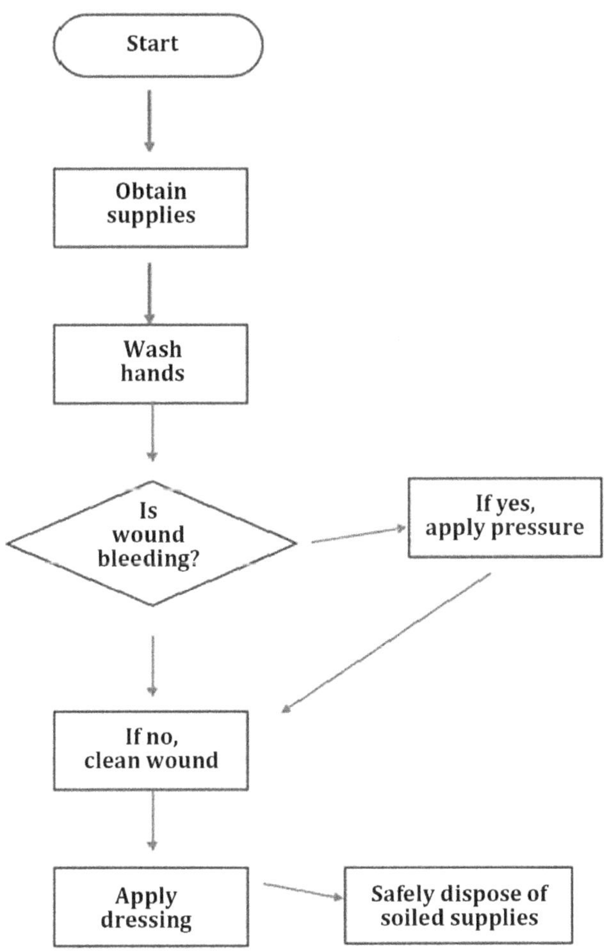

Assessing Learner Characteristics and Skills

Assessing the learner is founded on the theory that learners have varied skills and perspectives and as such recall, process, and construct, information in different ways while learning. Learning theory is foundational to the design process and in particular the assessment of learners. Instruction that is not geared toward the learner and supported by varied opportunities for learners to experience the learning at hand will do little to support the learner in achieving academic goals. Knowing learner characteristics is therefore perhaps the most critical facet of the design of instruction. Assessing learner characteristics will inform instructional strategies in the design while assessing learner prerequisite skills will address the sequence of instructional tasks as noted above. In order to know the learner and therefore have the background needed to develop relevant instruction, certain and specific data is needed about learners' skills and readiness for the learning task. Conducting an assessment of the learner can take many forms however a common method of data collection both in online learning environments as well as face to face learning environments is through a survey methodology. The data sought in the assessment of learners is also varied however generally, demographic data, entry level skills data, motivation, attitudes, and ability data are commonly desired (see Dick, Carey, & Carey, 2015). Focusing resources in knowing learners preferences for learning situations will support integration of strategies that align with the varied learning situations afforded through activities designed with varied learning theories in mind. a brief account is presented below of generally considered common theories that are referred to in the literature and that are foundational here.

Behaviorist Learning Theory

Most prevalent in the literature is the work of B. F. Skinner in operant conditioning. According to Skinner, learners have control over their responses as they learn and it is the consequences of past actions that can direct future actions of the learner. Benjamin Bloom later incorporated Skinner's behaviorist principles in his mastery learning approach by offering a sequence that the learner would ultimately move through in order to demonstrate mastery over a particular concept. In the typical Bloom's Taxonomy (Bloom, 1956) as it is referred to, the learner would move through six levels of complexity beginning with Knowledge, then Comprehension, then Application, then Analysis, then Synthesis, and finally Evaluation. There has been a move to a more 21st Century version of Bloom's Taxonomy that begins with Remembering, then Understanding, then Applying, then Analyzing, then Evaluating, then Creating. Much of the system of behavioral and performance objectives today are based in behaviorist principles.

Cognitivist Learning Theory

As what is considered a natural development beyond Behaviorist principles, the notion of information processing theories began to appear and most notably the Cognitivist learning theory. The Cognitivist theorists point to processes within the brain as information is received by the learner, considered cognitively, then stored for later use. This is sometimes compared to computer processing. Much of the information processing theory is based on the work of Atkinson and Shiffrin (1968) who proposed three types of memory, the sensory that takes in the information, the short-term memory or working memory, and the long-term memory that will retain any information that is encoded in the brain beyond the short-term memory for later use. The premise being that in order for long-term memory to retain information, there must be a certain level of processing and encoding that the brain accomplishes in order to retain the information and hence the learning. Linking new information to information already known by the learner is the general approach to incorporating the cognitive learning theory into the design of instruction.

Constructivist Learning Theory

Constructivist learning is built on the premise that the learner must build or construct his or her own learning by connecting information and making new meaning for him or herself (Jonassen, 1999). Constructivist principles include the social and environmental interactions beyond the information processing. Constructivist learning principles are based on a combination of concepts therefore within social learning. Many scholars include the work of Howard Gardner (1999) in his theory of multiple intelligences under the umbrella of Constructivist Learning Theory though equally as many scholars will contend that the Theory of Multiple Intelligences stands alone as its own significant learning theory. Learners are challenged in learning with a Constructivist approach as learners are presented with real world problems to work through that result in the application of new knowledge, built or constructed by the learner, to the problem at hand. It requires a level of integration and negotiation of the meaning with the world around the learner and in the social approach, the people within it.

While there does exist a more extensive list of learning theories in support of the design of instruction, incorporating the above theories into the design of learning strategies in response to data from the learner analysis will give greater support to the specific learners present at that given assessment. A learner analysis even if abbreviated should accompany all design of instruction to ensure that the design is appropriate for the learner in meeting learning goals.

Forming Objectives and Aligning Assessment

The development of assessments of learning must be closely aligned with stated objectives of the instruction. A disconnect between the objectives and the measure of outcomes renders the design weak and ineffective. Objectives inform the learner of specific competencies to be gained as a result of the instruction. Objectives should be written for achieving the required tasks as well as to supplement the tasks where needed through any prerequisite skills identified within the learner analysis. Learners must be made aware of each task and each objective to successfully move through the instruction. Likewise, learners must be aware of the means of assessment to measure their competency and performance related to stated objectives.

Visible alignment of the objectives with the assessment should be made available to learners prior to the delivery of instruction. While this does not mean revealing written test items, it does mean ensuring that test items are designed to specifically assess competencies stated in the objectives. Content not addressed in instruction would not have relative objectives and therefore would not be included in the assessment. In either learning environment, online, face to face, or blended, learning objectives are an initial starting point in the introduction to in instruction in which learners will encounter. Smaldino, Lowther & Russell, (2008) detail a method for the development of learning objectives in that each should include an identification of the learner or audience such as, *the LPN (licensed practical nurse) student,* followed by a specific statement of the behavior expected such as, *will be able to conduct an infection control inspection,* followed by a statement of the condition for which the learning will take place such as, *given the infection control checklist and clinical room assignment,* followed by the expected degree to which the performance must be completed such as, *with 100% accuracy.* Combined the statement would read, *LPN (licensed practical nurse) student will be able to conduct an infection control inspection, given the infection control checklist and a clinical room assignment with 100% accuracy.* When learning objectives are inclusive of the audience, behavior, conditions, and degree of accuracy, learners are supported in having specific statements pointing to what is to be learned and what is expected in performance.

In the nurse educator's instructional design course syllabus, it is equally important to include the objectives of the instruction as it is to include the means of assessment. Because feedback is critical to the development of the critical skill sets nurses must achieve (Bruno & Santos, 2010) scheduled feedback should also accompany the course schedule of assignments usually found within the syllabus. Giving learners a starting point within their course management system to directly view objectives sets a path for clear understanding of expectations. Similarly, planned measures of learner performance should be clearly visible at the start of instruction as well to notify learners of the type and frequency of assessments to expect in during instruction. If arrangements might be made in advance for a proctored assessment for online learners at a cooperating institution or facility to ensure guidelines of the administration of the assessment are adhered to, this information is pertinent for learners as well. Well-reasoned design of instruction leaves no room for confusion on expectations on the learner's part.

Instructional Strategies and Maintaining the Social Context

Instructional strategies should be designed alongside data collected from the assessment of the learner characteristics and skills. Instructional strategies for nurse educators should consist of a reasoned approach to reaching the learner through interaction and activity that requires participation and engagement, presents models, simulations, and demonstrations, and incorporates interim assessment. Each of these approaches in instructional strategies is linked through relevance for the learner supported through engagement with the content that is guided with frequent instructor/student and student/student interaction. When the content delivery is through an online learning environment, additional attention to the communication system within the environment further supports reaching learners regardless of the particular instructional strategy at hand. Setting up the learning management system to present content for learners should become a seamless navigation for learners through a course structure that is modular in form and is clearly marked with where to begin first. Setting up the course navigation in this way will support the knowable context needed for learners to engage with the content and with each other. Therefore, it is important for nurse educators to consider that computer mediated communications in online learning environments are often lacking in the subtle social cues learners rely on when communicating as they do when learning face to face (Slagter van Tryon & Bishop, 2006).

Social cues act as signals in the instructional communication system, and while they are relatively effortless to relay face-to-face, they become more difficult for learners to perceive online where spatio-temporal proximity is altered. Just as in face-to-face delivery of instruction, there are benefits in extended learner interactions and collaboration promoting successes in learning that reveal the social context while online is key in successful learning experiences as well (Biocca, Harms, & Burgoon, 2003; Kreijns, Kirschner, Jochems, & van Buuren, 2004). Yet, the extent to which learners in the online learning environment are able to overcome the oftentimes challenging mediated environment, and perceive themselves as socially connected to their peers, is not easy to achieve. Strategies for initiating and maintaining social connectedness online should be employed at the start of the instruction/course and must not wane as the instruction progresses. Nurse educators in online courses may need intentional facilitation of social cues to initiate and maintain the same development of academic social interactions online as are often experienced face-to-face from the first encounter to the last (see Pate, Smaldino, Mayall, & Luetkehans, 2009). Strategies for engagement can be as general as communicating expectations (Paul & Cochran, 2013) or more complex as within the expectations of highly structured group projects with high stakes outcomes (Chiong & Jovanovic, 2012). As a result, nurse educators that take a reasoned approach to initiating and maintaining the social context of the learning environment offer a heightened level of support for successful collaboration for the duration of the instruction.

The author has designed and developed an instrument entitled the "Social Perceptions in Learning Contexts Instrument (SPLCI)" (Slagter van Tryon & Bishop, 2012) a research tool for measuring social connectedness that is included at the close of this chapter (Appendix 1). Employing this tool to assess levels of perception of social connectedness is just one strategy for examining efforts in engaging students with each other while learning. The SPLCI is based on the "*E-mmediacy*" framework (Slagter van Tryon & Bishop, 2006) defined as feelings of social connectedness one has with fellow online participants (classmates, instructor, teaching assistant) through technology-mediated experiences that simulate episodic perception of immediacy. To support the developing social structure among learners, the following E-mmediacy guidelines can be followed to overcome barriers in the instructional communication system in order to achieve increased opportunity for relevance through social connections see (Table 1).

Ongoing Evaluation of the Design

Evaluation of the instruction itself, of the design and delivery, should take place continually to assess areas of opportunity for improvement. High quality instructional design becomes so because it is consistently revisited, revised and improved. Conducting this formative type of evaluation (see Dick, Carey & Carey, 2015) informs the design and this process has been known to take many forms. The research instrument, the SPLCI, noted above is one such tool for ongoing assessment of a particular facet of the

Table 1. E-mmediacy Guidelines Framework

	Increased Interactions	Comprehensive Technical Support	Persistent Follow Up
Status assessments	1. facilitate your students' status assessments by designing interactions that allow learners to observe individualizing social characteristics	2. facilitate your students' status assessments by providing the support needed to overcome technical barriers to perceiving individualizing social characteristics	3. Facilitate your students' status assessments by requiring ongoing interactions that help learners process individuating social characters more deeply
Norm development	4. Facilitate your students' norm development by designing interactions that allow learners to observe dynamic social behaviors	5. Facilitate your students' norm development by providing the support needed to overcome technical barriers to perceiving dynamic social behaviors	6. Facilitate your students' norm development by requiring ongoing interactions that help learners process dynamic social behaviors more deeply
Role differentiation	7. Facilitate your students' role differentiation by designing interactions that allow learners to observe salient social functions.	8. Facilitate your students' role differentiation by providing the support needed to overcome technical barriers to perceiving salient social functions	9. Facilitate your students' role differentiation by requiring ongoing interactions that help learners process salient social functions more deeply

Theoretical foundations for enhancing social connectedness in online learning environments Slagter van Tyron, P. J. Bishop, M. J. (2009). Distance Education 30(3), 291-315 instruction however a formal tool is not a requirement for assessment of the instruction or strategies. A subject matter expert (SME) is often included in a formative assessment to walk through the design checking for alignment in needs and tasks as well as alignment in objectives and assessments. Requesting the support of a colleague to examine instructional design work with a critical eye is a powerful first step in checking for relevance to learners and clarity in presentation. Further, learner feedback is an additional valuable check for clarity as learners are able to point to areas of the instruction that were immediate points of stress or confusion in presentation.

An ongoing assessment can be appropriately related to direct observations of learner interactions within the content and the strategies employed. Self-reflection and formative questions such as, "What segments of the instruction resulted in the most contact with learners for clarity?" and, "Did any problems arise within the technology as the instruction was delivered?" or, "Are there other options possible for altering delivery for a segment of the instruction that proved difficult due to technological barriers?" are questions that might be included in this iterative process of evaluation before during and after the design is complete. Ongoing anecdotal notes and journaling through the design and later delivery of instruction offer a wealth of detail and data for revisiting segments of the design for refinement. In either or all potential methods, the instructional design process is continual in that there is never a final product without multiple opportunities to revisit each design segment for clarity.

FUTURE RESEARCH DIRECTIONS

As nurse educators begin to enhance their expertise in their field with new expertise in instructional design, nurse educators might incorporate design research into their work. Just as Reeves (2005) called for design research that presents collaboration opportunities that are more socially responsible, nurse educators have a wide open and unique opportunity to contribute new design principles specific to the field in ways that progress the design of instruction in direct response to health care needs.

Research in allocation of resources in supporting nurse educators in the development of instructional design documents is needed to further understand the barriers they currently face in crossing into this interdisciplinary field. Additional research in educational benefits for the field of nursing in broadening the scope of study by providing high quality instructional design courses would also serve to support health care professionals in advancing the field.

Research that examines the benefits of collaborations among instructional designers and nurse educators is needed to detail areas of support each field might offer to the other as the interactions become more frequently prevalent among both fields. This volume is one such approach to this type of collaboration. Finally, research into barriers in transitions nurse educators face in migrating programs from the face to face learning environment to the online learning environment, for both educators and students in the field of nursing, would support a better understanding of opportunities in achieving learning goals.

CONCLUSION

This chapter sought to highlight the relevance of the instructional design process for the nurse educator by examining a preliminary set of instructional design guidelines to initiate direction in the systematic design and development of instruction. The overall goal of instruction for all learners is the successful achievement in learning and as such precision in the planning, development, and design of instruction is a universal need. Nurse educators have exceptionally intricate content to depart so therefore it reasons that high quality design can only serve to enhance the competencies in development of skills for their future nursing professionals. Narrative throughout this chapter pointed to relevance in the instructional design process through careful and purposeful coordination of all parts of the instruction with a well-reasoned and tightly woven integration of each segment in the final product. This approach is appropriately aligned with the interdisciplinary and interdependent environment of the healthcare professional and in particular, the field of nursing within the overall system of healthcare. This abbreviated approach to the design of instruction is intended therefore to be a starting point for nurse educator seeking a plan for meeting and exceeding core competencies as proposed by the NLN.

REFERENCES

Ashton, K. S. (2012). Nurse Educators and the future of nursing. *Journal of Continuing Education in Nursing*, *43*(3), 113–116. PMID:22263552

Atkinson, R. C., & Shiffrin, R. M. (1968). Human memory: A proposed system and its control processes. In K. W. Spence & J. T. Spence (Eds.), *The psychology of learning and motivation: Advances in research and theory* (Vol. 2, pp. 89–195). New York: AcademicPress.

Biocca, F., Harms, C., & Burgoon, J. K. (2003). Toward a more robust theory and measure of social presence: Review and suggested criteria. *Presence (Cambridge, Mass.)*, *12*(5), 456–480.

Bloom, B. S. (1956). *Taxonomy of educational objectives*. New York, NY: Longman.

Brown, A. H., & Green, T. D. (2016). *The essentials of instructional design: Connecting fundamental principles with process and practice*. New York: Routledge.

Bruno, I., & Santos, L. (2010). Written comments as a form of feedback. *Studies in Educational Evaluation*, *36*(3), 111–120.

Chiong, R., & Jovanovic, J. (2012). Collaborative Learning in Online Study Groups: An Evolutionary Game Theory Perspective. *Journal of Information Technology Education: Research*, *11*, 81–101.

Dick, W., Carey, L., & Carey, J. O. (2015). *The systematic design of instruction* (8th ed.). Boston, MA: Pearson.

Driscoll, M. P. (2005). *Psychology of learning for instruction* (3rd ed.). Boston, MA: Allyn & Bacon.

Egerton, E. O., McConnell, E. S., Corazzini, K., Kitzmiller, R. R., & Crook, J. O. (2010). Birds of a Feather: Introducing a Virtual Learning Community for Geriatric Nurse Educators. *Journal of Continuing Education in Nursing*, *41*(5), 203–209. PMID:20481420

Gardner, H. (1999). *Intelligence reframed: Multiple intelligences for the 21st century*. New York: Basic Books.

Hannafin, M. J., Hannafin, K. M., Land, S. M., & Oliver, K. (1997). Grounded practice and the design of constructivist learning environments. *Educational Technology Research and Development*, *45*(3), 101–117.

Johnson, A. (2008). A Nursing Faculty's Transition to Teaching Online. *Nursing Education Perspectives*, *29*(1), 17–22. PMID:18330417

Jonassen, D. (1999). Constructivism and computer-mediated communication in distance education. *American Journal of Distance Education*, *9*(2), 7–26.

Kreijns, K. M., Kirschner, P. A., Jochems, W., & van Buuren, H. (2004). Determining sociability, social space, and social presence in (a)synchronous collaborative groups. *Cyberpsychology & Behavior*, *7*(2), 155–172. PMID:15140359

Krouse, A. (2015). Instructional design: More important than ever! *The Journal of Nursing Education*, *54*(6), 304–305. PMID:26057423

Mayer, R. E. (2011). *Applying the science of learning*. Upper Saddle River, NJ: Pearson.

National League for Nursing. (2005). *Core competencies of nurse educators*. Available at http://www.nln.org/professional-development-programs/competencies-for-nursing-education/nurse-educator-core-competency

Pate, A., Smaldino, S., Mayall, H. J., & Luetkehans, L. (2009). Questioning the Necessity of Nonacademic Social Discussion Forums within Online Courses. *Quarterly Review of Distance Education*, *10*(1), 1–8.

Reeves, T. C., Herrington, J., & Oliver, R. (2005). Design research: A socially responsible approach to instructional technology research in higher education. *Journal of Computing in Higher Education*, *16*(2), 96–115.

Rossett, A. (1995). Needs assessment. In G. Anglin (Ed.), *Instructional technology: Past, present and future* (2nd ed.; pp. 183–196). Englewood, CO: Libraries Unlimited, Inc.

Slagter van Tryon, P. J., & Bishop, M. J. (2006). Identifying e-mmediacy strategies for webbased instruction: A Delphi study. *Quarterly Review of Distance Education*, *7*(1), 49–62.

Slagter van Tryon, P. J., & Bishop, M. J. (2009). Theoretical foundations for enhancing social connectedness in online learning environments. *Distance Education*, *30*(3), 291–315.

Slagter van Tryon, P. J., & Bishop, M. J. (2012). Evaluating social connectedness online: The design and development of the Social Perceptions in Learning contexts Instrument. *Distance Education*, *33*(3), 347–364.

Smaldino, S. E., Lowther, D. L., & Russell, J. D. (2008). *Instructional Technology and Media for Learning* (9th ed.). Upper Saddle River, NJ: Pearson.

Smith, P. L., & Ragan, T. J. (2004). *Instructional design* (2nd ed.). Hoboken, NJ: John Wiley & Sons.

KEY TERMS AND DEFINITIONS

Blended Learning: A combination of instructional delivery partially in a face-to-face and real time encounter and instructional delivery in partially in a distance delivery such as in the case of online learning.

Computer Mediated Communication: Interactions that do not take place face-to-face but are delivered over a varied channel such as text based, two way audio, or video.

E-Mmediacy: Feelings of social connectedness one has with fellow online participants (classmates, instructor, teaching assistant) through technology-mediated experiences that simulate episodic perception of immediacy.

Formative Assessment: The process of continual evaluation of all facets of instruction developed for a given educational purpose of editing and refining that instruction.

Instructional Design: A plan for a holistic approach to developing content, materials, strategies, and evaluation to address educational need.

Learning Management System: A Web based portal system for storing and delivering content for online and/or blended delivery of coursework.

Online Learning: Teaching and learning in an environment that is not set in a face-to-face modality but rather at a distance and with the support of Web based technologies.

Performance Assessment: A measurement of the current state of desired activity compared to the desired state of desired activity of a system, institution, group of individuals, or an individual.

Design Research: A research methodology where research within the design of instruction and during the process of instructional design is examined to inform design practice.

Spatio-temporal Proximity: Experience of distance between participants in an interaction where communication is mediated.

Systems Approach: Developing a product through the design principle that all parts are interdependent and are considered for their integral role in the overall product developed.

APPENDIX 1

Table 2. The Social Perception in Learning Contexts Instrument (SPLCI)

SPLCI /SA

Directions: Read each statement below and think about it in relation to your most recent class experience. Decide the extent to which you agree with that statement and circle the appropriate number in the column to the right of each statement that corresponds with your response.

I had enough information about the other class participants...

	Strongly Disagree	Disagree	Neutral	Agree	Strongly Agree	
1. to have a sense of how others would respond during interactions.	1	2	3	4	5	
2. to know if some of my fellow classmates were more interesting to me than others.	1	2	3	4	5	
3. to rate other's academic strengths/weaknesses.	1	2	3	4	5	
4. to decide who would be most **able** to help me if I had a course-related problem.	1	2	3	4	5	
5. to decide who would be most **willing** to help me if I had a course-related problem.	1	2	3	4	5	
6. to have a sense of how friendly others in the class were (friendly defined as warm or comforting).	1	2	3	4	5	
7. to determine who possessed the necessary technology to participate fully in this course.	1	2	3	4	5	
8. to determine who possessed the necessary technology skills to participate fully in this course.	1	2	3	4	5	
	SUM	SUM	SUM	SUM	SUM	SA/Total

☐ + ☐ + ☐ + ☐ + ☐ = ☐

continued on following page

Table 2. Continued

SPLCI /ND

Directions: Read each statement below and think about it in relation to your most recent class experience. Decide the extent to which you agree with that statement and circle the appropriate number in the column to the right of each statement that corresponds with your response..

I had enough information about the other class participants...

	Strongly Disagree	Disagree	Neutral	Agree	Strongly Agree	
9. to imagine what amount of interaction there would be if I were at a small seminar with this group of students.	1	2	3	4	5	
10. to know how much interaction to expect from the others in this course.	1	2	3	4	5	
11. to know how individuals in the class would respond if I told them I did not understand what we were studying.	1	2	3	4	5	
12. to determine how the others would respond if I did not communicate with them during class discussions for an extended amount of time.	1	2	3	4	5	
13. to determine if this group kept up with the course assignment due dates.	1	2	3	4	5	
14. to determine which individuals knew the class rules for how to behave and interact in the class.	1	2	3	4	5	
15. to determine which individuals knew how we were expected to interact with the instructor.	1	2	3	4	5	
16. to know what would happen if someone did not comply with expected group behaviors.	1	2	3	4	5	
17. to know more about them then just their names.						
	SUM	SUM	SUM	SUM	SUM	ND/Total
	☐ +	☐ +	☐ +	☐ +	☐ =	☐

continued on following page

Table 2. Continued

SPLCI /RD

Directions: Read each statement below and think about it in relation to your most recent class experience. Decide the extent to which you agree with that statement and circle the appropriate number in the column to the right of each statement that corresponds with your response.

I had enough information about the other class participants...

	Strongly Disagree	Disagree	Neutral	Agree	Strongly Agree	
18. to decide who would be the most effective leader of the group.	1	2	3	4	5	
19. to decide who was the most opinionated person in the group.	1	2	3	4	5	
20. to decide who was most likely to be frustrated with the learning environment.	1	2	3	4	5	
21. to decide who had the strongest work ethic in this course.	1	2	3	4	5	
22. to decide who would be the best motivator for the group.	1	2	3	4	5	
23. to determine who participated the least in the group.	1	2	3	4	5	
24. to select with whom I would work best.	1	2	3	4	5	
25. to group others into effective teams.	1	2	3	4	5	
26. that given a list of statements, I would be able to identify with confidence which person made which statement.						
	SUM	SUM	SUM	SUM	SUM	RD/Total

☐ + ☐ + ☐ + ☐ + ☐ = ☐

APPENDIX 2

Table 3. SPLCI Participant Scoring Grid

Participant # ________

Participant Status Assessments

SA Total

Very Low		Low			Moderat e			High			Very High	
8	**9**	-----	**20**	**21**	------	**27**	**28**	------	**35**	**36**	-----	**40**

Participant Norm Development

ND Total

Very Low		Low			Moderat e			High			Very High	
8	**9**	-----	**23**	**24**	------	**30**	**3**	------	**40**	**41**	-----	**45**

RD Total

Participant Role Differentiation

Very Low		Low			Moderat e			High			Very High	
8	**9**	-----	**23**	**24**	------	**30**	**3**	------	**40**	**41**	-----	**45**

Participant Full Scale

Full Scale Total

Very Low		Low			Moderat e			High			Very High	
24	**25**	----	**36**	**37**	------	**95**	**9**	----	**113**	**114**	----	**130**

Chapter 7
Online Applied Learning in Nursing Education

Beth Oyarzun
University of North Carolina – Wilmington, USA

Elizabeth A. Gazza
University of North Carolina – Wilmington, USA

ABSTRACT

The instructional design process, Analyze, Design, Develop, Implement, and Evaluate (ADDIE), along with a pedagogical approach was applied to the design and implementation of an online applied learning activity. The activity was delivered in an accelerated nursing leadership asynchronous online course within the fully online RN-BSN program at the University of North Carolina Wilmington (UNCW). Research associated with online applied and experiential learning, particularly in the area of nursing education, that guided the design is presented. The design process and the evaluation results are discussed with future implications.

INTRODUCTION

Enrollments in online programs offered by institutions of higher education continue to increase across the United States. In fall 2014, 5.8 million students enrolled in at least one online course with 1.85 million of those students completing all of their classes at a distance (Allen & Seamen, 2016). Enrollment in online nursing education programs also have increased. Undergraduate and graduate levels nursing programs are delivered online and a large number are degree completion programs, or registered nurse to Bachelor of Science in nursing (RN-BSN) programs. RN-BSN programs are of interest to registered nurses who initially completed an associate degree in nursing or diploma nursing program and now wish to earn a baccalaureate degree in nursing. From 2012 to 2013, enrollment in all types of RN-BSN programs increased by 15.2%, which marks the 11th year of enrollment increases (American Association of College Nursing [AACN], 2014). In 2014, a majority (59%; n=400) of the 679 RN-BSN programs in the US were delivered online (AACN, 2015). Other health-related disciplines, including social work (Council on Social Work Education [CSWE], 2016), occupational therapy (The American

DOI: 10.4018/978-1-5225-2098-6.ch007

Copyright © 2017, IGI Global. Copying or distributing in print or electronic forms without written permission of IGI Global is prohibited.

Occupational Therapy Association, Inc. [AOTA], 2016], physical therapy (American Physical Therapy Association [APTA], 2015), and medicine (American Medical Association [AMA], 2016), also utilize online instructional strategies to varying degrees for didactic instruction in undergraduate, graduate, and/or continuing education programs.

Preparing nurses and other healthcare professionals for clinical practice includes a combination of didactic instruction and clinical experiences where students safely apply what they are learning in various healthcare settings. This poses a persistent challenge in online learning where students in health-related educational programs often engage in online coursework at locations distant from faculty who facilitate learning. Smith, Passmore, and Faught (2009) interviewed online nursing instructors regarding the challenges and found that instructors are mainly concerned with authentic assessments that allow them to be able to judge the learner's ability to apply new skills in real world settings.

This chapter proposes an answer to the question, how can students apply what they are learning when faculty are not physically present to assess application of skills in various healthcare settings and in settings where patient safety is paramount? Using a case study approach, the chapter includes a description of a theory-based pedagogical approach and the instructional design process that integrated applied learning experiences into an accelerated online asynchronous course in an RN-BSN program. While the case is based in nursing education, the approach and process can be used by any online educational programs for health professionals.

BACKGROUND

Problem

Nursing education programs, along with other programs that prepare professionals in other health-related disciplines, require experiences where students apply concepts in practice settings. Practitioners cannot simply learn the theory of nursing or medicine, graduate, and safely care for patients; they need to have opportunities to apply concepts in practice under the watchful eye of faculty or other experienced professionals who can guide them while learning. This is particularly important when health care agencies need graduates who are work-ready and can safely and competently provide care. This is especially true given the shortage of quality health care professionals in the United States.

Nursing has used online education as a way to prepare nurses for advanced levels of practice. RN-BSN and graduate programs are online and serve as ways to prepare nurses for higher level positions such as leadership and management, nursing education, or Nurse Practitioner (NP). These education programs require skill development. As programs become more widely available to nurses, separated by geography where faculty cannot directly supervise but other qualified professionals can facilitate learning, there is a need to identify ways to include applied learning.

Applied Learning

Applied learning is a broad term that involves "principles and practices associated with engaged scholarship, communities of practice, civic engagement, experiential education, and critical pedagogy" (Schwartzman & Henry, 2009, pp. 4-5). While there are many learning theories associated with applied learning such as, service learning, project based learning, active learning, authentic learning, context-based learning, and learning by doing, for the purposes of this chapter, experiential learning theory is used to frame the case study that demonstrates integration of applied learning in online education programs for healthcare professionals.

From a theoretical perspective, applied learning is constructivist in nature and aligns with Kolb's Experiential Learning Theory in which experiential learning is defined as learning through experiences and reflection on those experiences (Kolb, 1984). "Learning is the process whereby knowledge is created through the transformation of experience" (Kolb, 1984, p. 38). Kolb's theory is based on a four stage learning cycle. The stages are concrete experience, reflective observation, abstract conceptualization, and active experimentation. Each stage requires the learner to complete a task. In the concrete experience, the learner should complete an activity. In the reflective observation phase, the learner reflects on the completed activity. In the abstract conceptualization stage, the learner should conceptualize what was observed. Lastly, in the active experimentation stage, the learner should plan how to test what was conceptualized. As a pedagogy, experiential learning focuses on the connection between theory and the authentic or real world including the knowledge and skills needed by individuals practicing in a particular discipline (Downing & Herrington, 2013).

Ash and Clayton (2009) highlight reflection as a critical component that ensures deep and meaningful thought that enhances the learning experience. Kolb, Boyatzin, and Mainemelis (2001) conducted a literature review of 1004 studies that cited experiential learning theory as the theoretical model. These studies included papers from the fields of education, management, computer science, psychology, medicine, nursing, accounting, and law. The research indicated support for the experiential learning theory's use for integrated learning.

Incorporating applied or experiential learning in healthcare settings has traditionally been done in clinical, practicums, internships, residencies. Students go to a clinical setting where there are real patients and apply what they have learned. More recently, simulation has been used in nursing and in interdisciplinary education. Experiential learning simulation design has been found to positively influence the development of nursing judgement and competency (Chmil, Turk, Adamson, & Larew, 2015). These valuable experiences can and should also be incorporated into online courses.

The use effectiveness of applied learning has been examined by nursing and other disciplines. One study aimed to evaluate the effectiveness of active learning strategies in undergraduate nursing education through descriptive, cross-sectional comparative design (Shin, Sok, Hyun, & Kim, 2014). The active learning strategies were based on experiential learning theory and included simulation, case studies, and reflective activities. The results showed that the nursing competency scores were significantly higher for those in the active learning group. Waltz, Jenkins, and Han (2014) conducted a review of the literature to identify evidence about the use and effectiveness of active learning in nursing and other health professions. Fifteen of 22 studies reported positive results with regard to effectiveness, yet the authors concluded the evidence was insufficient and identified the need for quality research on the topic.

While there is evidence to support the effectiveness of applied experiences in facilitating learning, most of the research has been conducted in traditional classroom and clinical settings. Integrating applied learning into the online environment has thus far received limited attention in nursing and other disciplines. Holtslander, Racine, Furniss, Burles, and Turner (2012) utilized the Four-Component Instructional Design (4C/ID) model to integrate authentic learning strategies and constructivist learning pedagogy into qualitative research methods in an online, asynchronous graduate level course for nursing, psychology, medical, and sociology students. The results of the project revealed that students were able to develop authentic research proposals indicating value in the applied learning approach.

The discipline of business provided an interesting study about the difference between online and traditional course delivery methods and specifically, the transfer of theory to the real world (Hassen, 2008). Study findings indicated that online students produced better results than traditional students in the application of classroom knowledge to the real word. Hansen (2008) attributed this to the stronger sense of community in the online environment that resulted from activities such as online chats and debriefings.

The National Society for Experiential Education (NSEE, 2009), is an organization founded in 1971 whose mission is to promote the use of experience as an integral part of education and as a result, to empower learners. NSEE (2009) identified seven principles to guide ethical practice specific to experiential education. Included in the principles is a commitment to use quality standards and practices in the placement and supervision of students who engage in experiential learning activities in the field, such as those completed by students in nursing and other health-related online programs. Additionally, NSEE (2013) identified eight best practices that guide the development and delivery of all experiential activities. The principles are:

1. **Intention:** All participants understand the purpose of the activity and there is purposefulness to the experience.
2. **Preparedness and Planning:** All participants have sufficient foundational knowledge for the experience and commit to focus on the intention through planning and goal setting.
3. **Authenticity:** The experience has a real world context or can be translated to a real world experience.
4. **Reflection:** The experience includes opportunities to analyze assumptions and consider the possible outcomes with regard to the past and future. Reflection is integral at all phases because it transforms the experience to a learning experience by allowing the learner to internalize the information.
5. **Orientation and Training:** All participants are provided with all necessary background information regarding participants, context, and environment of the experience.
6. **Monitoring and Continuous Improvement:** The experience should be structured yet flexible with a continuous feedback loop to provide support and encouragement.
7. **Assessment and Evaluation:** Outcomes and processes should be evaluated on initial intentions and final outcomes.
8. **Acknowledgment:** All participants are included in the recognition of the learning impact and accomplishments.

These eight principles give practical strategies for implementing Kolb's experiential learning theory. This case study adopted these strategies along with an instructional design process to guide the design of the activity. The instructional design process adopted is described in the following section.

Instructional Design

Instructional design is the systematic practice of creating instructional experiences which make the acquisition of knowledge more efficient, effective, and appealing (Merrill, Drake, Lacy, & Pratt, 1996). Analyze, Design, Develop, Implement, Evaluate (ADDIE) is an instructional design process that can be used to create and implement effective instruction in any setting (Branch, 2009). While there are many instructional design processes and models, many of them incorporate the ADDIE phases. The phases of the ADDIE process are described in more detail in the following sections.

- **Analysis:** The analysis phase of instructional design involves identifying instructional goals and gathering information about the learner characteristics and the learning environment. Before identifying the instructional goals designers often analyze learner performance to identify needs, which are gaps between current and desired performance. This process is also referred to as performance analysis, needs analysis, or needs assessment. "Needs analysis allows the designer to take a fresh and data-driven look at the work, the worker, and workplace, to base training recommendations on opinions, practices and work products – not on habit, whim or arbitrary decrees" (Rossett, 1999, p. 64). The results of the needs analysis help designers identify a list of needs, which are prioritized based on importance and used to develop instructional goals. Goals define the expected learning outcomes. Before identifying goals, learner characteristics are also explored. These characteristics may include learning styles, prior knowledge, and attitudes toward content. An analysis of the learning environment is also conducted in order to gain information regarding resources (hardware, software, instructional materials, etc.).
- **Design:** Once the needs and goals are identified and the learner/contextual analysis are complete, the next step is designing instruction. The design phase involves writing the
- performance objectives, sequencing the content based upon the previous analysis, and determining appropriate instructional strategies. In order to complete these tasks instructional designers use a taxonomy of learning to classify the desired learner outcomes into specific categories (e.g., Gagne, Bloom). Classifying the learner outcomes is the basis for analyzing tasks, formulating the performance objectives, identifying instructional strategies and assessment items. Once the objectives and assessment items are complete designers sequence the content of instruction using results of a task analysis. The result of the analysis and design phases is a design document or blueprint for the instruction that will be developed.
- **Develop:** The development phase involves producing all instruction materials based upon the design specifications, which could be print, audio-visual, electronic, or integrated technologies.
- **Implement:** The implementation phase involves delivering the newly developed material according to the established blueprint.
- **Evaluate:** The evaluation phase measures the effectiveness of the new instruction in two ways; formative and summative evaluation. Formative evaluation takes place in every phase while summative takes place after implementation.

While the issue of safety if of primary concern when it comes to applied learning, there is evidence to support the use of applied learning experiences in nursing and health professions education and in online environments (Waltz, Jenkins, & Han, 2014). Through the use of NSEE's (2013) eight principles of experiential learning as the framework and ADDIE as the instructional design process, it is possible to create and integrate applied learning experiences in online health-related programs. The following case serves as one example of how to design these experiences and overcome the challenges associated with integrating applied learning on online courses in practice disciplines. This case study adopted the ADDIE instructional design process and the NSEE best practices for designing experiential learning activities to design a Leadership and Management nursing practicum for a fully online leadership and management course. The course was delivered asynchronously.

SOLUTION AND RECOMMENDATIONS

Context of the Case Study

These NSEE principles and the ADDIE instructional design model were adopted as the frameworks for designing an applied learning experience that was incorporated into an accelerated online asynchronous leadership and management course in an RN-BSN program. The experience is referred to as the Leadership and Management Practicum. The project aligned with the institution's Quality Enhancement Plan (QEP). The plan promotes the use of applied learning in face-to-face and online courses and aims to improve the quality of learning for students and faculty. Internal grants support initiatives that align with the QEP, including the Leadership and Management Practicum.

The RN-BSN program, in which this case is focused, is a Commission on Collegiate Nursing Education (CCNE)-accredited, fully online accelerated highly-enrolled program. The program houses approximately 1,000 licensed nurses who complete fully online asynchronous 7 week courses during 6 semesters per year. The curriculum includes courses such as leadership and management, community-based care, research, health policy, and professional role responsibilities. The curriculum also includes practice experiences that aligned with the expectations of the AACN (2012), an organization that establishes quality standards for nursing education. This means that all enrolled students, including those participating in the Leadership and Management Practicum, had to engage in clinically-based practice experiences.

It is important to note that all students who are enrolled in the program are fully licensed registered nurses. Nearly all students are employed in nursing positions that align with their scope of practice and therefore, are immersed in a variety of clinical and health-related practice settings. This provides opportunities to safely utilize the work environment for well-planned applied learning experiences and allows for authenticity of experience.

An interdisciplinary team comprised of the nursing faculty member teaching the Leadership and Management in Health Care course, an instructional designer, and a career counselor collaborated to design and implement the Leadership and Management Practicum. The expertise of the interdisciplinary team in the areas of content, online education, course design, and career planning facilitated development of an applied learning project that aligned with NSEE's (2013) 8 principles of experiential learning.

Practice Experiences and the Instructional Design Process

Using the concepts of leadership and management, course objectives, and program outcomes as guides, a series of practice experiences were developed. The experiences were carefully selected to ensure the safe application of newly-learned concepts in practice settings. Details about the experiences are presented using ADDIE as framework and include support from NSSE's (2012) 8 Principles of Applied Learning and published evidence. While nursing was the focus on the practice experiences, the framework and the applied learning principles are applicable to online education for all health-related disciplines.

Analysis

Analyzing the goals, learning experiences, and learning environment is the first step in creating meaningful applied learning experiences in nursing education and in online programs that prepare practitioners in all health-related disciplines. One key outcome for the Leadership and Management in Health Care course is that students will be able to examine nursing leadership and management skills in a variety of settings using the knowledge, skills, and attitudes of professional nursing practice. Students who enroll in the course are registered nurses earning a Bachelor of Science degree in Nursing. As already noted, the course is delivered completely online, in an asynchronous format, and consists of 7 modules completed over 7 weeks. Students engage in the course from any geographic location in the world using the University-selected learning management system.

All students who enroll in the course have experience in nursing and nearly all of them are currently practicing in a healthcare setting in the geographic location where they reside. Since the concepts of leadership and management are not components of the education program they completed to become a registered nurse, the course provides them the first opportunity to learn about leadership and management theory and to apply theory in their clinical practice. The Leadership and Management Practicum ensured that all students had the opportunity to safely apply the theory to practice while being guided by course faculty. The practicum encompassed the cognitive, behavioral, and psychomotor domains and thus enhanced the learning experience for the student.

Design

Designing involves formulating objectives/outcomes, learning activities, and assessments of learning. This is true regardless of the disciplinary-focus of the health-related program being designed. Specific to the case example, in addition to meeting course objectives, the interdisciplinary team wanted the students to leave the course with an understanding of how they 'fit' into the realm of leadership and management in nursing and to realize their potential for serving in formal leadership and management positions in health care. In order to accomplish this, the following student learning outcomes specific to applied learning were identified, measured, and evaluated.

- **Student Learning Outcome 1:** Students will participate in a leadership and management applied learning experience to develop leadership and management skills that are needed to lead and manage in the health care settings where they practice, or could potentially practice, as registered nurses.
    - **Assessment 1:** Students will develop three goals formulated from the results of a leadership style inventory assessment for their development as a leader and manager in nursing and could be accomplished in 7 weeks.
    - **Learning Activities:** The Leadership and Management Practicum consisted of self-assessments, practice experiences, and critical reflective blogs. Through the initial blog, the Leadership Styles Blog, students addressed the results of the Leadership Style Inventory, how the results aligned with their own expectations and with those of an effective leader and manager, and the skills they felt they needed to focus on during the course. This activity aligned with the NSEE (2013) principle of intentionality, which includes an understanding of the purpose of the activity.
- **Student Learning Outcome 2:** Students will apply leadership and management theory in nursing practice through engagement in 7 clinical practice experiences.
    - **Assessment 2:** Course faculty evaluated written and video recorded assignments that reflect completion of the practice experiences.

Table 1. Seven Practice Experiences

Practice Experiences
2. In a healthcare setting, complete an analysis of the organizational system using organization and management theory as the framework.
2. Analyze a recent experience in clinical practice to determine if and how you adhered, or did not adhere to your core values and how you demonstrated ethical leadership.
3. Engage in a simulation activity where you function in the role of the leader of the unit where you practice nursing. Complete the Leadership Skills Questionnaire (Northouse,2015) to determine strengths and weaknesses with regard to your ability to leader and manage.
4. Interview a nurse manager who is responsible for fiscal management of the unit where you work and analyze the budgeting process used by that manager. Integrate information about health care financing and budgeting into a class discussion about health care financing.
5. Apply results of the Task and Relationship Questionnaire (Northouse, 2015) while engaging in clinical practice throughout a work week and build a relationship with at least one other health care provider.
6.While in clinical practice apply results from the Setting the Tone Questionnaire (Northouse, 2015) learned about setting the tone and implement at least one strategy to improve the tone on the unit where you practice.
7. (Culminating experience) Prepare application materials (resume and cover letter) for a and participate in a simulated interview (Video recorded) for hypothetical management position in nursing. Integrate your own leadership and management abilities and the theory you have been learning about in this course into the application and interview.

  - **Learning Activities:** The seven practice experiences are listed in Table 1. A written or video reflective blog was included with 6 of the practice experiences. The blog activity required that students reflect on their ability to apply leadership and management concepts in practice and included an interaction component among classmates. Blogging has been reported to enhance learning (Halic, Lee, Paulus, & Spence, 2010), help students to synthesize their thoughts, transition from student to practicing professional and for faculty to monitor learning (Reed & Edmunds, 2015). Additionally, blogging has been found to help students learn from peers' viewpoints and has enhanced their professional development (Lin & Shen, 2013). Collectively, the practice experiences and blogging activities aligned with the NSEE (2013) principles of preparedness and planning, authenticity, orientation and training, monitoring and continuous improvement, reflection, assessment and evaluation.
- **Student Learning Outcome 3:** Students will integrate leadership and management theory into their clinical practice and plan for ongoing development beyond course completion.
  - **Assessment 3**: Through the final reflective blog, students wrote and shared with classmates and faculty an analysis of their performance in the simulated application and interview, the critical reflections on achievement of the 3 goals identified at the start of the applied learning experience, and plans for continued application of new knowledge to clinical practice and ongoing development. In addition, course faculty reviewed and evaluated the application and interview assignments.
  - **Learning Activities**: The final reflective blog post consisted of a critical analysis of student performance in the simulated interview assignment, critical reflection on achievement of the 3 goals intentionally identified at the start of the course, and plans for ongoing development upon course completion. They also reviewed and responded to blog posts made by classmates. This aligned with the NSEE (2013) principles of assessment and evaluation, monitoring and continuous improvement, authenticity, reflection, and acknowledgement.

Table 2. Linkages between Components and Principles

Applied Learning Component	NSEE Principle
Goal Setting	Intention
Self-Assessments	Preparedness and Planning
Reflective Blogs	Reflection and Authenticity
Practice Experiences	Orientation and Training
Facilitation/Interaction	Orientation and Training, Monitoring and Continuous Improvement
Evaluation	Assessment and Evaluation

In summary, the project plan ensured that all NSEE (2013) principles were incorporated into the Leadership and Management Practicum. Table 2 shows the linkage between the planned activities and the respective NSEE principle.

Develop

Assembling an interdisciplinary team that includes educators, instructional designers, and content experts can facilitate the development and delivery of robust applied learning experiences regardless of the focus of the health-related program. The development phase is where faculty must consider components of the clinical settings that can be accessed and utilized in a way to ensures safety of all participants.

In the case example, each member of the interdisciplinary team was responsible for developing components of the practicum. The curriculum for the 3-credit online course was developed by the nursing faculty member. Learning objectives were identified for each module and linked to course and program outcomes. Each practice experience was linked to a modular objective. Practice experiences were selected based on the people, policies, and resources the practicing registered nurse had access to in their workplace, and the safety of engaging with those variables. Using the blueprint for instruction, learning activities, teaching strategies, instructions, and evaluation mechanisms for each applied learning activity were developed within the course in the institution's learning management system.

The instructional designer created supportive handouts and tutorials about the LMS tools that students used to complete the activities, including blogs and the streaming media storage service. The blog tool was used for the seven blog entries with some being textual and others video. The culminating simulated interview assignment required submission of a 30-minute video recording. Several needs were identified during initial testing of the streaming media software. First, the videos needed to be housed in a secure location since there was identifiable individuals talking about themselves. Second, the instructor preferred that the videos be downloadable for recordkeeping purposes. The university-adopted streaming media storage service that was integrated into the LMS was the only option that met all the criteria. The instructional designer tested the solution and completed detailed instructions for uploading the videos. The instructional designer offered support and consultation on video development and upload for the students.

The third member of the interdisciplinary team, a career counselor, developed resources for creating an effective resume and established a process for offering consultation on resume development and interview skills. All students had the opportunity to submit a draft version of the application materials to the career counselor in order to receive individual guidance about the best way to present oneself as a leader and manager in nursing. Integration of leadership and management theory into the application materials was essential.

Implement

Once design is complete, it is time to implement the applied learning experience in the online course. Carefully designed, meaningful experiences can safely be implemented in practice settings and without the direct supervision of faculty. The Leadership and Management Practicum was successfully implemented for the first time in the Fall, 2014 with 28 students in one section of the Leadership and Management in Healthcare course, The practicum has become a standard component of the all sections of the course.

Evaluate

Student achievement of the objectives related to the applied learning experiences was evaluated through the use of standardized rubrics. Overall effectiveness of the practicum evaluated using the three student outcomes.

- **Student Learning Outcome 1 Assessment:** Through the initial blog, the Leadership Styles Blog, students addressed three prompts, including their goals for leadership development in the course. Using a standardized rubric, course faculty reviewed students' responses to the three prompts and confirmed the three goals identified by the student were appropriate for development as a leader and manager in nursing and could be accomplished in 7.5 weeks. All 28 students submitted a blog post for this assignment. The mean score on this assignment was 2.96 (0-3 possible score range). This indicates students were successful in articulating their expectations and intentionally identified the goals they wanted to achieve through the applied experiences in the course.
- **Student Learning Outcome 2 Assessment:** Students applied leadership and management theory in nursing practice through engagement in 7 clinical practice experiences.
  All 28 students completed all 7 clinical learning experiences. Results of the Management Position Application Assignment reflected a mean score of 19.14 points (0-20 possible range). Results of the Leadership and Management Interview Assignment reflected a mean score of 39.11 (0-40 possible range). These data seem to indicate that the clinical practice experiences, reflective blog posts, resume preparation activities, and interview activities were effective at facilitating student integration of leadership and management theory into practice and ultimately, serve as evidence of student learning.
- **Student Learning Outcome 3 Assessment:** Students planned for ongoing development as a leader and manager beyond completion of the course. All students wrote and submitted a final critical reflective blog post. The mean score for this assignment was 5.7 (0-6 possible range). All students reflected on the progress made toward achieving the 3 goals they identified in the first activity in the course with a majority indicating they achieved those goals. All students identified appropriate plans for ongoing development as a leader and manager in nursing. They also reviewed and commented on plans posted by their classmates as a way to make a positive impact on nursing beyond the score of their course.

Discussion

The evaluation data supports the idea that applied learning experiences can effectively and safely be implemented with teacher guidance in health-related online education programs such as the one in nursing. This is congruent with the findings of Breen and Jones (2015) who found positive results after designing and implementing an experiential activity into another RN-BSN course. The desired outcomes were for learners to obtain broader knowledge that extended beyond technical competence.

The experiences must be thoroughly planned with consideration for the people, policies, and resources. Utilizing resources within a health care setting where the student is employed allowed for an authentic learning experience and careful selection of the activities ensured safety of all participants. While this particular case involved nursing education, the principles of ADDIE and applied learning translate to all health-related disciplines that use online education at the undergraduate, graduate, or continuing education levels. For example, an education instructor may use these same methodologies to develop an educational leadership practicum requiring the learners to produce resumes and interview for a principle job.

An unanticipated outcome of this applied learning experience was the level of engagement demonstrated by the students. It is extremely telling that 100% of the class participated in the ungraded reflective blog activities. This could indicate that intentionality of the experience increased participation by the students although further exploration of their engagement is warranted. Results of project evaluation indicate effectiveness of the blogs in facilitating learning, which is consistent with findings of Halic, Lee, Paulus, and Spence (2010) and Reed and Edmunds (2015).

One challenge of the practicum was full achievement of the 3 goals intentionally established by students in module 1 within a 7-week time frame. Interestingly, at the beginning of the course, most students did not see themselves as leaders and managers. The final reflections indicated that many students recognized their potential; that they have the beginning skills needed to lead and manage and that with continued development, they could assume formal roles. This aligns with findings of Lin and Shen (2013). Additionally, this was an extremely rewarding outcome for the interdisciplinary team to witness and one that could have a positive impact on nursing practice.

Following implementation, the interdisciplinary team identified three process-related challenges of the project. First, students in a health-related online programs have varying technical abilities. In order to ensure technology is used as a tool rather than as the focus on the learning activity, thorough directions are needed for the use of high-technology tools such as video streaming. Students initially spent more time on use of the software than on the assignment. Directions and support are essential and should be routine components of applied learning experiences either online or face-to-face.

Secondly, this model used in the sample case may not be scalable in nursing or other health-related education programs. As class size increases, it becomes more challenging for one career counselor to review resume drafts and one instructional designer to support video development and submission. Ideally, all students would benefit from submitting a resume and cover letter to a career counselor and individualized technology support. Additional support options need to be explored to continue to provide individualized support to faculty and students.

Lastly, presence, persistence, and vigilance are key in applied learning experiences. Regardless of the health-related discipline using online delivery, faculty must be actively engaged in order to facilitate individual student development through the clinical experiences and reflective blog posts. This can be challenging in highly-enrolled online courses in health-related disciplines.

FUTURE RESEARCH DIRECTIONS

The outcomes of the applied learning practicum indicate that experiential learning can occur in online nursing courses. The designed practice experience was specific to nursing and for licensed nurses who were employed in practice settings. While the principles of applied learning and ADDIE are applicable to all health-related disciplines, effectiveness of a similar approach in other disciplines requires further exploration.

This practicum project did not include measures of effectiveness of the quality student support provided by the instructional designer or career counselor. The project team planned on providing high quality, individualized support since this applied learning experience and the team wanted to increase the likelihood of the experience being successful. The appreciation from the students indicates that this could be a topic for future research and rethinking how universities should support their distance learners. One consistent issue in distance education is retention (Allen & Seamen, 2016). Providing high quality, individualized support could help improve retention rates.

Lastly, long term effects of applied learning experiences could provide more evidence about how applied learning in nursing and other health-related disciplines education improves practice and competency development practicing professional. This would require longitudinal research study that would evaluate effectiveness over time.

CONCLUSION

Applied learning experiences may be effective an instructional strategy for nursing and other health-related disciplines provided that the experiences are designed well and students have sufficient support. Learning and applied learning theory and instructional design processes offer strategies to guide interdisciplinary teams as they integrate applied learning experiences that are aligned with learning outcomes and student needs.

The project detailed in this chapter outlined one successful example of an applied learning experience using ADDIE instructional design process and NSEE's (2013) 8 principles that guide ethical practice specific to experiential education. The results indicate that applied learning can help students realize their potential specific to leadership and management and as a result, positively impact nursing practice.

REFERENCES

Allen, I. E., & Seaman, J. (2016). *Online Report Card: Tracking Online Education in the United States*. Babson Park, MA: Babson Survey Research Group and Quahog Research Group. Retrieved July 20, 2016 from http://onlinelearningsurvey.com/reports/onlinereportcard.pdf

American Association of College Nursing. (2014). *2014 annual report of the American Association of College Nursing*. Retrieved August 5, 2016 from http://www.aacn.nche.edu/aacn-publications/annual-reports/AnnualReport14.pdf

American Association of Colleges of Nursing. (2012). *White paper: Expectations for practice experiences in the RN-baccalaureate curriculum*. Retrieved October 26, 2016, from http://www.aacn.nche.edu/aacn-publications/white-papers/RN-BSN-White-Paper.pdf

American Association of Colleges of Nursing. (2015). *Degree Completion Programs for Registered Nurses: RN to Master's Degree and RN to Baccalaureate Programs*. Retrieved March 30, 2015 from http://www.aacn.nche.edu/media-relations/fact-sheets/degree-completion-programs

American Medical Association. (1995-2016). *Education center.* Retrieved October 26, 2016, from https://www.ama-assn.org/ama/pub/education-careers/education-center.page?

American Occupational Therapy Association, Inc. (2016). *Distance education entry-level occupational therapy (OT) educational programs.* Retrieved October 26, 2016, from http://www.aota.org/~/media/Corporate/Files/EducationCareers/Schools/DistanceEd/Distance_Education_Top_Percentage_OT_2014-2015.pdf

American Physical Therapy Association. (2015). *APTA Learning Center.* Retrieved October 26, 2016, from http://learningcenter.apta.org/default.aspx

Ash, S. L., & Clayton, P. H. (2009). Generating, deepening, and documenting learning: The power of critical reflection in applied learning. *Journal of Applied Learning in Higher Education, 1*, 25-48. doi: 10.1097/NNE.0000000000000159

Branch, R. M. (2009). *Instructional design: The ADDIE approach* (Vol. 722). Springer Science & Business Media. doi:10.1007/978-0-387-09506-6

Breen, H., & Jones, M. (2015). Experiential learning: Using virtual simulation in an online RN-to-BSN program. *The Journal of Continuing Education in Nursing, 46*(1), 27-33. doi:http://dx.doi.org.liblink.uncw.edu/10.3928/00220124-20141120-02

Chmil, J. V., Turk, M., Adamson, K., & Larew, C. (2015). Effects of an experiential learning simulation design on clinical nursing judgment development. *Nurse Educator*, *40*(5), 228–232. doi:10.1097/NNE.0000000000000159 PMID:25763781

Council on Social Work Education. (2016). *Accreditation: Online and distance education*. Retrieved October 26, 2016, from http://www.cswe.org/Accreditation/Information/OnlineandDistanceEducation.aspx

Downing, J., & Herrington, J. (2013, December). *Applied learning in online spaces: Traditional pedagogies informing educational design for today's learners.* Paper presented at the 30th Ascilite Conference, Sydney, Australia.

Halic, O., Lee, D., Paulus, T., & Spence, M. (2010). To blog or not to blog: Student perceptions of blog effectiveness for learning in a college-level course. *The Internet and Higher Education*, *13*(4), 206–213. doi:10.1016/j.iheduc.2010.04.001

Holtslander, L. F., Racine, L., Furniss, S., Burles, M., & Turner, H. (2012). Developing and piloting an online graduate nursing course focused on experiential learning of qualitative research methods. *The Journal of Nursing Education*, *51*(6), 345–348. doi:10.3928/01484834-20120427-03 PMID:22533499

Kolb, D. (1984). *Experiential learning: experience as the source of learning and development*. Englewood Cliffs, NJ: Prentice Hall.

Kolb, D. A., Boyatzis, R. E., & Mainemelis, C. (2001). Experiential learning theory: Previous research and new directions. *Perspectives on Thinking, Learning, and Cognitive Styles, 1*, 227-247.

Lin, K. Y., & Shen, Y. F. (2013). The nursing students attitude toward using blogs in a nursing clinical practicum in Taiwan: A 3-R framework. *Nurse Education Today*, *33*(9), 1079–1082. doi:10.1016/j.nedt.2012.03.019 PMID:22520239

Merrill, M. D., Drake, L., Lacy, M. J., & Pratt, J. (1996). Reclaiming instructional design (PDF). *Educational Technology*, *36*(5), 5–7.

National Society for Experiential Education. (2009). *Eight principles of good practice for all experiential learning activities.* Retrieved August 17, 2016 from http://www.nsee.org/8-principles

National Society for Experiential Education. (2013). *Guiding principles of ethical practice.* Retrieved August 17, 2016 from http://www.nsee.org/guiding-principles

Northouse, P. G. (2015). *Introduction to leadership concepts and practices* (3rd ed.). Thousand Oaks, CA: Sage.

Reed, S. J., & Edmunds, D. (2015). Use of a blog in an undergraduate nursing leadership course. *Nurse Education in Practice*, *15*(6), 537–542. doi:10.1016/j.nepr.2015.07.010 PMID:26299700

Rossett, A. (1999). Knowledge management meets analysis. *Training & Development*, *53*, 62–68.

Schwartzman, R., & Henry, K. (2009). From celebration to critical investigation: Charting the course of scholarship in applied learning. *Journal of Applied Learning in Higher Education*, *1*, 3–23.

Shin, H., Sok, S., Hyun, D. S., & Kim, M. J. (2015). Competency and an active learning program in undergraduate nursing education. *Journal of Advanced Nursing, 71*(3), 591–598. doi: 101111/jan.12564

Smith, G. G., Passmore, D., & Faught, T. (2009). The challenges of online nursing education. *The Internet and Higher Education*, *12*(2), 98–103. doi:10.1016/j.iheduc.2009.06.007

Waltz, C. F., Jenkins, L. S., & Han, N. (2014). The use and effectiveness of active learning methods in nursing and health professions education: A literature review. *Nursing Education Perspectives*, *35*(6), 392–400. doi:10.5480/13-1168

KEY TERMS AND DEFINITIONS

Applied Learning: An approach to learning that is project based and reflective allowing learners to engage in authentic practical applications of skills while under in the direct guidance of instructors.

Experiential Learning: An approach to learning situated in real world scenarios that connect theory with practical application of skills to advance learner development and expertise for professional roles.

Nursing Education: Foundational theory and practical medical experience learners engage in for the purpose of critical preparation for the responsibilities of care and expertise of duties as licensed professionals in all fields of nursing.

Online: A mode of delivering education through Web-based applications where learners and instructors are separated by time and space.

Chapter 8
Teaching Residents How to Teach

Heidi Kromrei
Detroit Medical Center, USA

William L. Solomonson
Oakland University, USA

Mark S. Juzych
Wayne State University, USA

ABSTRACT

In this chapter, the context of medical education is reviewed in terms of how to teach in the health care setting, commonly used instructional strategies, and the clinical learning environments of the medical student and resident trainees. Although accreditation bodies require residents to teach, and it is an activity that is assigned, it is often not delivered by the sponsoring institution. Key terms in education, learning theories, and instructional strategies are presented. In particular, strategies for medical educators to prepare residents to teach effectively in their residency program are provided. Finally, an instructional development plan for residents, with supporting worksheets and examples, is presented.

INTRODUCTION

A core task of residency is to teach medical students as well as patients, families, students, and other health professionals. Nevertheless, very little, if any, evidence-based practical instruction is provided to residents to perform this task well. It is common for residents who have high levels of subject matter expertise, but no background in adult learning theory, instructional strategies, or instructional design, to be tasked with teaching. This issue can be addressed by instilling residents with a basic knowledge of learning theories and/or approaches to instruction for certain types of learners as well as by providing tools to help develop instruction. To this end, foundational concepts, instructional models, and instructional strategies for use in a residency teaching setting are presented.

The goal of this chapter is to provide medical educators, such as program directors, faculty, and chief residents, with basic instructional frameworks and tools to develop the teaching competencies of residents. The learning objectives of the chapter are for learners to:

DOI: 10.4018/978-1-5225-2098-6.ch008

Copyright © 2017, IGI Global. Copying or distributing in print or electronic forms without written permission of IGI Global is prohibited.

- Review the contextual setting of medical education.
- Understand key terms: learning theory, pedagogy, andragogy, behaviorism, and cognitivism.
- Recognize effective instructional strategies for medical education settings.
- Develop or assist in the development of a plan for teaching residents to teach.

BACKGROUND

The process of educating physicians in the United States is both complex and highly regulated. Before entering into a residency program, allopathic undergraduate medical students in the United States must graduate from a Liaison Committee on Medical Education (LCME)-accredited medical school. After graduation, students are matched with a graduate medical school to complete their residency training. Graduate medical education (GME) typically requires an additional three to seven years of education, depending on the medical student's specialization. Allopathic residency and fellowship programs are accredited by the Accreditation Council for Graduate Medical Education (ACGME). Approximately 700 sponsoring institutions, such as hospitals, universities, medical centers and medical schools, are evaluated for accreditation by ACGME. These institutions sponsor approximately 9,600 individual residency training and fellowship programs, which also are evaluated and accredited by ACGME (2016).

These two regulatory agencies that accredit medical schools and residency programs in the United States mandate that residents be trained to teach and assess medical students and others, as noted above. The LCME requires that:

Residents who supervise or teach medical students and graduate students... must be familiar with the educational objectives of the course or clerkship and be prepared for their roles in teaching and assessment.... There should be central monitoring of the level of residents' participation in activities to enhance their teaching and assessment skills. There should be formal evaluation [of these skills] with opportunities provided for remediation... if needed. (LCME ED-24, 2016, pp. 10-11)

In 2001, approximately 50% of ACGME-accredited programs surveyed reported some formal teaching training for residents (Morrison et al., 2001). LCME mandates that institutions that offer medical education programs must be prepared to describe policies and programs designed to teach residents how to teach and assess the performance of medical students in addition to noting how resident participation in these training programs is monitored. Further, the ACGME considers teaching skills to be a core resident competency and expects that residents will develop the ability to teach patients, families, students, visiting resident rotators, and other health professionals (ACGME, 2016). Analyses of "residents-as-teachers" programs show positive outcomes related to the perceptions of participants but limited evidence of program effectiveness (Hill, Yu, Barrow, & Hattie, 2009). Despite requirements and expectations that residents are taught how to teach medical students and others, many medical schools and residency programs report non-compliance with this requirement, and those that are compliant are often unable to ascertain program effectiveness.

Aside from the accreditation requirement for residents to teach, there are inherent benefits of teaching for residents. First, as most instructors will verify from personal experience, teaching a course is one of the best methods to improve retention of the subject matter. Further, as Wamsley, Julian, and Wipf (2004) have noted, over time, residents experience an improvement in their teaching confidence, self-assessment of teaching behaviors, and student evaluations. In sum, the act and quality of resident teaching is important not only to the sponsoring institutions and residency training programs for accreditation and evaluation purposes but also to the resident for education and development in becoming a competent practicing physician.

THE CONTEXTUAL ENVIRONMENT OF MEDICAL EDUCATION

Historical evidence suggests that the practice of medicine dates back at least 8,000 years but that the first recorded systematic modern education of physicians occurred in about the 10th century in modern Italy (de Divitiis, Cappabianca, & de Divitiis, 2004). The curriculum of the *schola medica salernitana* included poetic verses in Latin of physician precepts as well as a physician's reference book, replete with guidelines for both caring for patients and treating families with respect. Although it is not exactly clear how medical students were trained in the 10th century, it can be assumed that reading, memorization, and some sort of didactics occurred even at this early stage of medical education. In modern times, educational research and practice have had an impact on medical education in myriad ways, from over a century of journal clubs to over four decades of problem-based learning. Presented below are some of the major instructional strategies utilized in today's graduate medical education settings in which residents commonly find themselves in teaching roles.

Instructional Strategies in Medical Education

One-Minute Preceptor Model (OMP)

The intent of the OMP is to help the teacher to diagnose both the student and the patient (Irby, Aagaard, & Teherani, 2004). The OMP provides the teacher with a script, which follows a five-step process, as follows:

1. Obtain a commitment from the student as to what he or she thinks is occurring with the patient.
2. Probe for the underlying reasoning on the part of the student as to what leads to his or her conclusion.
3. Teach the student a general rule.
4. Provide positive feedback.
5. Correct mistakes. The student's performance on Steps 1 and 2 will drive the general rule taught in Step 3. The OMP is generally viewed to be an efficient and effective instructional method in clinical settings. Table 1 displays the five-step process for implementing OMP (Irby et al., 2004).

Traditional Preceptor Model (TP)

The traditional preceptor model (TP) is more narrowly focused on patient diagnosis. The preceptor asks a series of questions about the patient to diagnose the patient's problem (Irby et al., 2004). Although it

Table 1. The one-minute preceptor: Five-step process (Adapted from Irby et al., 2004)

Step	Description	Action
1	Get a commitment	Ask the leaner to articulate his or her diagnosis or plan
2	Probe for supporting evidence	Evaluate the learner's knowledge or reasoning
3	Teach general rules	Teach the learner common take-home points that can be used in future cases, aimed preferably at an area of weakness for the learner
4	Reinforce correct actions	Reinforce what was done well; provide positive feedback
5	Correct mistakes	Provide constructive feedback with recommendations for improvement

can function well in a confirmative way to assess correct/incorrect diagnoses, one criticism of the TP is that it does not allow for an effective understanding of the decision-making process of medical students.

SNAPPS

Used commonly in the outpatient setting, SNAPPS, an acronym for summarize, narrow, analyze, probe, plan, and select, is a collaborative model for case presentations. It links "learner initiation and preceptor facilitation in an active learning conversation" (Wolpaw, Wolpaw, & Papp, 2003, p. 893). Table 2 presents the SNAPPS six-step process:

Simulations

1. **High Fidelity:** Simulation involves the immersion of a student in a realistic scenario created within a physical space that replicates all or part of the real environment (Doherty-Restrepo & Tivener, 2014). High-fidelity simulations replicate real-world settings and situations to such a high degree that a suspension of disbelief can occur in the medical student, and he or she can be fully "immersed" in the simulation. For example, computer-based human-patient simulators recreate physiological signs and symptoms based on educational goals, using a realistic mannequin. High-fidelity simulations typically include a debriefing session to reinforce learning objectives through reflection and consideration of alternative actions in the future.
2. **Low Fidelity:** Low-fidelity simulation includes the use of instructional tools such as partial anatomical models, role-playing with peers, and simpler mannequins with low-fidelity capabilities

Table 2. SNAPPS Process (Wolpaw et al., 2003)

Step	Action
1	Summarize the case history and findings
2	Narrow the differential to two or three possibilities
3	Analyze the differential by comparing and contrasting the possibilities
4	Probe the preceptor by asking questions about any uncertainties, difficulties, or alternative approaches
5	Plan the management for the patient's medical issues
6	Select a case-related issue for self-directed learning

(Doherty-Restrepo & Tivener, 2014). One critique is that these elements do not provide medical students with the level of fidelity to become "immersed" in the simulation. However, for basic factual and conceptual content, such as gross anatomy and physiology, low-fidelity simulations can be effective instructional strategies.

Objective Structured Clinical Examinations (OSCEs)

These programs offer a way to evaluate medical students' clinical competence in an objective manner, using well-prepared clinical components. OSCE components may include such topics as auscultation of the heart, taking a medical history, interpreting an ECG, or determining a diagnosis (Harden & Gleeson, 1979). These components are assessed in order and are the focus of each station in the examination. The medical student travels from station to station for a specified amount of time at each, with typically no more than 20 stations total included in the evaluation.

SOAPS

SOAPS provide teachers with a critical evaluation method of an oral case presentation (Green, 2006). SOAPS is an acronym for the five parts of the method: (a) Story represents how well the student describes the details of the patient's case; (b) Organization represents how well the student presents the facts so that they are easily understood; (c) Argument is the effectiveness of the presentation for the diagnosis, limited differential, and/or plan; (d) Pertinence concerns the alignment of the content of the presentation to the facts of the case and the elimination of those that are not pertinent; and (e) Speech is the fact that the case presentation is verbal and that verbal presentation has an identifiably different effect than does a written presentation.

Feedback

Research has shown that feedback is a powerful variable that has an impact on learning outcomes (Clark, 2008). In medical education, this manifests in many ways, often in information being given to students in regard to their performance on a given task. Feedback that is provided immediately and that incorporates specific information can have a profound impact on student learning. The use of feedback is not for evaluative purposes but, rather, to guide future behaviors in a given activity in the correct manner. As noted by Ende (1983), "Once the nature of the feedback process is appreciated, however, especially the distinction between feedback and evaluation and the importance of focusing on the trainees' observable behaviors rather than on the trainees themselves, the educational benefit of feedback can be realized" (p. 777). Ende provided guidelines for providing feedback for medical educators, in that it should:

1. Be undertaken with the teacher and trainee working as allies, with common goals.
2. Be well-timed and expected.
3. Be based on first-hand data.
4. Be regulated in quantity and limited to behaviors that are remediable.
5. Be phrased in descriptive, non-evaluative language.
6. Deal with specific performances, not generalizations.
7. Offer subjective data, labeled as such.

8. Deal with decisions and actions, rather than assumed intentions or interpretations.

Audio-Visual Strategies

It is common for medical students to prefer watching video lectures to attending lectures in person, and students expect technology to allow for a high-speed playback of video lectures to reduce time spent watching them. In this regard, the use of video in lectures has been the subject of research for over a decade, with results that show no decrease in learning or slight increases (Bridge, Jackson, & Robinson, 2009). As such, the use of PowerPoint, YouTube, and other tools has become ubiquitous in medical education. These tools provide teachers with endless variations and content delivery options to create high-quality instruction. Although PowerPoint, or a similar presentation tool, helps to capture and present content in a professional manner, by itself, it does not offer distinct instructional advantages. In fact, the "misuse" of PowerPoint, for example by presenting "walls of text" on a slide and simply reading it to students, can impede learning (Clark & Mayer, 2011). Instead, instructional models, such as multi-media learning theory, should be used to help design effective audio-visual presentations. Further, guides that focus on presentation quality are readily available to teachers.

Lecture

The traditional lecture has been a cornerstone of instruction in medical education from time immemorial, and the utilization of technology for learning is no longer an innovational ideal; rather, it is an expectation of millennial learners. Although many medical schools and residency programs still structure curricula and program didactics, using passive lecture techniques, others are transitioning to recording live lectures and offering students an opportunity to view them online. Many medical school lecture halls are nearly empty, as this generation of learners opts to watch "streaming" lectures by themselves or with other medical students. Some researchers are calling for online mini-lectures in "flipped classroom" settings (Prober & Heath, 2012), which call for students to view content online and participate in problem- and case-based learning or other interactive activities during classroom time. Preparing educational presentations and developing flipped classroom activities to teach medical students or visiting resident rotators is a rich teaching opportunity for residents, who can reinforce their own learning of specialty content through developing such presentations and activities.

Conferences

Attendance at medical conferences plays an important role in the education of the resident and medical student. Conferences allow students, as presenters, to disseminate information, such as the results of research study required by the residency program, and become part of the community of research contributors to the field. As attendees, conferences allows students to gain knowledge through attending relevant presentations, to network with colleagues, and to discern the culture of profession practice. Finally, conferences provide an opportunity for students to become more engaged with the organization that is running the conference and to explore membership and potential volunteer positions in the future.

Journal Club

Journal clubs have been used as an instructional strategy in North American since at least 1875 (Linzer, 1987). Residency programs typically schedule journal club meetings for students to discuss and review articles in current medical journals for the potential of applying the articles' findings in clinical settings. Residents and fellows, and occasionally medical students, are typically charged with preparing a presentation for the selected article and facilitating discussion and critique of the content with attending faculty, residents, and medical students. One additional instruction use of journal clubs is to nurture the "critical appraisal skills" of the presenters and other learners.

Morbidity and Mortality (M&M) Sessions

These sessions allow residents and faculty to discuss cases in which patient M&M occurred. In these sessions, students can review the actions taken in the cases, discuss any errors, and increase their conceptual understanding of the situation and outcomes. M&M sessions also can model career-long learning for medical education learners (Ferguson et al., 2016).

Problem-Based Learning (PBL)

Hmelo-Silver (2004) defined PBL as "focused experiential learning organized around the investigation, explanation, and resolution of meaningful problems" (p. 236). PBL is characterized by four features (Clark, 2008):

1. A student-centered approach that relies on the learner to identify and review knowledge needed to resolve a case;
2. Use of an authentic problem introduced to the tutorial group prior to any preparation or study;
3. Synchronous, small-group, collaborative work supported by a faculty facilitator, combined with self-directed study to investigate learning issues that arise from problem discussion; and
4. Use of the problem and tutorial discussion of the problem as vehicles to identify the required knowledge (facts and concepts) as well as problem-solving skills to resolve it.

PBL differs from "traditional" strategies in that it places students into small groups, uses cases as instructional prompts, and incorporates student self-study to explore and determine answers to the case problem. Thus, students are self-directed and learn from each other as part of the group dynamic. Teachers act more as guides than is seen a traditional model. This approach parallels other modern approaches to instruction, such as discovery, enquiry, experiential, and constructivist learning (Neville, 2009).

Contextual Environments for Medical Education

Decades of research have shown that the environment in which learning occurs can have a profound impact on learning outcomes. Indeed, the learning environment should be a core consideration in the design of instruction. Resident-teachers must provide instruction to medical students in a variety of clinical learning environments. The majority of interactions between resident-teachers and medical students take place in the hospital and ambulatory clinic settings, where medical students are often supervised and taught by residents. These clinical learning environments are varied and differ by locale (e.g., urban, suburban, rural), institutional affiliation (e.g., academic medical center, community or university hospital), patient population characteristics (e.g., insured/uninsured, race, culture, gender, educational level, socioeconomic status), and other variables.

Clinical learning environments in medical education typically include inpatient (i.e., hospital wards and operating rooms), outpatient (e.g., ambulatory clinics, outpatient surgery centers), and community settings and classrooms. These clinical learning environments include patients in need of care provided by a health care team that will vary significantly in both size and experience, depending on the setting. Medical student involvement in the ambulatory setting can vary greatly, from one-on-one instruction with a resident to a larger team structure. Hospital clinical teaching sites in academic medical centers may include single-specialty or interdisciplinary patient care teams inclusive of medical students, residents, fellows, and other health care students (e.g., nursing, pharmacy, social work, nutritionist) in addition to rotating residents from other programs and medical students from other institutions. A small community hospital patient care team may include a faculty member, resident, and medical student.

Medical *teaching rounds* vary in content and approach, and the roles of the resident-teacher and medical student also vary, depending on structure and setting. *Bedside rounds* may include a traditional teaching format whereby the admitting medical student or resident presents to his or her teacher and team in front of the patient. In *table rounds*, the admitting medical student or resident presents the patient to the teacher and team during a meeting prior to rounding on the patient floor. *Hall rounds* call for the admitting medical student or resident to present the patient to his or her teacher and team in the hall prior to patient encounter. A surgical program's *morning report* may include a presentation from the resident who was on call the night before, reviewing the patient x-rays, workup, and plan prior to seeing the patient with the rounding team. Faculty either confirm or adjust the plan, post-patient exam. Each of these and other rounding protocols offer a rich opportunity for the employment of both cognitive and behavioral instructional strategies.

Residents and fellow-teachers also provide a significant portion of formal didactics to medical students and other residents. Journal club, M&M, grand rounds, and board examination preparation sessions are routinely dependent on presentations and facilitation by residents and fellows. Residents begin teaching and supervising medical students as early as their first day in the program. Complex teaching environments such as these are challenging for the experienced teacher and even more so for the newly enrolled resident or fellow-teacher who is aiming to master the knowledge and skills required of his or her medical specialty while simultaneously acting as a teacher to medical students and junior residents.

LEARNING THEORIES, INSTRUCTION, AND INSTRUCTIONAL STRATEGIES

Instruction deals directly with improving learners' knowledge, skills, or abilities (KSAs). It is the deliberate arrangement of learning events to facilitate a learner's acquisition of KSAs to support learning objectives. An instructional strategy is a specific technique that teachers use to actively engage students in the learning process. For example, role-play is an effective instructional technique to allow residents to practice discussing a diagnosis and discussing treatment options with a patient.

A learning theory is a set of general principles or ideas that relate to how we interpret, process, and retain information. These theories help us to frame our thinking around the design of instruction and to approach ways to understand how learning occurs in adult learners, who come with their own set of experience and knowledge. Learning theories include principles, guidelines, or beliefs about how learning takes place. Many learning theories are supported by research, and others are more philosophical in nature. Learning theories can be descriptive, working to explain how something occurs. They also can be prescriptive, offering procedures and frameworks for designing instruction with predictive learning outcomes.

In working with residents to improve their teaching skills, the authors have found that presenting a comparison of pedagogy and andragogy is particularly effective. The primary reason for this is that pedagogy is the educational approach with which many already are familiar, and, thus, it can be used as a starting point to conceptualize andragogy. Although neither approach is particularly complex, the philosophical framework of andragogy and, specifically, the idea of residents as adult learners who bring with them a rich mélange of prior experiences, knowledge, and skills helps to crystallize residents' perspective of their learners as self-directed participants. Further, in making the transition from the undergraduate medical education classroom context to clinical learning environments, there is an expectation that students will take responsibility for their own learning and become self-motivated, lifelong learners. The principles of andragogy reinforce these expectations for both the undergraduate medical education student and resident-teacher.

Table 3. provides a comparison of the approaches of pedagogy and andragogy. *Pedagogy* is considered to be the art, science, or profession of teaching. Although, in a historical sense, the term has been focused on the application of teaching children (Greek: *Pedo* or *paedo* means "relating to children"), it is widely used in educational settings to broadly refer to any approach of educators to teaching. In the traditional view of pedagogy, the learner is assumed to have little experience upon which to base new learning. Hence, the learner is viewed as being dependent on the teacher, who is ultimately responsible for the learner's success or failure. This makes the role of the teacher to be of prime importance and influence on learning. In pedagogy, the teacher, or the overarching system of education, evaluates the learner's performance. *Andragogy* is the art and science of helping adults to learn (Knowles, Holton, & Swanson, 2014). A core aspect of this help is the understanding on the part of the teacher that adult learners bring a wealth and diversity of prior experience and knowledge. The role of the teacher as the prime influence on learning is greatly diminished, as the learner and his or her peers are also key resources in learning. In effect, the learner is ultimately responsibility for learning, not the teacher. Thus, self-evaluation is typically the approach used to assess learning outcomes.

It is important to note that andragogy considers an adult learner as being part of a lifelong learning process somewhere along a continuum of being more or less self-directed and dependent on the learning situation and familiarity with the content, context, and pre-existing subject knowledge, as well as

Table 3. Pedagogy and andragogy

Pedagogy	Andragogy
The art, science, or profession of teaching	The art and science of helping adults learn
Learner has little experience	Learner brings volume/quality of experience
Experience of instructor is most influential	Adults bring diversity of experience; are rich resources for one another
The learner is dependent	The learner is self-directed
Teacher is responsible for what is learned	Learner is responsible for what is learned
Teacher evaluates learning	Self-evaluation is a characteristic approach

on other factors. Along this continuum, several factors have an impact on resident-teachers' approach to teaching medical students and junior residents.

Concept of the Medical Student Learner

During the process of maturation, a person moves from dependency toward increasing self-directedness, but at different rates for different people and in different dimensions of life. As part of the teaching process, resident-teachers have a responsibility to encourage and nurture this movement in medical students and junior resident learners. Adults have a deep psychological need to be generally self-directing, but they may be dependent in certain temporary situations. This dependency is particularly poignant for third-year medical students and first-year residents or interns, who are entering the clinical learning environment with little or limited experience in the role of physician.

Role of Medical Students' Experience

As medical students grow and develop, they accumulate an increasing reservoir of experience that becomes a progressively rich resource for learning, for themselves and for others. Further, in practical fields such as medicine, people tend to better retain the learning that they gain from experience as compared to learning settings that simply provide a description of activities. Accordingly, the primary techniques in medical education are experiential ones, such as laboratory experiments, discussion, problem-solving cases, and field experiences.

Readiness to Learn

People become ready to learn something when they experience a need to learn it to cope more satisfyingly with real-life tasks and problems. The resident-teacher has a responsibility to create conditions and provide tools and procedures for helping learners discover their "need to know." Learning programs should be organized around life-application categories and sequenced according to the learners' readiness to learn.

Orientation to Learning

Learners see education as a process of developing increased competence to achieve their full potential in life. They want to be able to apply whatever knowledge and skill they gain today to living more effectively tomorrow. Medical students want to learn, then apply. Accordingly, learning experiences should be organized around competency-development categories, such as the six core competencies identified by the ACGME (medical knowledge, patient care, practice-based learning, interpersonal and communication skills, professionalism, and systems-based practice). Competencies, once established, are easy to evaluate. The establishment of competencies reinforces the performance-centric aspect of medical education as well as students' orientation to learning.

Motivation to Learn

As learners shift to being more self-directed as a result of accumulated knowledge and experience, there is a natural shift from the need for extrinsic motivation as provided by the teacher or system to intrinsic motivation. Typically, by the time a medical student has entered residency, his or her intrinsic motivation is well established. Nevertheless, the modes and strategies used by resident-teachers help to establish the path and behaviors to becoming a lifelong learner for other residents and can set expectations for progressively intrinsic motivation.

Behavior-Based Instructional Strategies for Resident Teaching

Behaviorism, resulting largely from the seminal work of Skinner in the mid-20th century, has provided a rich set of strategies that are still relevant to resident teaching today. These strategies include shaping, chaining, and fading.

Shaping

Shaping is the reinforcement of sequential steps toward the desired (goal) behavior. Each success is reinforced immediately, and then the next goal is established. This process then continues until the ultimate goal is reached. In medical education, an example of shaping can be found in a medical student's development of a patient presentation and the resulting "shaping" of presentation behavior by the resident-teacher or faculty member. The inclusion of necessary information is positively reinforced by a senior learner (i.e., resident or faculty), and when unable to provide the necessary information, the student may rely on senior colleagues to provide answers that elude them or to supplement their knowledge using evidence-based online tools. In shaping, reinforcement is delivered immediately, based on the desired response. The desired outcome is that the medical student is able to provide a cohesive patient presentation that relays the pertinent information for the patient's care.

Chaining

Chaining is used to establish complex behaviors that are comprised of discrete, simpler behaviors already known to the learner. Each step may be acquired through shaping, and then steps are linked together in sequence to form complex behaviors. Surgical simulators are an excellent medium for employment of this strategy. Each surgical step may be repeated multiple times until the learner gains proficiency under the direction of a senior resident or faculty member. As each sequential step is mastered, new steps are introduced for practice toward mastery. Low-fidelity simulations, for example, can benefit from chaining strategies, as students can practice simple suturing and knot techniques with simulation kits and build their repertoire of more complex sutures over time with frequent practice and feedback. Simulated environments are ideal for chaining strategies, as they allow for frequent practice and error reduction without harm to patients. Learners may progress from simulation to actual patient care once deemed efficient enough to practice under direct supervision.

Fading

Fading occurs when the desired behavior of the learner continues to be reinforced as the discriminate cues are gradually withdrawn. For example, verbal cues can be gradually reduced as performance proficiency increases. Non-verbal fading can occur as well, and procedural text-based job aids can be used until tasks are mastered. In medical education, examples of fading can be found in the level of verbal and physical support provided during procedures and diagnoses. The instructor should begin to fade support with small cases, simple procedures, and common diagnoses as the learner gains confidence and knowledge. Instructors should reduce verbal repetition of steps to make a diagnosis and should request that the learner fill in first or next steps. If job aids are utilized, their use can be minimized over time as the student masters the content, whereby the instructor regresses from describing each step/ task. Procedural physical support also should be withdrawn over time as learner competence increases, with the instructor's first modeling procedures, then allowing the student to perform the first and then subsequent steps as the student becomes proficient.

Behavior-Based Performance Management

These strategies can be very effective in helping to achieve desired performance outcomes. Additionally, behavior-based strategies are especially suited for a struggling learner as a form of formal remediation or probation. Ideally, they should be used as part of an instructional "tool set" to be implemented, as they support specific objectives. Having a strategy for the creation of goals and ways to support students' accomplishment is important. Below are the steps for creating a goal-specific, behavior-based instructional management program (Driscoll, 2004).

Step 1: Set behavioral goals.
Step 2: Determine appropriate reinforcers.
Step 3: Select appropriate procedures for changing behaviors.
Step 4: Implement procedures and record results.
Step 5: Evaluate progress and revise as necessary.

See the Behaviorist-Based Instructional Strategies Worksheet (Worksheet 1) in Appendix 1 for an example of a job aid that can assist residents in creating a Behavior-Based Instructional Management Program.

Cognitive-Based Instructional Strategies for Resident Teaching

Cognitive-based instructional strategies focus on the support and development of mental models or schemas in learners. These schemas are, in essence, "bits" of information that help the learner to formulate the ways in which they understand their world. Cognitive-based instructional strategies are based in an information-processing perspective and concern ways to maximize learners' selection of appropriate information, processing, retention, and transfer.

Modeling

In modeling, an expert performs a specific activity as the student observes. Through observation, a student builds a conceptual model of the process (schema-building). This is a steppingstone for the student to be able to perform the behavior. In medical education, medical students frequently assume the observer role prior to participating in the care of the patient during their clinical rotations. This modeling structure is inherent in the medical education hierarchy, in which a third-year medical student is paired with a resident or attending physician. Pairings create opportunities for residents and fellows to reinforce their own learning through instructional planning and strategies to teach medical students while reinforcing their fund of knowledge as they assume the role of teacher through the modeling of exemplary behaviors.

Coaching

Coaching involves the resident-teacher's observing the student, providing feedback, hints, or reminders, and then assignment of new tasks. The teacher aims to bring students closer to an expert level of performance. Hospital and clinical settings provide ample opportunity for employment of coaching techniques in medical education. Ambulatory clinic, pre- and post-operative patient encounters, procedural and operative encounters, and didactic settings all allow for observation of student participation in patient care, the opportunity to question the students' decision making and/or treatment planning, teacher provision of constructive feedback, and the provision of instructions for additional knowledge seeking to enhance the medical students' performance (e.g., additional reading, practice suturing, simulation activities).

Scaffolding

Scaffolding can be thought of as any instructional support mechanism that helps a student along the path to achieving a goal. The resident-teacher can provide support, suggestions, assistance, reciprocal teaching, or physical support. Support is provided for only the specific part of the task that the student cannot yet manage. Similar to fading, there is a gradual removal of these supports over time. Thus, an accurate diagnosis of the student's skill level is required of the resident-teacher. In medical education, scaffolding strategies are particularly suitable for the operating room (OR). For example, the teacher begins by providing cognitive "think aloud" strategies while performing the procedure to educate students on the physical aspects of the procedure as well as the knowledge recall and decision-making processes required. The instructor gradually reduces verbal descriptions and physical support in the OR as the students' skills progress. As students become more competent, they should begin to provide their own cognitive "think-aloud" strategies to junior learners and begin to assume the role of teacher.

Articulation

This strategy requires students to verbally communicate with or respond to a resident-teacher in an attempt to verify that the student's level of understanding and knowledge are relevant to the topic being discussed. The resident-teacher calls on students to articulate knowledge, reasoning, and problem solving as well as asks questions (e.g., to compare and contrast). The resident-teacher also can ask students to perform a think-aloud, which allows for insights into students' thought processes beyond factual knowledge. In addition, the resident-teacher can ask a student to assume the role of critic. In medical education, an example of articulation is a surgical case discussion at the scrub sink or in the surgical staff room, whereby the student articulates the differential diagnosis, pathophysiology, and surgical plan for the patient to the teacher. The resident-teacher may ask the student to compare this case to another, contrasting diagnosis, pathophysiology, and surgical plan. The student also may be asked to provide a list of potential complications for this type of case, comparing potential reactions or prescribed indications should such complications arise.

Reflection

Reflection allows students to have an abstracted replay of events. The student may compare his or her problem-solving process with others' processes. The resident-teacher should supply expert feedback in this process to enhance learning. In medical education, an example of reflection is asking the student to review the most challenging and/or meaningful case of the day, reflecting on his or her decision-making processes, reactions, emotions, lessons learned, and things to be done differently should such a case appear again. This reflection can be face-to-face or recorded in a journal or portfolio format for later review and discussion. It is important for the student and teacher to discuss student reflections, as guidance and examples should be provided by the instructor for reinforcement of ideal behaviors, to aid in retention, and to provide constructive feedback for improvement.

Exploration

In exploration, the resident-teacher "pushes" the student into active problem solving. Pushing the student with exploration is critical, as it moves the student into areas outside his or her comfort zone. The resident-teacher needs to "fade" in problem solving, based on the specific goals of the instruction and content. In medical education, an example of exploration may be found in the teaching of strategies when students are "on call." When a student calls a senior colleague for guidance when he or she is on call, an opportune teaching moment evolves. The instructor may force and strengthen critical problem-solving skills by pushing the student to explore potential diagnoses, treatment strategies, and communication plans. This teaching strategy empowers the student to recall medical knowledge and to call upon previous learning and experiences to reach conclusions that, at first, seemed out of reach. Feedback must be provided, but is withheld until the student has reached the limits of his or her knowledge and capabilities.

See the Cognitive-Based Instructional Strategies Worksheet (Worksheet 2) in Appendix 2 for an example of a job aid that can assist residents in creating a Cognitive-Based Instructional Management Program.

DEVELOPING A RESIDENT TEACHING PLAN

Kern, Thomas, and Hughes (2010) developed a six-step process to help medical education administrators develop a sound medical education curriculum. This structure provides a valuable resource for analyzing a residency program's current state of preparedness to teach residents to teach. The authors have adapted Kern et al.'s format by adding descriptions and questions to assist in designing a formal curriculum to train residents to teach others. The steps of the process are presented below.

Step 1: Problem Identification and General Needs Assessment.

Step 2: Needs Assessment of Targeted Members.
Step 3: Goals and Objectives.
Step 4: Instructional Strategies.
Step 5: Implementation.
Step 6: Evaluation and Feedback.

The first step ensures that the residency program identifies the general need for a "Teaching Residents How to Teach" curriculum. This is followed by the second step, a needs assessment of the medical education stakeholders who are affected by resident-teachers. In the third step, the goals and objectives are designed and developed in alignment with the identified needs of the residency program and its stakeholders. The fourth step entails the design and development of appropriate instructional strategies. It is essential that current program instructional strategies be compared with ideal instructional strategies for the medical specialty when completing this step. Clinical learning environment contexts also must be considered when designing these strategies, with the aim of facilitating utilization of appropriate and efficient teaching methods for individual program characteristics. The fifth step of the process is the implementation of the "Teaching Residents to Teach" curriculum and requires identification of resource availability and allocation, barriers to implementation, and identification of plans to communicate the curriculum to program stakeholders. The sixth and final step of the curriculum development process is the development and implementation of a curriculum evaluation plan and provision of feedback to improve individual participant and program curriculum performance. Table 4 presents this six-step process for the development of a "Teaching Resident How to Teach" curriculum.

See the Six-Step Approach to Developing a Curriculum to Train Residents to Teach (Worksheet 3) in Appendix 3 for an example of a job aid that can assist residency programs in creating a curriculum

FUTURE RESEARCH DIRECTIONS

Resident preparedness to teach medical students is required by both undergraduate and graduate medical education accreditation authorities. Fulfillment of an accreditation requirement must not be the only aim in developing a curriculum to teach residents to teach, however; rather, the goals for the educational process must be to train outstanding resident-teachers who are actively engaged in developing and evolving their teaching skills in a meaningful and purposeful way. The ultimate aim should be to cultivate lifelong learning skills and intrinsic motivation for continued participation in expanding the teaching capabilities of our future physician workforce.

There are many published works that provide a description of specific instructional strategies in the clinical learning environment, including those that pertain to effective feedback (Gigante, Dell, & Sharkey, 2010), teaching rounds (Irby & Wilkerson, 2008; Ramani, 2003), teaching models (Furney et al., 2001), simulation (Pian-Smith et al., 2009), operating room teaching (Roberts, Brenner, Williams, Kim, & Dunnington, 2012), and evidence-based teaching skills (Smith et al., 2000). Programs developed to teach residents to teach, however, are fewer and often specialty-specific (Edwards, Kissling, Brannan, Plauche, & Marier, 2008; Jewett, Greenberg, & Goldberg, 1982; White, Bassali, & Heery, 1997). Translational research that engages subject-matter experts in both instructional technology and clinical teaching are needed to establish and share best practices for teaching residents to teach in clinical learning environments and contexts.

Table 4. Six-Step approach to developing a curriculum to train residents to teach (adapted from Kern et al., 2010)

Step	Step Description	Residency Program Questions
1. Problem Identification and General Needs Assessment	Describe the problem and determine the general need to "Teach Residents to Teach" 3. Medical education accreditation agencies (i.e., Accreditation Council for Graduate Medical Education and Liaison Committee on Medical Education) require that residents receive instruction on how to teach 4. Residents must learn to be effective teachers in multiple settings	• What is currently being done by our program to teach residents how to teach? • What personal and environmental factors affect our ability to teach residents to teach (e.g., availability of teaching experts, faculty time, internal/external resources available)? • Ideally, what should be done by whom?
2. Needs Assessment of Targeted Members	Conduct a needs assessment of stakeholders affected by resident-teachers in the clinical learning environment 6. Identify the learners who are taught by your program's residents 7. Identify the needs of each learner group 8. Define the role of resident-teachers in your program 9. Define the needs and expectations of program administration and faculty relative to resident teaching 10. Determine the needs of your resident-teachers	.........• Whom will our residents teach (e.g., medical student, junior residents, residents rotating from other programs, patients, families, other healthcare team members)? • What must our residents teach to whom? • How will the program align faculty and resident-teacher roles and responsibilities? • Do our residents have previous training and experience in teaching others? • What existing proficiencies exist: cognitive, affective, psychomotor skills and abilities? • What is the current performance level of our resident-teachers? • What are the perceived deficiencies and learning needs of our resident-teachers? • What are the preferences and experiences of our residents-teachers and students regarding different learning strategies? • What are the characteristics of the learners/curriculum/clinical learning environment? • What are the needs of our learners, and what must they know (e.g., medical students, patients, residents)? • What resources are available to our resident-teachers? • What resources are available to our learners?
3. Goals and Objectives	Develop a reasonable number goals and objectives for the "Teaching Residents to Teach" curriculum 5. Ensure that these goals and objectives are SMART (Specific, Measurable, Achievable, Realistic, and Time-Bound) 6. Ensure that these goals and objectives align to the needs identified in Step 2 7. Ensure that these goals and objectives address deficits identified in the previous curriculum 8. Ensure that these goals and objectives consider all of the clinical learning contexts in which residents will teach	• Is each goal and objective SMART? • What outcomes need to be accomplished (goals) in our teaching residents to teach program? • How will these outcomes be measured? • What objectives support the goal(s)? • Which objectives align to the needs identified in Step 2? • Which objectives address deficits identified in Step 2? • What indicators can be used to assess accomplishment of goals? • Are all of the residency program learning contexts identified and addressed?
4. Instructional Strategies	Determine the ideal instructional strategies for teaching residents to teach, considering your program's clinical learning environment contexts 6. Select curriculum content to teach residents to teach 7. Use Worksheets #1 and #2 to identify relevant instructional strategies 8. Select appropriate instructional strategies for each clinical learning environment context and desired KSAs 9. Identify current best teaching practices in your specialty and program 10. Determine which current strategies are ineffective	• What varieties of instructional methods can be used? • Which specific instructional methods can be used: Readings, lectures, discussion, PBL, programmed learning; learning projects; role models; demonstration, artificial models, role plays, standardized patients, clinical experiences; audio/video review of learner; group learning; behavioral interventions? • What are the ideal instructional strategies in our medical specialty? • What are the successful instructional strategies used in our program? Inefficient strategies? • What are the key differences between our current and the ideal approach to teaching residents to teach? • Which instructional strategies in our program should be abandoned? Which should be retained and enhanced?
5. Implementation	Implement your "Teaching Residents to Teach" curriculum 7. Procure support for curriculum implementation 8. Identify and procure resources 9. Identify and address barriers to implementation 10. Introduction of curriculum 11. Administration of curriculum 12. Refinement of curriculum over several cycles	• What resources support this curriculum? • How and when can these resources be obtained? • What are the administrative mechanisms to support the curriculum? • What barriers to curriculum implementation exist, and how can they be addressed? • How should the curriculum be communicated and to which program stakeholders?
6. Evaluation and Feedback	Design, develop and implement an evaluation plan to assess curriculum outcomes and provide feedback for improvement 5. Assess performance of the resident-teachers 6. Assess performance of the curriculum 7. Identify ethical concerns 8. Collect and analyze data; report results	• Who are the users, uses, and resources for evaluation? • How will formative and summative evaluation work at individual and program levels? • What are the resources, evaluation questions, and evaluation design? • What are the measurement methods and instruments?

This chapter presented an approach that can be used across medical specialties to design, develop, implement, and evaluate curricula to "Teach Residents to Teach" while taking into consideration the unique aspects of a department's clinical learning environment context. Future research directions for the development of "Teach Residents to Teach" curricula should include reports of the outcomes of such tailored educational programs that aim to identify best practices that can be utilized to enhance future program curriculum development in medical specialties as well as provide templates for general application.

CONCLUSION

Medical schools must ensure that medical students are taught by qualified faculty and residents who participate in activities that aim to enhance their teaching and assessment skills. LCME reported that "resident preparation" was one of the most common noncompliance citations seen in full survey reports from 2010 to 2013 (Barzansky, 2013). Residents provide a significant proportion of medical student teaching in the clinical learning environment (Wilson, 2007) and, as such, hold an opportunity to have a significant impact on the clinical rotation and didactic teaching culture as well as medical student learning outcomes. Implementing a formal program to teach residents how to teach could have longitudinal effects on the medical education teaching environment in addition to instilling a generation of physician-teachers with a sound foundation of evidence-based teaching practices.

If residents are engaged in becoming effective teachers, the clinical learning environment is improved in multiple ways. First, clinical rotation educational experiences and didactics are enhanced through utilization of appropriate and efficient instructional strategies. Second, employment of effective teaching strategies by residents provides opportunity to increase their own retention of essential medical knowledge while simultaneously improving medical student educational experiences, medical knowledge, and patient care skills. Finally, training multiple cohorts of effective resident-teachers creates the potential to enhance the departmental teaching culture and to increase all stakeholders' investment in creating and maintaining a robust clinical learning environment. The proposed approach to develop curriculum aimed to teach residents to become effective teachers utilizes principles of adult learning theory and acknowledges unique aspects of individual clinical learning environments to design tailored, evidence-based curriculum for residency programs.

REFERENCES

Accreditation Council for Graduate Medical Education. (2016). *What we do.* Retrieved May 21, 2016, from http://www.acgme.org/What-We-Do/Overview

Barzansky, B. (2013). *Medical school preparation for LCME accreditation.* Wayne State University School of Medicine. Retrieved June 6, 2015, from http://www.lcme.med.wayne.edu/intro.pdf

Bridge, P. D., Jackson, M., & Robinson, L. (2009). The effectiveness of streaming video on medical student learning: A case study. *Medical Education Online*, *14*(0), 11. doi:10.3402/meo.v14i.4506 PMID:20165525

Clark, R. C. (2008). *Building expertise: Cognitive methods for training and performance improvement.* San Francisco, CA: John Wiley & Sons.

Clark, R. C., & Mayer, R. E. (2011). *E-learning and the science of instruction: Proven guidelines for consumers and designers of multimedia learning*. San Francisco, CA: John Wiley & Sons. doi:10.1002/9781118255971

de Divitiis, E., Cappabianca, P., & de Divitiis, O. (2004). The schola medica salernitana: The forerunner of the modern university medical schools. *Neurosurgery*, *55*(4), 722–745. doi:10.1227/01.NEU.0000139458.36781.31 PMID:15458581

Doherty-Restrepo, J. L., & Tivener, K. (2014). Current literature summary: Review of high-fidelity simulation in professional education. *Athletic Training Education Journal*, *9*(4), 190–192. doi:10.4085/0904190

Driscoll, M. P. (2004). *Psychology of learning for instruction* (3rd ed.). Needham Heights, MA: Pearson.

Edwards, J. C., Kissling, G. E., Brannan, J. R., Plauche, W. C., & Marier, R. L. (1988). Study of teaching residents how to teach. *Academic Medicine*, *63*(8), 603–610. doi:10.1097/00001888-198808000-00003 PMID:3398015

Ende, J. (1983). Feedback in clinical medical education. *Journal of the American Medical Association*, *250*(6), 777–781. doi:10.1001/jama.1983.03340060055026 PMID:6876333

Ferguson, C., Inglis, S. C., Newton, P. J., Middleton, S., Macdonald, P. S., & Davidson, P. M. (2016). Education and practice gaps on atrial fibrillation and anticoagulation: A survey of cardiovascular nurses. *BMC Medical Education*, *16*(1), 1–10. doi:10.1186/s12909-015-0504-1 PMID:26758627

Furney, S. L., Orsini, A. N., Orsetti, K. E., Stern, D. T., Gruppen, L. D., & Irby, D. M. (2001). Teaching the one-minute preceptor. *Journal of General Internal Medicine*, *16*(9), 620–624. doi:10.1046/j.1525-1497.2001.016009620.x PMID:11556943

Gigante, J., Dell, M., & Sharkey, A. (2010). Beyond good job: How to give effective feedback. *Pediatrics*, *127*(2), 205–207. doi:10.1542/peds.2010-3351 PMID:21242222

Green, E. H. (2006). *SOAPS to SAFER: A model for teaching and evaluating oral case presentations.* Retrieved April 24, 2016, from https://www.med.unc.edu/aging/fellowship/current/presentations/giving-feedback-on-oral-presentations/making-soaps-safer

Harden, R. M., & Gleeson, F. A. (1979). Assessment of clinical competence using an objective structured clinical examination (OSCE). *Medical Education*, *13*(1), 39–54. doi:10.1111/j.1365-2923.1979.tb00918.x PMID:763183

Hill, A. G., Yu, T. C., Barrow, M., & Hattie, J. (2009). A systematic review of resident-as-teacher programmes. *Medical Education*, *43*(12), 1129–1140. doi:10.1111/j.1365-2923.2009.03523.x PMID:19930503

Hmelo-Silver, C. E. (2004). Problem-based learning: What and how do students learn? *Educational Psychology Review*, *16*(3), 235–266. doi:10.1023/B:EDPR.0000034022.16470.f3

Irby, D. M., Aagaard, E., & Teherani, A. (2004). Teaching points identified by preceptors observing one-minute preceptor and traditional preceptor encounters. *Academic Medicine*, *79*(1), 50–55. doi:10.1097/00001888-200401000-00012 PMID:14690997

Irby, D. M., & Wilkerson, L. (2008). Teaching rounds: Teaching when time is limited. *BMJ: British Medical Journal*, *336*(7640), 384–387. doi:10.1136/bmj.39456.727199.AD PMID:18276715

Jewett, L. S., Greenberg, L. W., & Goldberg, R. M. (1982). Teaching residents how to teach: A one-year study. *Academic Medicine*, *57*(5), 361–366. doi:10.1097/00001888-198205000-00002 PMID:7069756

Kern, D. E., Thomas, P. A., & Hughes, M. T. (Eds.). (2010). *Curriculum development for medical education: a six-step approach*. Baltimore, MD: JHU Press.

Knowles, M. S., Holton, E. F. III, & Swanson, R. A. (2014). *The adult learner: The definitive classic in adult education and human resource development*. New York, NY: Routledge.

Liaison Committee on Medical Education. (2016). *Functions and structure of a medical school*. Retrieved May 14, 2016, from http://lcme.org/publications/

Linzer, M. (1987). The journal club and medical education: Over one hundred years of unrecorded history. *Postgraduate Medical Journal*, *63*(740), 475–478. doi:10.1136/pgmj.63.740.475 PMID:3324090

Morrison, E. H., Friedland, J. A., Boker, J., Rucker, L., Hollingshead, J., & Murata, P. (2001). Residents-as-teachers: Training in US residency programs and offices of graduate medical education. *Academic Medicine*, *76*(10Supplement), S1–S4. doi:10.1097/00001888-200110001-00002 PMID:11597856

Neville, A. J. (2009). Problem-based learning and medical education forty years on. *Medical Principles and Practice*, *18*(1), 1–9. doi:10.1159/000163038 PMID:19060483

Pian-Smith, M. C., Simon, R., Minehart, R. D., Podraza, M., Rudolph, J., Walzer, T., & Raemer, D. (2009). Teaching residents the two-challenge rule: A simulation-based approach to improve education and patient safety. *Simulation in Healthcare*, *4*(2), 84–91. doi:10.1097/SIH.0b013e31818cffd3 PMID:19444045

Prober, C. G., & Heath, C. (2012). Lecture halls without lectures—a proposal for medical education. *The New England Journal of Medicine*, *366*(18), 1657–1659. doi:10.1056/NEJMp1202451 PMID:22551125

Ramani, S. (2003). Twelve tips to improve bedside teaching. *Medical Teacher*, *25*(2), 112–115. doi:10.1080/0142159031000092463 PMID:12745516

Roberts, N. K., Brenner, M. J., Williams, R. G., Kim, M. J., & Dunnington, G. L. (2012). Capturing the teachable moment: A grounded theory study of verbal teaching interactions in the operating room. *Surgery*, *151*(5), 643–650. doi:10.1016/j.surg.2011.12.011 PMID:22244182

Smith, C. A., Ganschow, P. S., Reilly, B. M., Evans, A. T., McNutt, R. A., Osei, A., & Yadav, S. et.al. (2000). Teaching residents evidence-based medicine skills. *Journal of General Internal Medicine*, *15*(10), 710–715. doi:10.1046/j.1525-1497.2000.91026.x PMID:11089714

Wamsley, M. A., Julian, K. A., & Wipf, J. E. (2004). A literature review of resident-as-teacher curricula. *Journal of General Internal Medicine*, *19*(5 Pt. 2), 574–581. doi:10.1111/j.1525-1497.2004.30116.x PMID:15109328

White, C. B., Bassali, R. W., & Heery, L. B. (1997). Teaching residents to teach: An instructional program for training pediatric residents to precept third-year medical students in the ambulatory clinic. *Archives of Pediatrics & Adolescent Medicine*, *151*(7), 730–735. doi:10.1001/archpedi.1997.02170440092016 PMID:9232050

Wilson, F. C. (2007). Teaching by residents. *Clinical Orthopaedics and Related Research*, *454*, 247–250. doi:10.1097/BLO.0b013e31802b4944 PMID:17091017

Wolpaw, T. M., Wolpaw, D. R., & Papp, K. K. (2003). SNAPPS: A learner-centered model for outpatient education. *Academic Medicine*, *78*(9), 893–898. doi:10.1097/00001888-200309000-00010 PMID:14507619

KEY TERMS AND DEFINITIONS

Accreditation Council for Graduate Medical Education (ACGME): An internationally recognized accreditation authority for graduate medical education residency and fellowship programs in the United States.

Andragogy: The art and science of helping adults learn.

Instruction: The deliberate arrangement of learning events to facilitate a learner's acquisition of knowledge, skills, or abilities to support learning objectives.

Instructional Strategies: Specific techniques that teachers use to support students' in the selection, interpretation, retention, and transfer in the learning process.

Liaison Committee on Medical Education (LCME): The nationally recognized accreditation authority for medical education programs that lead to the medical doctor (M.D.) degree in the United States and Canada.

Learning Theory: A set of general principles or ideas that relate to how we interpret, process, and retain information.

Objective Structured Clinical Examinations (OSCEs): These programs offer a way to evaluate medical students' clinical competence in an objective manner, using well-prepared clinical components.

One-Minute Preceptor Model (OMP): This helps the teacher to diagnose both the student and the patient and provides the teacher with a script that follows a five-step process.

Pedagogy: The art, science, or profession of teaching.

Problem-Based Learning (PBL): Focused experiential learning organized around the investigation, explanation, and resolution of meaningful problems.

SOAPS: A critical evaluation method of an oral case presentation. SOAPS is an acronym for story, organization, argument, pertinence, and speech.

SNAPPS: A collaborative model for case presentations. SNAPPS is an acronym for summarize, narrow, analyze, probe, plan, and select.

APPENDIX 1

Table 5. Worksheet 1: Behavior–Based Instructional Strategies

Instructional Strategy	Description of the Strategy	Where and When can/do I use It? In What Clinical/Didactic Setting? List Faculty Members and Resident Best Practices
Shaping	• Reinforcement of successive approximations to goal behavior • Closer approximation to the goal should not be reinforced until the previous goal has been firmly established • Reinforcement is delivered immediately contingent upon the desired response	
Chaining	• Used to establish complex behaviors made up of discrete, simpler behaviors already known to the learner • Each step may be acquired through shaping, then steps are linked together in sequence to form complex behaviors	
Fading	• The desired behavior continues to be reinforced as the discriminate cues are gradually withdrawn • Gradual reduction of verbal cues as proficiency increases • Written job aids that can be used until tasks are mastered	
Behavior Management Program	• Set behavioral goals • Determine appropriate reinforcers • Select appropriate procedures for changing behavior • Implement procedures and record results • Evaluate progress and revise as necessary	

(Adapted from Driscoll, 2004)

APPENDIX 2

Table 6. Worksheet 2: Cognitive-Based Instructional Strategies

Instructional Strategy	Description of the Strategy	Where and when can/do I use it? In what clinical/didactic setting? List Faculty Members and Resident Best Practices
Modeling	• Expert performance, student observes • Student builds conceptual model of the process • Student learns behavior	
Coaching	• Teacher observes student and offers hints, feedback, reminders, new tasks • Teacher aims to bring student performance closer to expert	
Scaffolding	• Teacher provides support, suggestions, assistance, reciprocal teaching, or physical support • Teacher executes parts of the task that student cannot yet manage • Gradual removal of support over time • Requires accurate diagnosis of current skill level	
Articulation	• Teacher elicits student to articulate knowledge, reasoning, and problem-solving and ask questions (e.g. comparisons), • Teacher asks student to think aloud • Teacher asks student to assume role of critic	
Reflection	• Abstracted replay of events • Student compares problem-solving process with others' processes • Expert feedback in this process enhances learning	
Exploration	• Teacher pushes student into problem solving • Forcing is critical, • Teacher must "fade" in problem solving	

(Adapted from Driscoll, 2004)

APPENDIX 3

Table 7. Worksheet 3: Six-Step Approach to Developing a Curriculum to Train Residents to Teach

Step	Description of My Plan	Resources Needed
1. Problem Identification and General Needs Assessment		
2. Needs Assessment of Targeted Learners		
3. Goals and Objectives		
4. Instructional Strategies		
5. Implementation		
6. Evaluation and Feedback		

(adopted from Kern et al., 2010)

Chapter 9
Interprofessional Education

Rebecca Moote
Regis University, USA

ABSTRACT

Interprofessional education (IPE) is recognized as an important component in the education of healthcare students. The goal of bringing students together to learn with, from, and about each other is to ultimately impact collaborative practice and improve patient care. Over the last 20 years there has been increased focus on the design and implementation of IPE experiences. Several IPE collaborative organizations and IPE centers have been formed to provide evidence-based recommendations and guidelines. Strategies have been created for designing and implementing high quality IPE activities, developing faculty in IPE, overcoming student stereotypes, determining assessment strategies, and identifying barriers to IPE. This chapter will focus on each of these elements and provide specific recommendations on how to create and implement IPE that improves student learning.

INTRODUCTION

In 2001, the Institute of Medicine (IOM) published the Quality Chasm report stating that "the health care delivery system has floundered in its ability to provide consistently high-quality care" (Institute of Medicine, 2001, p. 2). In a follow-up report, the IOM commented further on one component as a tool to address the problem. That report focused on health care education and recognized the need for a focus on interprofessional education (IPE). The report stated: "All health professionals should be educated to deliver patient-centered care as members of an interdisciplinary team" (Greiner & Knebel, 2003, p. 45).

IPE and the training of students to function as an interprofessional team is crucial to enhance the provision of quality health care (Remington, Foulk, & Williams, 2006). Students who participate in IPE are more likely to be collaborative practitioners (Bridges, Davidson, Odegard, Maki, & Tomkowiak, 2011). High-quality IPE experiences require strategic instructional design. In and of itself, interprofessional education has unique pedagogical principles and nuances. Faculty members and administrators must consider several specific components throughout the creation and implementation process. These relate to design methodology, faculty development, student preparation, barriers to IPE, and assessment techniques. Each of these important components will be discussed in detail in this chapter.

DOI: 10.4018/978-1-5225-2098-6.ch009

Copyright © 2017, IGI Global. Copying or distributing in print or electronic forms without written permission of IGI Global is prohibited.

Design Methodology

Designing IPE activities can be a daunting, yet exciting task. It can be thrilling to work with faculty across professions and create an opportunity that elevates the individual professional experience. In order to create an IPE student event or program, there are several things to consider including: how should students interact; which competencies and objectives to focus on; who should be involved; which topic to choose; and how to integrate with established curricula.

Setting and Environment

In designing IPE experiences, faculty members should consider the context of their academic setting. The academic environment of the school or college will influence the IPE opportunities available to a program (Buring, Bhushan, Brazeau, et al., 2009; Kahaleh, Danielson, Franson, Nuffer, & Umland, 2015). Institutions with a medical center will often have a wide variety of professions that may be interested in IPE curricula. Stand-alone schools may have to identify IPE partners in the community or at other academic institutions. One of the first steps to creating an IPE experience or program is identifying the interested or key partners. For that reason, it may prove least cumbersome to begin IPE work with the individual professions within an institution. Faculty members may already have established relationships with other professions at their own institutions from which to base IPE discussions and interest. Once identified, discussions regarding programmatic needs, opportunities, and interest in IPE should begin (Buring, Bhushan, Brazeau, et al., 2009; Kahaleh et al., 2015).

A variety of teaching methodologies have been used successfully in IPE. Examples of interactive learning methods include seminar-based discussions, visits to patients/clients, problem-based or team-based learning, simulation including role playing and simulated clinical learning environments, and interprofessional clinical placements (Oandasan & Reeves, 2005a; Reeves, Goldman, & Oandasan, 2007). Oandasan et, al. recommend small group learning settings as effective IPE teaching environments. Most IPE programs report that they create groups of 5-10 students (Oandasan & Reeves, 2005a; Reeves et al., 2007). Anderson et, al. found that students particularly enjoyed IPE experiential activities that incorporated direct patient care (Anderson, Smith, & Hammick, 2015). Langton describes five different ways to format IPE activities. IPE could be inserted into new or existing curricula as one or more modules. It could be incorporated into clinical practice or work. It could be done as an online component in conjunction with other courses. Or it could be part or all of a program of common curricula across all professions (Langton, 2009).

Some suggest that it is important to the learning environment that the number of professional students represented be balanced (Kahaleh et al., 2015; Oandasan & Reeves, 2005a; Reeves et al., 2007). If there is a larger number of any profession represented per group, it is possible that they will dominate the interaction. While it is not essential to have equal numbers, there should be some effort to balancing student numbers to ensure that one profession will not dominate the group or activity (Horsburgh, Lamdin, & Williamson, 2001; Reeves et al., 2007). If possible, maintaining group consistency across activities is also recommended. This has been suggested to enhance interactions but may be too logistically challenging for some institutions (Oandasan & Reeves, 2005a; Ruiz, Ezer, & Purden, 2013).

Competencies and Objectives

In 2009, representatives from nursing, pharmacy, osteopathic medicine, dentistry, public health, and medicine convened to create the Interprofessional Education Collaborative (IPEC) (Interprofessional Education Collaborative [IPEC] Expert Panel, 2011). They released an expert panel report on core competencies for interprofessional collaborative practice. They defined interprofessional education as: "When students from two or more professions learn about, from and with each other to enable effective collaboration and improve health outcomes" (World Health Organization, 2011). Core IPE competencies, now referred to as Interprofessional Collaboration, were created. The competencies include: Values/ Ethics for Interprofessional Practice, 2) Roles/Responsibilities; 3) Interprofessional Communication; 4) Teams and Teamwork (IPEC, 2016). These competencies can be used to aid creation of IPE activities and assessment of learning outcomes. The outcome of the IPEC has been widely disseminated and cited. An update report in 2016 reaffirmed the core competencies and addressed the role of IPE in response to the Triple Aim and the Patient Protection and Affordable Care Act in 2010 (IPEC, 2016).

The purpose of the IPEC competencies is to enhance profession-specific competencies. The competencies are intentionally general, allowing each profession to incorporate them into the context of their individual accreditation standards (IPEC, 2016). In 2014, the IPEC-sponsoring professions (listed above) formed the Health Professions Accreditors Collaborative (HPAC). The HPAC endorsed the IPEC competencies as "fundamental to educational programs in the health professions" (IPEC, 2016).

While the core competencies are over-arching and general in scope, IPE activities may also have explicit objectives related to healthcare or clinical topics (Reeves et al., 2007). It is important that activities are relevant to students' future practice and this is often achieved by basing the activity on healthcare content (Oandasan & Reeves, 2005a; Reeves et al., 2007). However, the focus of IPE activities should not be on learning clinical content. Rather, objectives for an IPE event should be focused on providing students the opportunity to practice collaboration. It is not enough to have students work in parellel to solve a problem, termed multi-professional learning (Oandasan & Reeves, 2005a). They must work together.

Representation of Professions

Each invested profession should have faculty representation in the design, implementation, and assessment phases of an IPE activity. If a profession will be participating in the IPE activity, faculty members of that profession should be involved in the creation and planning of the event (Oandasan & Reeves, 2005b). This will foster a collaborative environment among faculty that can serve as a model for students. When beginning IPE content development, it is sometimes more attainable to start with two professions. This decreases the number of logistical and scheduling barriers. As other professions are added to an IPE activity, an initial meeting to fully review the content is necessary. All professions involved should have an opportunity to participate in creation and modification of content. With each profession added, the activity most likely will require revisions. Setting this precedent early in the process will demonstrate the value of all involved professions.

Determining which professions are involved in an IPE activity can be challenging. The mandate for IPE curricula in accreditation standards is explicit (IPEC, 2016). However, it may not always be feasible to incorporate all professions at an institution into every IPE activity (Buring, Bhushan, Brazeau, et al., 2009). Potential impacting factors to consider include scheduling, curricula, and adequate space (Buring, Bhushan, Broeseker, et al., 2009). Scheduling constraints and curricular logistics can be significant barriers to creating IPE experiences. As more professions are incorporated, the potential for more complex logistics may occur. It is important to also ensure that adequate facilities are available to facilitate face-to-face interactions, if this is a need of the activity. A final consideration includes timing the IPE activity. As professions are incorporated into an IPE activity, the time required for the activity may increase. The interprofessional model values joint decision-making and "each team member is empowered to assume leadership on patient care issues appropriate to their expertise" (Buring, 2009, p. 2).

Therefore, as each profession is incorporated into an event, it is possible that the discussion or interaction time will need to be prolonged. The design of the activity should maximize student collaboration with each involved profession. The activity should be such that students achieve a more optimal outcome together than any profession could achieve in isolation. Despite these barriers, significant value can be added to an IPE activity with the incorporation of additional professions. Faculty members must evaluate each activity, its place in individual professional curricula, and the potential barriers to participation (Buring, Bhushan, Brazeau, et al., 2009; Kahaleh et al., 2015).

Topic

The assignment should play to the professional strengths of each represented group. At the end of the activity, each profession should have gained valuable insight into the unique contribution of the professions involved. Students should be able to provide examples of how collaboration will enhance their practice and patient outcomes. To do this, IPE events should focus on interprofessional student interaction and the design of the activity should enable group dynamics that have professional balance and stability. The activity should also have relevance and status (Reeves et al., 2007). One of the challenges of IPE is to balance a focus on clinical or concept learning with IPE learning. When creating an IPE event, an emphasis should be placed on the learning process just as much as the content involved (Sargeant, 2009).

The primary goal of making a student-learning event IPE is to develop students who have the knowledge, skills, and attitudes to practice effective collaboration to enhance patient outcomes (Buring, Bhushan, Broeseker, et al., 2009; Oandasan & Reeves, 2005a). IPE learning functions most effectively as a means to accomplishing this goal, rather than an end in itself. IPE does not need to be the explicit topic focus but rather an implicit curricular theme (Abu-Rish, Pfeifle, Jones, Hall, & Zierler, 2016; Hall & Zierler, 2015). Faculty members should consider knowledge, skills and attitudes in creating IPE topics (Anderson et al., 2015). The activity should build awareness and respect for the other professions. Students should have an opportunity to evaluate and develop skills for collaboration and communication across professions (Sargeant, 2009).

There are several specific topics that lend themselves more naturally to IPE. Topics that are well suited for IPE include those that focus on patient-centered care, collaboration, evidence-based practice, and critical thinking skills (Buring, Bhushan, Brazeau, et al., 2009; Ruiz et al., 2013). Health-care ethics is a curricular component to many professional degrees and may have fewer barriers to implementing IPE (Buring, Bhushan, Brazeau, et al., 2009; Kahaleh et al., 2015). Other topics include: medication adherence, communication skills, health-care systems, emergency preparedness, evidence-based medicine, public health, global health, patient safety, medication safety, end of life/palliative care (Buring, Bhushan, Brazeau, et al., 2009; Ruiz et al., 2013).

Regardless of the topic, there are some essential components that all IPE activities should have. At the start of the activity, time should be provided to allow students to introduce themselves and provide information about their program. This can be as short as ten minutes and will potentially relieve any tension or angst concerning IPE. It can often generate energy in the room as conversation builds. At the end of each IPE activity, a timely debrief should occur to capture student perception of IPE. Reflection has also been frequently suggested as an important component to IPE (Bridges et al., 2011; Oandasan & Reeves, 2005a; Sargeant, 2009). These can be both individual and group reflections. Some examples of reflection opportunities for students include group discussions; reflection papers, posters, or presentations; structured reflection forms or assessments (Bridges et al., 2011).

Curricular Incorporation

How should IPE be incorporated into established curricula across multiple professions? There are multiple ways to insert IPE activities into curricula. Activities could be stand-alone events incorporated into courses, complete interprofessional courses, single day events, or seminars (Bridges et al., 2011; Chen et al., 2015; Ho et al., 2008; Kahaleh et al., 2015). There are benefits and challenges associated with each. Stand-alone events embedded in a course may be the most logistically feasible at the onset of IPE curricular creation. Faculty members may be more willing to begin with this approach because the workload is potentially more manageable. It is one event in one course. Embedding IPE content into a course as a single activity may help faculty focus on the IPE elements of the experience. The activity can be used to complement the course content, rather than competing with it (Buring, Bhushan, Brazeau, et al., 2009). A potential limitation to the stand-alone approach is lack of reinforcement of IPE content through multiple interactions.

To create a complete interprofessional course, consider courses that are common curricula across all professions. Ethics and professional development are examples. The benefit to this approach is that no extra time in curricula would be required. However, it may be daunting to create the amount of IPE content necessary for a complete course (Kahaleh et al., 2015). Seminars and single day events have the benefit of status. Students may naturally perceive IPE as important to their profession if it is given designated time in the form of seminars or full day events. Student perception of IPE has been suggested to be an important consideration in implementing IPE (Oandasan & Reeves, 2015a). The logistics of planning a seminar and single day events may be challenging at some institutions.

When is the best time to introduce interprofessional interactions to students? There are two distinct views regarding this, both with supporting evidence. The first suggests that IPE should be incorporated early in professional training (Bridges et al., 2011; Horsburgh et al., 2001). Early exposure to IPE can help influence the development of positive perceptions of other healthcare professions (Horak, O'Leary, & Carlson, 1998; Leaviss, 2000). Horak et al found that students early in their training were more flexible thinkers and more willing to work with other disciplines. (Horak et al., 1998) It may also help prevent the creation of negative stereotypes and attitudes towards other professions (Stull & Blue, 2016). If this method is chosen, the IPE activity and content should be appropriate for the learning stage of the students involved. One recommendation may be to focus on communication and team-building skills towards early learners (Horsburgh et al., 2001). Hind et al studied the perceptions of healthcare students in the first 6 weeks of their pre-licensure programs (Hind et al., 2003). Overall, students demonstrated a strong identity to their individual profession and a willingness to engage in IPE.

In evaluating the correlation of stereotypes to professional identity, several interesting findings emerged: 1) Students who identified strongly and positively with their own professional group also had a strong sense of professional identity. It is not surprising that if a student has a good understanding of their own profession that this would translate to a strong feeling of connectedness with their profession.

2) Students who identified strongly and positively with their own professional group viewed other professions positively. This did surprise investigators, as the hypothesis was that a strong personal sense of one's own profession would create a negative stereotype towards other professions. The investigators hypothesized that this could be due to students identifying with other professional students as being a part of a larger group, such as healthcare students or students from the same institution. 3) Students who had a strong sense of professional identity were more positive towards IPE. This finding supports the assumption that a strong professional identity creates a secure student who is not threatened by interaction with other professional students who might have similar roles (Hind et al., 2003).

Proponents of placing IPE later in student programing feel that the concept of professional identity should drive placement in the curriculum (Gilbert, 2005). Students need to have a sense of their unique professional identify prior to IPE engagement. In the beginning of their professional education, students tend to be very focused on developing an understanding of their own discipline (Gilbert, 2005). Placement of IPE after an introductory course on profession-specific roles and responsibilities should be considered. In order for a profession to demonstrate the value of their perspective and skills in a group, they should be able to articulate those perspectives and have some level of professional skill. By starting IPE too early, students may have developed an incomplete understanding of their full scope of practice as a profession and may not be able to communicate or demonstrate that scope to the other professions with whom they interact (Anderson et al., 2015).

To examine the influence of professional identity on student attitudes towards IPE, Stull et al studied a group of first-year students from 10 different professions (n=864). After five small group meetings over the course of a semester, changes in student attitudes toward IPE were examined. The study found that student attitudes toward their own profession and other professions declined after the intervention. Authors suggested that this is the result of Kegan's Theory of Self. In order to develop beyond the first stage of professional identity, according to Robert Kegan's Theory of Self, students must be exposed to challenges of their attitudes and experiences (Stull & Blue, 2016). If students lack a strong professional identity, it can create role insecurity and make it difficult to learn and work collaboratively with other professions. During the first early exposure to IPE, students may see shared roles and responsibilities as a threat. They may also place a high value on individual autonomy (Stull & Blue, 2016).

It is possible that the ideal IPE incorporation into the curriculum is across all years of learning (Anderson et al., 2015; Bridges et al., 2011; Horsburgh et al., 2001; McNair, 2005). This allows the student to have exposure throughout their education. If possible, IPE learning should be timed during or right after a uniprofessional course that addresses scope of practice and professional identity. If this method is selected, Anderson et al recommend a theoretical IPE focus. This creates a foundation of understanding that can be used to build upon in clinical application. It also provides students an opportunity to expound on the learning and knowledge gained from previous experiences (Bridges et al., 2011). It may also increase interest and willingness to engage as advanced students. Advanced students have been exposed to clinically challenging patients or scenarios and may appreciate their limitations. They may have an increase appreciation for collaboration as a result of this.

Faculty Development

Faculty development in IPE should begin early in the IPE development process (Buring, Bhushan, Brazeau, et al., 2009). Many studies have identified that faculty development is key to providing sustainable and high quality IPE (Buring, Bhushan, Brazeau, et al., 2009; Hall & Zierler, 2015; Ho et al., 2008; Shrader,

Mauldin, Hammad, Mitcham, & Blue, 2015). Faculty members often become the champions for IPE and creating a collaborative faculty community early in the process can generate enthusiasm and excitement for IPE design and implementation (Ho et al., 2008). The goals of an IPE faculty development program should be to 1) create a positive attitude towards and a common understanding of IPE, 2) develop competence in creation of curricula and facilitation skills in IPE, and 3) ensure a strong theoretical foundation in group and team dynamics (Buring, Bhushan, Brazeau, et al., 2009; Davis, Clevenger, Posnock, Robertson, & Ander, 2015; Oandasan & Reeves, 2005a).

Faculty Perceptions and Attitudes

Not all faculty members are initially convinced of the value and effectiveness of IPE (Buring, Bhushan, Brazeau, et al., 2009; Colyer, 2008; Lawlis et al., 2014). Faculty members may also be reluctant to engage in IPE due to increased workload and lack of protected time for IPE (Buring, Bhushan, Brazeau, et al., 2009). A recent article assessed faculty perceptions, knowledge, and attitudes towards IPE and interprofessional practice (Hinderer et al., 2016). Seventy-one faculty from three campuses of two rural public US universities participated in a 23-item survey. Faculty represented medical lab science, nursing, pharmacy, physical therapy, physician assistant, rehabilitation, and respiratory therapy. The study demonstrated positive IPE perceptions despite a lack of IPE awareness in over 85% of survey participants. The majority felt others undervalued their profession and that their colleagues did not attempt to learn about their contributions. They also reported lack of confidence in ability to teach IPE and reported low IPE knowledge. This study demonstrates the need to provide faculty members an environment to discuss differences and common goals in education. The process of creating and implementing shared IPE curricula can increase a faculty member's sense of value among colleagues. Faculty development for IPE can also provide an opportunity to address stereotypes and enhance collegiality.

Perhaps one of the most important attributes of an effective IPE facilitator is enthusiasm for IPE. IPE facilitators should serve as role models and champions of IPE among faculty peers and students (Anderson et al., 2015; Buring, Bhushan, Brazeau, et al., 2009; Ho et al., 2008; Lawlis et al., 2014; Oandasan & Reeves, 2005a). These attributes can create a positive and engaging environment. This characteristic can often mitigate the foreseeable challenges of stereotyping and scope of practice issues that can arise. Additionally, it is important that faculty members be open to discussing the difficult issues. One study found that former students reported negative views regarding other professions that were encouraged by their instructors (Leaviss, 2000). The most uncomfortable issues include: power and hierarchy, differences in the philosophy of professional practice, leadership, role blurring, communication, and differences in teaching methodology or pedagogy (Buring, Bhushan, Brazeau, et al., 2009; Oandasan & Reeves, 2005a; Silver & Leslie, 2009; Smith et al., 2015). If students are asked to confront some of these dynamics in the classroom, faculty members should be willing to do the same. Faculty members need to be self-aware of their own perceptions as they prepare and conduct IPE sessions. It is not enough to identify differences but also be able to demonstrate respect and value for these differences (Abu-Rish et al., 2016; Buring, Bhushan, Brazeau, et al., 2009; Silver & Leslie, 2009). Faculty members who are able to do this will be also be able to create experiences with students that reflect this sentiment and it will create an environment for students to arrive at similar conclusions.

Facilitation

Teaching IPE involves collaboration with multiple faculty members across various disciplines, which requires unique skills. Because IPE facilitation requires specific teaching skills and strategies, faculty development is critical to successful IPE (Abu-Rish et al., 2016; Anderson et al., 2015; Buring, Bhushan, Brazeau, et al., 2009; Davis et al., 2015; Hall & Zierler, 2015; Kahaleh et al., 2015; Oandasan & Reeves, 2005a; Ruiz et al., 2013; Sargeant, 2009; Silver & Leslie, 2009). Some examples of IPE facilitation strategies that promote student-driven interprofessional interaction include: open-ended questions, positive reinforcement, and allowing space for student interactions (Ruiz et al., 2013). Faculty facilitation and expertise has been directly linked to the success of an IPE experience (Hall & Zierler, 2015; Ruiz et al., 2013). A skilled IPE facilitator should demonstrate the following attributes and characteristics (Buring, Bhushan, Brazeau, et al., 2009; Oandasan & Reeves, 2005a; Silver & Leslie, 2009):

- Self-awareness.
- Respect and value for professional differences.
- Consciousness and knowledgeable regarding group dynamics.
- Ability and skill with managing power and hierarchy issues.
- Group facilitation and team teaching experience.
- Group conflict resolution skills.
- Clinical expertise related to the specific practice setting.
- Capable of connecting theory to practice.

Many studies have focused on the area of faculty development in facilitation (Buring, Bhushan, Brazeau, et al., 2009; Davis et al., 2015; Hall & Zierler, 2015; Ruiz et al., 2013; Sargeant, 2009; Silver & Leslie, 2009). One of the most important is creating a supportive environment for the students to express their views and question their stereotypes (Oandasan & Reeves, 2005a; Ruiz et al., 2013; Sargeant, Hill, & Breau, 2010). There is a delicate balance between students respecting each other's professional identities and promoting team collaborative practice. True collaborative practice may challenge student perceptions and force them to confront competing tensions between scopes of practice and professional roles/responsibilities. Facilitators should strive to create such an environment. A second goal of effective IPE facilitation is recognition by students as a role model in interacting with other faculty and students (Hall & Zierler, 2015). Lastly, facilitators should be willing to critically self-reflect on their facilitation abilities. One way to do this is using the Interprofessional Facilitation Scale (IPFS) (Sargeant et al., 2010). See Appendix 1. The Scale focuses on how well the facilitator encourages interprofessional interaction and how well the facilitator describes the benefits of IPE. It may be uncomfortable for faculty peers to provide open and honest feedback to other peer facilitators. This assessment tool can provide structured feedback to faculty members. Sargeant et al. (2010) suggest using this tool in IPE faculty development workshops and continuing education.

Factors Impacting Faculty

When planning a faculty development session, it is important to consider several different contexts. In its very nature, IPE is impacted by micro-, meso-, and macrofactors. These should be considered prior to creation of the session. The micro-factors involved include the learner, educator and learning context.

Examples of micro-factors include student numbers and enrollment; attitudes and beliefs faculty may have regarding other professions; preconceived ideas regarding IPE practices; scheduling and logistical issues; and different teaching styles (Buring, Bhushan, Brazeau, et al., 2009; Ho et al., 2008). The meso-factors include leadership and administration (Cahn, 2014). Administration and faculty leaders should strive to create an internal culture that is supportive of IPE initiatives. As discussed in a later section of this chapter, leadership among faculty and administrative support are essential to the sustainability and thriving of IPE at an institution. Administrative factors include lack of financial resources, inflexible curricula, and professional boundaries (Ho et al., 2008). The macro-factors include accreditation and institutional structures (Cahn, 2014; Gilbert, 2005; Lawlis et al., 2014). A focus on accreditation is included below. Examples of institutional factors that could support faculty interest in IPE include: awards and recognition, portfolios to stimulate curricular change, IPE faculty positions (Ho et al., 2008). While not all faculty members may be aware of the issues involved in each of these layers, an IPE faculty development course should provide a context to discuss issues surrounding each of these factors (Abu-Rish et al., 2016; Silver & Leslie, 2009).

Accreditation standards have not always promoted IPE. In a 2013 study, the accrediting documents for the following professions were evaluated: dentistry, medicine, nursing, occupational therapy, pharmacy, physical therapy, physician assistant, psychology, public health, and social work (Zorek & Raehl, 2013). Of the 21 documents analyzed, more than half contained two or fewer statements on IPE. Nursing and pharmacy together contained 77% of all the statements. The authors concluded that there is a need for common IPE language and common standards in accrediting documents (Zorek & Raehl, 2013). In 2014, the HPAC was formed with the goal of discussing IPE initiatives and communicating with stakeholders. The Collaborative hopes to better prepare students to practice collaboratively (IPEC, 2016). Accreditation can act as a powerful impetus for change at an institutional level (Ho et al., 2008). Standardization of these accreditation elements to all healthcare professions can elevate the focus of IPE at administrative levels. It may also stimulate avenues for funding research and development of IPE.

Potential Topics for Faculty Development

There are many different topic options for creation of an IPE faculty development exercise. Some institutions have created one-day events and there are some programs that occur over a year (Abu-Rish et al., 2016; Hall & Zierler, 2015; Sargeant et al., 2010; Shrader et al., 2015). It is important to allow time for faculty reflection at the end of development training (Hall & Zierler, 2015; Shrader et al., 2015). Providing an opportunity for faculty members to reflect on what they have learned can help translate knowledge to personal application (Hall & Zierler, 2015). Peer reflection and mentoring has been found to be very rewarding in IPE faculty development (Hall & Zierler, 2015).

Below are some suggestions of potential focus areas for faculty development.

1. One of the initial interactions with the group might include a discussion or activity related to baseline knowledge of the other professions. In many cases, faculty members may not appreciate the various differences between professions or even be aware of a lack of knowledge. This type of activity can create a sense of curiosity and interest in each profession. It may also alleviate any initial tension in the group regarding IPE.
2. Providing an overview of IPE concepts and theory (Hall & Zierler, 2015; Shrader et al., 2015). This will ensure that everyone is in agreement on what the definition and key knowledge principles

of IPE are. The IPEC Core Competencies should be included in this introduction (Hall & Zierler, 2015). A discussion regarding the impact of the IPEC Core Competencies on accreditation standards and curriculum (discussed below) can help to identify mutual concerns and opportunities for IPE incorporation (Kahaleh et al., 2015).

3. Another potential topic for faculty development is curricular discussion (Hall & Zierler, 2015; Ho et al., 2008). It is important to create curricular outcomes and identify common educational outcomes (Kahaleh et al., 2015). If one of the purposes of an IPE development workshop is to identify IPE opportunities, it may be helpful to have faculty members discuss similar curricular threads or areas that they have considered incorporating IPE. If the purpose of the IPE workshop is to prepare established programming, it may be helpful to spend time working on those activities. An expert IPE faculty member should have the ability to use professional differences to demonstrate high performance team collaboration (Buring, Bhushan, Brazeau, et al., 2009). This can generate rich discussion among the professions.
4. Time dedicated to facilitation skills may also be helpful (Buring, Bhushan, Brazeau, et al., 2009; Shrader et al., 2015). Despite the level of faculty expertise or time spent in the classroom, IPE group facilitation can require an intentional modification of personal teaching techniques. What has been successful in the classroom for one profession may not translate to another (Lawlis et al., 2014). Also, teaching philosophies and styles may differ between faculty members of different professions (Buring, Bhushan, Brazeau, et al., 2009). A discussion on the teaching methods that are ideal for IPE could be helpful (Silver & Leslie, 2009).
5. Discussion on programmatic goals. What changes do faculty members want to see in their students? How would you measure IPE success? This topic will relate directly to assessment techniques, not only of student outcomes but faculty and program outcomes as well (Buring, Bhushan, Brazeau, et al., 2009).

Faculty development should not end after a single development event or introductory training for IPE. Rather, faculty development should occur throughout exposure to IPE. The most productive development will occur in teaching IPE, reflecting on the experience, and making substantive changes in response to that reflection (Bridges et al., 2011; Buring, Bhushan, Brazeau, et al., 2009).

Student Preparation for IPE

Just as it is important to prepare faculty members prior to IPE engagement, it is also important to prepare students. Faculty members should be aware of attitudes and stereotypes that students will bring with them into an IPE environment. Faculty role modeling collegiality and open dialogue regarding difficult issues will create a supportive environment for students to engage with each other. The goal is to create the "psychological safety" necessary for students to feel comfortable speaking up in a team setting (Weaver, Salas, King, 2011). In order to create this setting, faculty members should consider specific orientation and information that students will need to feel prepared and ready during IPE activities.

Attitudes and Stereotypes

Several studies have identified that students do bring stereotypes of other professions and collaborative practice into IPE interactions (Anderson et al., 2015; Gilbert, 2005; Hean, Clark, Adams, & Humphris,

2006; McNair, 2005; Oandasan & Reeves, 2005b). Factors that may impact the development of those stereotypes include age, previous work experience, and profession (Hammick, Freeth, Koppel, Reeves, & Barr, 2007; Horsburgh et al., 2001; Oandasan & Reeves, 2005b). Students may also have a reluctance regarding IPE interactions. This can stem from a desire to maintain professional identity and distance from other professions. Many students may see value in their ability to do it alone (Hammick et al., 2007). The goal of IPE is not to dissolve professional identity but for students to appreciate the value that other professions bring to their personal practice. A strong professional identity does not necessarily present a barrier to engaging in IPE. It is merely important for students to identify the stereotypes and perceptions they have regarding other professions. Once identified, an honest examination and discussion of those stereotypes and how they impact attitudes and behaviors can occur. An ideal IPE activity will create a space for that discussion to happen (Stull & Blue, 2016). Creating a space for students to reflect on teamwork and stereotypes may help counteract preconceived attitudes and assumptions (Anderson et al., 2015).

Orientation

Prior to engagement in IPE activities, students must be oriented to IPE. The ideal format of an IPE orientation would be in an interprofessional session with students and faculty from other professions. Faculty should model respect and appreciation for the various roles, responsibilities, and contributions of other professions during this event. Students should be provided with reasons for the incorporation of IPE into their education and how this will impact their practice. IPE activities should be directly relevant to a student's future practice (Oandasan & Reeves, 2005a; Reeves et al., 2007). Consideration should be given to pre-assessment of students prior to IPE engagement in order to assess change over time during pre-licensure training (Stull & Blue, 2016). Assessment of students in IPE will be discussed in more detail in Evaluation of IPE.

Specific Information Provided to Students

Before each IPE activity, students should be notified of the different professions that will be participating. Prior knowledge of which professions will be present may give students the opportunity to think about differences in roles and responsibilities. It may also help them consider what they don't know about that profession and be prepared to ask questions. In some cases, it may be helpful to provide current level of education. Due to scheduling or other logistics, students of different educational levels are often involved in IPE activities together. While this may not present any issues from a teaching perspective, it may prevent confusion or frustration among students if the year of each student is conveyed prior to the activity. For example, combining first-year pharmacy students with third-year physical therapy students can create an imbalance in student expectations of each other. The physical therapy students may expect the pharmacy students to have the same clinical experience as they do. If students are aware that their professional experience will be varied, they are able to better align those expectations with students' educational level and preparedness (Chen et al., 2015; Kahaleh et al., 2015).

The dynamics of roles and responsibilities needs to be considered prior to the IPE event. This is an IPEC Core Competency and an area of potential tension between professions (Gilligan, Outram, Levett-Jones, 2014; IPEC, 2016; Stull & Blue, 2016). Faculty members should decide how to address this tension. Students early in their professional training may not completely grasp their profession role

(Anderson et al., 2015). It may behoove faculty members to discuss the student role in the IPE activity before the interaction with other professions. This approach might mitigate any confusion related to overlapping roles or scope of practice. This approach was found to be successful in training IPE faculty for facilitation and could potentially be extrapolated to training students for IPE interaction (Hall & Zierler, 2015). An alternative approach might also be argued. Faculty members might provide students with the objectives of the IPE event and allow the professions to engage in discussion around roles and responsibilities (Kahaleh et al., 2015). This can allow for open dialogue among students to identify complementing expertise as well as limitations to individual professions.

It is important for faculty members to consider course logistics when preparing students. The nature of IPE may create nervousness or angst prior to engagement with other professions. Ensuring that all students are treated equitability will alleviate frustration among students. In some cases, students may have pre-assignment work or preparation prior to IPE interactions. It is important that all professions are aware of the assignment requirements and have equal opportunities to prepare. This will avoid any negative perceptions of a profession that can occur if one group comes unprepared. Some students may feel a reluctance to participate based on program or class issues. Examples include inequalities in assessment, disparities in profession-specific teaching, and perceived redundancy to previous course content (Hammick et al., 2007; Oandasan & Reeves, 2005a; Reeves et al., 2007). These issues can be overcome by careful curricular review by faculty members, equitable grading across professions and in relation to profession-specific education, and demonstration of the relevance of IPE to profession-specific learning.

SOLUTIONS AND RECOMMENDATIONS

Barriers to IPE

There are several barriers to IPE that must be addressed at a faculty and administrative level. These include scheduling, cost, and administrative support (Abu-Rish et al., 2016; Buring, Bhushan, Broeseker, et al., 2009; Gardner, Chamberlin, Heestand, & Stowe, 2002; Gilbert, 2005; Hammick et al., 2007; Ho et al., 2008; Kahaleh et al., 2015; Lawlis et al., 2014).

Scheduling

Scheduling is perhaps one of the most challenging barriers to IPE (Cahn, 2014; Gilbert, 2005; Ho et al., 2008; Lawlis et al., 2014). This is an issue whether an IPE event is planned within one university or across institutions. Each profession and academic unit has a unique and often complex structure and curriculum. The demands of accreditation and internal systems can jeopardize a unit's flexibility and/or ability to modify curricula to accommodate IPE (Hammick et al., 2007). If possible, one solution is to create an IPE dedicated time across academic programs. This ensures that all faculty and students are available at the same time and can alleviate specific timing issues. (Kahaleh et al., 2015) Another potential solution is scheduling IPE during the summer or other times that are not as academically busy. Some programs create a block schedule of IPE instead of separate events throughout the semester (Anderson et al., 2015). Regardless of the strategy an institution chooses to take, it is helpful, if not essential, to have key IPE faculty contacts within each profession. Having an invested IPE faculty member as a resource and contact can help navigate curricular and scheduling issues for each profession. A faculty-driven

IPE scheduling meeting a semester or year prior to IPE events can resolve many scheduling conflicts. It may also be helpful to have curricular oversight from each school/college to ensure that individual outcomes are achieved and that mapping of the curriculum is considered. This investment of faculty time, for both scheduling needs as well as IPE implementation, is a crucial component to the success of IPE and is discussed below.

Cost

Funding for IPE is one of the most consistently demonstrated barriers to IPE (Chen et al., 2015; Gilbert, 2005; Lawlis et al., 2014). Optimal IPE incorporation into curricula can lead to increased cost to an institution and thus can create a barrier to IPE (Abu-Rish et al., 2016; Gilbert, 2005; Lawlis et al., 2014). IPE is cost intensive for several reasons. First is an increase in faculty cost. The increase in faculty cost may arise from protected time for faculty to create, facilitate, and assess IPE activities (Kahaleh et al., 2015; Silver & Leslie, 2009). The ideal IPE activity places students in an environment where they learn with, from, and about each other. Interprofessional faculty representation during this event is optimal (Abu-Rish et al., 2016; Bridges et al., 2011; Gilbert, 2005; Kahaleh et al., 2015; Ruiz et al., 2013). This goes against predefined notions of student to faculty teaching ratios. In order to provide ideal IPE, these ratios need to be reconsidered.

There is added value in having multiple faculty perspectives involved in teaching IPE and clinical content. This has been demonstrated in clinical settings and makes logical sense in a classroom setting as well (Gardner et al., 2002; Gilbert, 2005; Silver & Leslie, 2009). Some specific patient populations, patients infected with human immunodeficiency virus (HIV) for example, benefit from interprofessional collaborative care. It therefore makes logical sense that there is a benefit to teaching students about provision of this care in an interprofessionally facilitated format (Gilbert, 2005). Thus, an activity that could be created, facilitated, and assessed by one faculty from one profession will now require multiple faculty members (Kahaleh et al., 2015; Silver & Leslie, 2009). Second is the cost of faculty time for IPE training. There will be an associated cost to the institution to provide faculty development time. As described above, this is a critical step in creating a strong IPE program and the faculty need for development is clearly proven (Anderson et al., 2015; Buring, Bhushan, Brazeau, et al., 2009; Lawlis et al., 2014). Thirdly, there is an increased faculty workload associated with IPE that will result in indirect costs to the institution. IPE curricular creation and development inherently takes more time as groups of faculty members must meet to discuss objectives, assessments, curricular threads, and outcomes (Abu-Rish et al., 2016; Buring, Bhushan, Brazeau, et al., 2009; Kahaleh et al., 2015). Buring et al (2009) suggests that the time for IPE course development is approximately three times that of a uniprofessional course.

There are several potential solutions to the issue of high cost with IPE. Seeking internal and external funding is essential. Administrative support for IPE should be demonstrated by provision of internal funding. One potential solution, according to Ho et al. (2008), is for professional development programs to combine funds from discipline-specific sources to support IPE efforts. The creation of a robust evaluation and assessment of IPE should produce research and scholarship. Scholarly efforts often lead to funding sources. For the issue of cost related to faculty workload and time allocation, creation of collaborative faculty groups may help offset the cost. Streamlining efforts and reducing redundancy can maximize faculty time and efforts (Lawlis et al., 2014).

Administrative Support

In a study of IPE centers in the US and Canada, significant administrative support was listed as the driving force to creation of the IPE centers (Chen et al., 2015). University support at an administrative level is key to the creation and sustainability of IPE (Ho et al., 2008; Oandasan & Reeves, 2005b). According to Ho et al. (2008), administration can "set the direction for change, establish structures and parameters for implementation, allocate human and fiscal resources, and stimulate interest and commitment across a variety of stakeholders" (p. 937). Administration should be involved as invested stakeholders in the initial planning and creation of IPE. (Ho et al., 2008) Administrative support is not merely financial, although this is a critical component (Buring, Bhushan, Broeseker, et al., 2009; Hall & Zierler, 2015; Oandasan & Reeves, 2005b; Shrader et al., 2015; Silver & Leslie, 2009).

Support for IPE programming should also include providing protected faculty time and recognition of this work (Gilbert, 2005; Silver & Leslie, 2009). Incorporation of IPE work in faculty rank and promotion should be considered (Ho et al., 2008; Shrader et al., 2015). There must also be support in prioritization of space to hold IPE programming and assistance with scheduling logistics (Buring, Bhushan, Broeseker, et al., 2009). One approach to increasing administrative support is research and scholarship related to IPE, discussed below. Securing funding and recognition through research elevates the profile of an institution and can be helpful in sustaining administrative support. Administrators are also more likely to support organizational change towards IPE if they have been consulted in the initial planning. They must also be convinced that such change will aid in achieving the institution's overall goals and mission (Ho et al., 2008).

FUTURE RESEARCH DIRECTIONS

Consideration of IPE evaluation should begin as early as possible (Kahaleh et al., 2015; Reeves, Boet, Zierler, & Kitto, 2015). Outcomes of new IPE content would ideally be considered at the beginning of the process. This should be a collaborative process with all professions represented (Kahaleh et al., 2015). Evaluation could focus on any of the following outcomes: teamwork knowledge and skills; determining the effects of the IPE activity on learner attitudes, knowledge, and skills; changing behaviors of the learners; communication; demonstration of the patient's role as the center of interprofessional care; the impact of co-facilitation on teaching delivery; debriefing and facilitation impact on learner outcomes (Reeves et al., 2015; Thistlethwaite, 2012). If the goal of the evaluation is future publication in a peer-reviewed journal, consideration should be given to current IPE literature. There are many articles focused on the change in learner attitudes and knowledge. However, there is still a strong need for the evaluation of IPE impact on collaborative healthcare practice and patient outcomes (Lutfiyya, Brandt, & Cerra, 2016; Oandasan & Reeves, 2005b; Reeves et al., 2015; Thistlethwaite, Kumar, Moran, Saunders, & Carr, 2015).

According to Lutfiyya et al. (2016), the following gaps exist in the evaluation of IPE:

- Team effectiveness
- Identification and application of educational best practices
- Tools for measuring IPE and collaborative practice
- Health-related outcomes

Common questions used to create and evaluate an IPE activity include:

- What is the impact of IPE on student's knowledge, behavior, attitudes, and skills?
- What is the impact of IPE on students' collaborative behavior?
    - How will behavioral change be measured?
    - How will changes in behavior be determined?
- How does the delivery of IPE impact outcomes?
    - What is the impact of co-facilitation?
    - What is the impact of debriefing and facilitation? (Reeves et al., 2015; Thistlethwaite et al., 2015)

There are two models frequently used to create an IPE assessment framework. Several studies recommend use of Kirpatrick's model of educational outcomes (Anderson et al., 2015; Reeves et al., 2015; Thistlethwaite et al., 2015). It has four levels of assessment: 1) reaction, 2) learning, 3) behavior, and 4) results. It has been modified to fit IPE (Thistlethwaite et al., 2015). (See Appendix 2) It is useful for examining and measuring student change. The Biggs' 3 P Model is also popular (Anderson et al., 2015). It takes into consideration the "presage" factors and "process" factors and their impact on student outcomes. Presage factors include student characteristics, teaching context, and preparation. Process factors include student orientation, teaching style, and pedagogic content.

In 2015, the Institute of Medicine released a report that focused on the assessment of IPE. The report analyzed available data and made recommendations for the best methods of measuring the impact of IPE on healthcare (IOM, 2015). It identified gaps in the IPE literature; there is a paucity of evidence to demonstrate IPE impact on "patient, population and system outcomes" (IOM, 2015, p. 2). One of the steps to remedy the situation is to create a conceptual model for measuring IPE impact. The report recommended a mixed-methods research approach, which combines qualitative and quantitative outcomes (IOM, 2015). The report provides an example of this method – comparative effectiveness research. It defines comparative effectiveness research as: "the generation and synthesis of evidence that compares the benefits and harms of alternative methods to prevent, diagnose, treat, and monitor a clinical condition or to improve the delivery of care" (p. 58). The report also provided an extensive evaluation of currently available methods for measuring IPE impact. Thirty-nine studies are compared in Appendix 1 of the report for readers to evaluate (IOM, 2015, p. 67). This report can be incredibly useful for faculty members seeking the appropriate measurement tool for evaluating IPE outcomes.

The National Center for Interprofessional Practice and Education website (https://nexusipe.org/advancing/assessment-evaluation) contains an up-to-date repository of IPE assessment tools. Nationally recognized IPE leaders have created several resources at this site to assist in review and selection of tools. One such resource is a primer created by the National Center titled "Evaluating Interprofessional Education and Collaborative Practice: What Should I Consider When Selecting a Measurement Tool?" (Schmitz & Cullen, 2015). This is an excellent assessment resource for both the novice and experienced IPE faculty member. Careful consideration should be taken when selecting a tool. While a tool may be validated, it may not assess the specific outcomes and objectives for a particular IPE activity or curriculum. Creating the framework of assessment first and then evaluating available tools will prevent incorrect selection of quantitative instruments. Kahaleh et al. (2015) recommend selecting no more than two instruments in order to avoid assessment burn out.

CONCLUSION

Interprofessional education can be an incredibly satisfying experience for faculty members and students. The unique design and methodology of IPE has the potential to reinvigorate established courses and generate enthusiasm for new curricula. Faculty members and administration interested in IPE have numerous resources available to aid in creating novel IPE opportunities for students. By recognizing the particular complexities of IPE and creating an assessment approach to evaluating outcomes, faculty members can overcome barriers to IPE and provide students with the skills and attitudes necessary to provide collaborative practice to their patients.

REFERENCES

Abu-Rish, E. B., Pfeifle, A., Jones, M., Hall, L. W., & Zierler, B. K. (2016). Findings from a mixed-methods study of an interprofessional faculty development program. *Journal of Interprofessional Care*, *30*(1), 83–89. doi:10.3109/13561820.2015.1051615 PMID:26576839

Anderson, E., Smith, R., & Hammick, M. (2015). Evaluating an interprofessional education curriculum: A theory-informed approach. *Medical Teacher*, *38*, 385–394. PMID:26079669

Bridges, D. R., Davidson, R. A., Odegard, P. S., Maki, I. V., & Tomkowiak, J. (2011). Interprofessional collaboration: Three best practice models of interprofessional education. *Medical Education Online*, *16*(0), 6035. doi:10.3402/meo.v16i0.6035 PMID:21519399

Buring, S. M., Bhushan, A., Brazeau, G., Conway, S., Hansen, L., & Westberg, S. (2009). Interprofessional Education Supplement Keys to Successful Implementation of Interprofessional Education : Learning Location, Faculty Development, and Curricular Themes. *American Journal of Pharmaceutical Education*, *73*(4), 60. doi:10.5688/aj730460 PMID:19657493

Buring, S. M., Bhushan, A., Broeseker, A., Conway, S., Duncan-Hewitt, W., Hansen, L., & Westberg, S. (2009). Interprofessional education: Definitions, student competencies, and guidelines for implementation. *American Journal of Pharmaceutical Education*, *73*(4), 59. doi:10.5688/aj730459 PMID:19657492

Cahn, P. S. (2014). In and out of the curriculum: An historical case study in implementing interprofessional education. *Journal of Interprofessional Care*, *28*(2), 128–133. doi:10.3109/13561820.2013.872607 PMID:24383409

Chen, F., Delnat, C. C., & Gardner, D. (2015). The current state of academic centers for Interprofessional Education. *Journal of Interprofessional Care*, *29*(5), 497–498. doi:10.3109/13561820.2014.1002908 PMID:25586071

Colyer, H. (2008). Embedding interprofessional learning in pre-registration education in health and social care: Evidence of cultural lag. *Learning in Health and Social Care*, *7*(3), 126–133. doi:10.1111/j.1473-6861.2008.00185.x

Davis, B. P., Clevenger, C. K., Posnock, S., Robertson, B. D., & Ander, D. S. (2015). Teaching the teachers: Faculty development in inter-professional education. *Applied Nursing Research*, *28*(1), 31–35. doi:10.1016/j.apnr.2014.03.003 PMID:24852452

Gardner, S. F., Chamberlin, G. D., Heestand, D. E., & Stowe, C. D. (2002). Interdisciplinary didactic instruction at Academic Health Centers in the United States: Attitudes and barriers. *Advances in Health Sciences Education: Theory and Practice*, *7*(3), 179–190. doi:10.1023/A:1021144215376 PMID:12510140

Gilbert, J. H. V. (2005). Interprofessional learning and higher education structural barriers. *Journal of Interprofessional Care*, *19*(sup1), 87–106. doi:10.1080/13561820500067132 PMID:16096148

Gilligan, C., Outram, S., & Levett-Jones, T. (2014). Recommendations from recent graduates in medicine, nursing, and pharmacy on improving interprofessional education in university programs: A qualitative study. *BMC Medical Education*, *14*(1), 52–62. doi:10.1186/1472-6920-14-52 PMID:24636554

Greiner, A., & Knebel, E. (2003). *Committee on the Health Professions Education Summit. Health Professions Education: A Bridge to Quality*. The National Academic Press.

Hall, L. W., & Zierler, B. K. (2015). Interprofessional Education and Practice Guide No. 1; Developing faculty to effectively facilitate interprofessional education. *Journal of Interprofessional Care*, *29*(1), 3–7. doi:10.3109/13561820.2014.937483 PMID:25019466

Hammick, M., Freeth, D., Koppel, I., Reeves, S., & Barr, H. (2007). A best evidence systematic review of interprofessional education: BEME Guide no. 9. *Medical Teacher*, *29*(8), 735–751. doi:10.1080/01421590701682576 PMID:18236271

Hean, S., Clark, J. M., Adams, K., & Humphris, D. (2006). Will opposites attract? Similarities and differences in students perceptions of the stereotype profiles of other health and social care professional groups. *Journal of Interprofessional Care*, *20*(2), 162–181. doi:10.1080/13561820600646546 PMID:16608718

Hind, M., Norman, I., Cooper, S., Gill, E., Hilton, R., Judd, P., & Jones, S. C. (2003). Interprofessional perceptions of health care students. *Journal of Interprofessional Care*, *17*(1), 21–34. doi:10.1080/1356182021000044120 PMID:12772467

Hinderer, K. A., Klima, D., Truong, H.-A., Rangel, A. G., Brown, V., Talley, W., & Joyner, R. L. Jr et al.. (2016). Faculty Perceptions, Knowledge, and Attitudes Toward Interprofessional Education and Practice. *Journal of Allied Health*, *45*(1), 1E–4E. PMID:26937886

Ho, K., Jarvis-Selinger, S., Borduas, F., Frank, B., Hall, P., Handfield-Jones, R., & Rouleau, M. et al. (2008). Making interprofessional education work: The strategic roles of the academy. *Academic Medicine*, *83*(10), 934–940. doi:10.1097/ACM.0b013e3181850a75 PMID:18820523

Horak, B. J., OLeary, K. C., & Carlson, L. (1998). Preparing health care professionals for quality improvement: The George Washington University/George Mason University experience. *Quality Management in Health Care*, *6*(2), 21–30. doi:10.1097/00019514-199806020-00003 PMID:10178156

Horsburgh, M., Lamdin, R., & Williamson, E. (2001). Multiprofessional learning : The attitudes of medical, nursing and pharmacy students to sharnces, Health Education, Keywordsed learning. *Medical Education*, *35*(9), 876–883. doi:10.1046/j.1365-2923.2001.00959.x PMID:11555226

Institute of Medicine Committee on Quality of Health Care in America. (2001). *Crossing the Quality Chasm: A New Health System for the 21st Century*. Retrieved May 30, 2016, from http://www.ncbi.nlm.nih.gov/pubmed/25057539

Institute of Medicine (IOM). (2015). *Measuring the impact of interprofessional education on collaborative practice and patient outcomes*. Washington, DC: The National Academies Press.

Interprofessional Education Collaborative Expert Panel. (2011). *Core competencies for interprofessional collaborative practice: Report of an expert panel*. Washington, DC: Interprofessional Education Collaborative.

Interprofessional Education Collaborative Expert Panel. (2016). *Core competencies for interprofessional collaborative practice: 2016 update*. Washington, DC: Interprofessional Education Collaborative.

Kahaleh, A. A., Danielson, J., Franson, K. L., Nuffer, W. A., & Umland, E. M. (2015). An interprofessional education panel on development, implementation, and assessment strategies. *American Journal of Pharmaceutical Education*, *79*(6), 78. doi:10.5688/ajpe79678 PMID:26430265

Langton, H. (2009). Interprofessional education in higher education institutions: models, pedagogies, and realities. In P. Bluteau & A. Jackson (Eds.), *Interprofessional Education: Making it Happen* (pp. 37–58). Basingstoke, UK: Palgrave Macmillan.

Lawlis, T. R., Anson, J., & Greenfield, D. (2014). Barriers and enablers that influence sustainable interprofessional education: A literature review. *Journal of Interprofessional Care*, *28*(4), 305–310. doi: 10.3109/13561820.2014.895977 PMID:24625198

Leaviss, J. (2000). Exploring the perceived effects of an undergraduate multiprofessional education intervention. *Medical Education*, *34*(6), 483–486. doi:10.1046/j.1365-2923.2000.00678.x PMID:10792692

Lutfiyya, M. N., Brandt, B. F., & Cerra, F. (2016). Reflections From the Intersection of Health Professions Education and Clinical Practice. *Academic Medicine*, *91*(6), 766–771. doi:10.1097/ACM.0000000000001139 PMID:26959223

McFadyen, A. K., Webster, V., Strachan, K., Figgins, E., Brown, H., & McKechnie, J. (2005). The Readiness for Interprofessional Learning Scale: A possible more stable sub scale model for the original version of RIPLS. *Journal of Interprofessional Care*, *19*(6), 595–603. doi:10.1080/13561820500430157 PMID:16373215

McFadyen, A. K., Maclaren, W. M., & Webster, V. S. (2007). The Interdisciplinary Education Perception Scale (IEPS): an alternative remodelled sub-scale structure and its reliability. *Journal of Interprofessional Care, 21*(4), 433–443.

McNair, R. P. (2005). The case for educating health care students in professionalism as the core content of interprofessional education. *Medical Education*, *39*(5), 456–464. doi:10.1111/j.1365-2929.2005.02116.x PMID:15842679

Oandasan, I., & Reeves, S. (2005a). Key elements for interprofessional education. Part 1: The learner, the educator and the learning context. *Journal of Interprofessional Care*, *19*(sup1s1), 21–38. doi:10.1080/13561820500083550 PMID:16096143

Oandasan, I., & Reeves, S. (2005b). Key elements of interprofessional education. Part 2: Factors, processes and outcomes. *Journal of Interprofessional Care*, *19*(sup1s1), 39–48. doi:10.1080/13561820500081703 PMID:16096144

Reeves, S., Boet, S., Zierler, B., & Kitto, S. (2015). Interprofessional Education and Practice Guide No. 3: Evaluating interprofessional education. *Journal of Interprofessional Care*, *29*(4), 305–312. doi:10.3109/13561820.2014.1003637 PMID:25671416

Reeves, S., Goldman, J., & Oandasan, I. (2007). Key factors in planning and implementing interprofessional education in health care settings. *Journal of Allied Health*, *36*(4), 231–235. PMID:18293805

Remington, T. L., Foulk, M. A., & Williams, B. C. (2006). Evaluation of evidence for interprofessional education. *American Journal of Pharmaceutical Education*, *70*(3), 66. doi:10.5688/aj700366 PMID:17136186

Ruiz, M. G., Ezer, H., & Purden, M. (2013). Exploring the nature of facilitating interprofessional learning: Findings from an exploratory study. *Journal of Interprofessional Care*, *27*(6), 489–495. doi:10.3109/13561820.2013.811640 PMID:23859380

Sargeant, J. (2009). Theories to aid understanding and implementation of interprofessional education. *The Journal of Continuing Education in the Health Professions*, *29*(3), 178–184. doi:10.1002/chp.20033 PMID:19728383

Sargeant, J., Hill, T., & Breau, L. (2010). Development and testing of a scale to assess interprofessional education (IPE) facilitation skills. *The Journal of Continuing Education in the Health Professions*, *30*(2), 126–131. doi:10.1002/chp.20069 PMID:20564701

Schmitz, C. C., & Cullen, M. J. (2015, March 20). *Evaluating interprofessional education and collaborative practice: What should I consider when selecting a measurement tool?* Retrieved from https://nexusipe.org/informing/resource-center/evaluating-ipecp

Shrader, S., Mauldin, M., Hammad, S., Mitcham, M., & Blue, A. (2015). Developing a comprehensive faculty development program to promote interprofessional education, practice and research at a freestanding academic health science center. *Journal of Interprofessional Care*, *29*(2), 165–167. doi:10.3109/13561820.2014.940417 PMID:25051084

Silver, I. L., & Leslie, K. (2009). Faculty development for continuing interprofessional education and collaborative practice. *The Journal of Continuing Education in the Health Professions*, *29*(3), 172–177. doi:10.1002/chp.20032 PMID:19728382

Smith, C. S., Gerrish, W. G., Nash, M., Fisher, A., Brotman, A., Smith, D., & Dreffin, M. et al. (2015). Professional equipoise: Getting beyond dominant discourses in an interprofessional team. *Journal of Interprofessional Care*, *29*(6), 603–609. doi:10.3109/13561820.2015.1051216 PMID:26652633

Stull, C. L., & Blue, C. M. (2016). Examining the influence of professional identity formation on the attitudes of students towards interprofessional collaboration. *Journal of Interprofessional Care*, *30*(1), 90–96. doi:10.3109/13561820.2015.1066318 PMID:26833108

Thistlethwaite, J. (2012). Interprofessional education: A review of context, learning and the research agenda. *Medical Education*, *46*(1), 58–70. doi:10.1111/j.1365-2923.2011.04143.x PMID:22150197

Thistlethwaite, J., Kumar, K., Moran, M., Saunders, R., & Carr, S. (2015). An exploratory review of pre-qualification interprofessional education evaluations. *Journal of Interprofessional Care*, *29*(4), 292–297. doi:10.3109/13561820.2014.985292 PMID:25431833

Weaver, S. J., Salas, E., & King, H. B. (2011). Twelve best practices for team training evaluation in health care. *Joint Commission Journal on Quality and Patient Safety*, *37*(8), 341–349. doi:10.1016/S1553-7250(11)37044-4 PMID:21874969

World Health Organization. (2011). *Framework for action on interprofessional education and collaborative practice*. Geneva: World Health Organization.

Zorek, J., & Raehl, C. (2013). Interprofessional education accreditation standards in the USA: A comparative analysis. *Journal of Interprofessional Care*, *27*(2), 123–130. doi:10.3109/13561820.2012.718295 PMID:22950791

KEY TERMS AND DEFINITIONS

Collaborative Practice: Health professionals providing patient care as a team, demonstrating respect and value for each profession, and consulting with each other to improve patient outcomes.

Facilitation: The skill of leading a group of individuals through learning experiences, not as a "sage on the stage", but as a humble yet experienced role model.

Interprofessional Education: When students from two or more professions learn with, from, and about each other.

Interprofessional Education Collaborative (IPEC): A group formed in 2009 to promote interprofessional education efforts across multiple professions.

APPENDIX 1

Table 1. The Interprofessional Facilitation Scale (IPFS)

Item	Scale				Measurement of
1. Described why interprofessional education is important.	1	2	3	4	Contextualized IPE
2. Explained how interprofessional collaboration can enhance patient-centered practice.	1	2	3	4	
3. Role-modeled positive interactions with other health professionals and how professionals can work together, for example, by working collaboratively with a co-facilitator.	1	2	3	4	
4. Created a learning environment in which the principles of interprofessional education were demonstrated or clearly explained (eg, did not focus on 1 provider group; acknowledged all professionals' contributions; acknowledged, respected, celebrated diversity in group)	1	2	3	4	Encouraged IPE Interaction
5. Openly encouraged participants to learn from other health providers' views, opinions, and experiences (eg, asked questions that generated free exchange of ideas, openness, and sharing among all professions).	1	2	3	4	
6. Used learning and facilitation methods that encouraged participants from different professions to learn with, from, and about each other (eg, icebreaker games, case studies, group discussions).	1	2	3	4	
7. Invited other professions to comment and share their experiences/perspectives as questions or comments were made in the large group.	1	2	3	4	
8. Used appropriate facilitator skills to keep discussion topics on track.	1	2	3	4	
9. Acknowledged and respected others' experiences and perceptions.	1	2	3	4	
10. Encouraged members of all professions to contribute to decisions and seek opinions from others in the group during case or patient discussions and decision-making activities.	1	2	3	4	
11. Asked participants to share their professional opinions, perspectives, and values relative to patient care and collaborative practice.	1	2	3	4	
12. Identified professional differences in a positive manner as participants offered their professional experiences and perceptions.	1	2	3	4	
13. Asked health professionals to indicate their profession and discuss each other's roles and responsibilities in the delivery of patient care.	1	2	3	4	
14. Listened to and acknowledged participants' ideas without judgment or criticism.	1	2	3	4	
15. Asked questions to encourage participants to consider how they might use each others' professional skills, knowledge, and experiences.	1	2	3	4	
Scale: 1=poor, 2=fair, 3=good, 4=excellent					

(Sargeant et al., 2010)

APPENDIX 2

Table 2. Kirkpatrick's Model of Educational Outcomes for IPE

1. Reaction	Learners' views on the learning experience and its interprofessional nature.
2a. Modification of attitudes/perceptions	Changes in reciprocal attitudes or perceptions between participant groups. Changes in perception or attitude towards the value and/or use of team approaches to caring for a specific client group.
2b. Acquisition of knowledge/skills	Including knowledge and skills linked to interprofessional collaboration.
3. Behavioral change	Identifies individuals' transfer of interprofessional learning to their practice setting and changed professional practice.
4a. Change in organizational practice	Wider changes in the organization and delivery of care.
4b. Benefits to patients/clients	Improvements in health or well-being of patients/clients

(Oandasan & Reeves, 2005b)

Chapter 10
Introducing Collaborative Care:
Teaching Basics of Interprofessional Education in an Online Environment

Joy Doll
Creighton University, USA

Karen A. Paschal
Creighton University, USA

Anna Maio
Creighton University, USA

Katie Packard
Creighton University, USA

Ann Ryan Haddad
Creighton University, USA

Meghan Potthoff
Creighton University, USA

Margaret Jergenson
Creighton University, USA

Kathryn N. Huggett
University of Vermont, USA

Martha Todd
Creighton University, USA

ABSTRACT

This chapter describes the development and implementation of an innovative course in interprofessional education (IPE), which ensures a large number and variety of health professions students have the appropriate foundations to collaborate. A description of the institution and the process of implementing interprofessional education is followed by a presentation of challenges and then solutions to address them in the creation of the course. Future research avenues in interprofessional education will be explored. This chapter will provide practical application of concepts for other institutions attempting to design and implement introductory interprofessional education for large numbers of students.

DOI: 10.4018/978-1-5225-2098-6.ch010

Copyright © 2017, IGI Global. Copying or distributing in print or electronic forms without written permission of IGI Global is prohibited.

INTRODUCTION

Interprofessional education (IPE) has been identified not only as an ethical obligation for health care delivery, but is now being recognized by accrediting bodies as critical to health sciences education (Interprofessional Education Collaborative, 2016; Zorek & Raehl, 2013). Academic institutions are now called upon to ensure students know how to work effectively in teams to promote collaborative care (Interprofessional Education Collaborative Expert Panel, 2011). Health sciences educators are challenged to develop graduates who are identified as "collaboration ready" for clinical practice (Gilbert, Yan & Hoffman, 2010). Concurrently, higher education delivery is changing with online learning and increased class sizes (Bower 2016; Kena, et al., 2015; Morrison, 2000; Association of American Medical Colleges, 2016). Integrating interprofessional education for all of an institution's learners presents unique challenges to academic instutions, raising questions such as:

- Where do educators begin in ensuring students have the appropriate foundations to begin to collaborate?
- How do educators offer a quality interprofessional learning experience to a multitude of learners?
- Where in the curriculum is it best to begin to introduce the concepts of interprofessionalism?

In this chapter, the authors will focus on an innovative, online course introducing the basic concepts of interprofessional education and interprofessional collaborative practice to a large number of learners from across multiple professions.

BACKGROUND

Creighton University, a Jesuit, Catholic university in the midwest, offers seven health sciences programs including Dentistry, Emergency Medical Services (EMS), Medicine, Nursing including both undergraduate and graduate programming, Occupational Therapy, Pharmacy and Physical Therapy. In 2012, Creighton announced a strategic initiative to address the need for IPE focused on addressing emerging disciplinary accreditation requirements.(Interprofessional Education Collaborative Expert Panel, 2011).

At Creighton, an IPE Steering Committee with faculty from each of the seven programs was charged with completing an inventory of IPE offerings and developing a proposal for an interprofessional (IP) infrastructure and additional IP courses/activities to meet IPE accreditation standards for each discipline. The inventory revealed there were substantial grass roots efforts for IPE in small pockets within the university but expansion of the current offerings would be required to meet the needs of an IPE curriculum for all health professions students. The inventory identified mostly voluntary interprofessional service learning activities and a couple interprofessional electives in which small groups of students participated. Despite the small number of offerings, the inventory revealed a strong faculty passion and desire for IPE, but many barriers in place that prevented its expansion.

It should be noted that Creighton has a long history of participation in interprofessional education including past funding from the Health Resources and Services Administration (HRSA). Yet, many of the existing service activities highlighted in the inventory and infrastructure did not meet the requirements of providing IPE to all students. The School of Pharmacy and Health Professions had progressed the farthest with multiple professions and an infrastructure to support interprofessional community engagement activities. But the structure still faced difficulties with scheduling to ensure all students would have opportunities to be involved in these experiences. This infrastructure supported only occupational therapy, pharmacy and physical therapy programs and occasionally included other professions when scheduling made interprofessional collaboration possible.

The inventory also revealed that other IPE activities were integrated in courses where some, but not all learners, were exposed to interprofessional collaboration. Lastly, a small group of passionate faculty had developed elective IPE courses but only a small number of students chose to participate in them. Many barriers existed to student participation in these IPE elective courses including scheduling, varying tuition structure, and faculty availablity to teach the courses. Part of the charge of the IPE Steering Committee was to develop a comprehensive IPE curricular plan for all health sciences students at the institution expanding current activities and building infrastructure to support IPE for all students.

Following the inventory and the recognition that more development of IPE was needed at Creighton, the IPE Steering Committee was tasked with developing a plan for IPE for approximately 900 students a year across the 7 professions. Furthermore, several of the programs include distance learners throughout the United States without direct access to the campus. These distance learners also need to meet accreditation standards for IPE. The best practices of distance learning were reviewed in creation of the ideal methods for offering IPE.These complexities led the IPE Steering Committee to determine that an innovative, self-paced online course might be a viable option. Although such a course would not meet all the disciplinary accreditation requirements, it would be a good starting point and provide a foundation for future IPE activities to be developed.

Therefore, the first step of unifying IPE efforts at Creighton would be to develop this required course for all health sciences students to introduce the concepts of interprofessional collaboration. This approach seemed critical to ensure all students had similar knowledge prior to engaging in IPE experiences. This was considered important because the IPE inventory had revealed students had varied IPE experiences at different stages in their curricula. It was recognized these students might not be adequately prepared and not truly benefit from the IPE experiences currently offered. A baseline experience could help minimize this issue.

The IPE Steering Committee developed a syllabus for a course which became entitled IPE 400 Introduction to Collaborative Care. The overall goal of the course was to provide basic instruction to all health professions students on the following topics: introduction to interprofessional collaborative care; understanding the roles and responsibilities of team members; and describing teams and team dynamics related to health care.

Since IPE accreditation is a significant issue for many academic insitutions, the authors felt the process of developing and implementing IPE 400 Introduction to Collaborative Care was important to disseminate to others struggling with similar issues. This chapter will discuss the steps of the course development including course design, course implementation and course evaluation. The intent of this chapter is to identify and describe best practices in the pedagogy of designing a large-scale self-paced distance course for diverse learners from multiple health professions. Lessons learned may assist other educators with strategies to garner administrative support to implement wide-scale IPE and pedagogical approaches to implement a similar approach at their institutions.

MAIN FOCUS OF THE CHAPTER

Issues, Controversies, Problems

Currently, academic institutions are required by accrediting bodies to develop robust and impactful interprofessional education (Zorek & Raehl, 2013). Many academic institutions educate a variety of health professions of which each profession has unique accreditation guidelines for IPE. The diversity in requirements challenges institutions to develop IPE for the masses. In the development of the content for the course, the first challenge also presents a significant irony of interprofessional education accreditation. Despite the core definition of interprofessional collaboration being about deliberative collaboration, each profession has defined their accreditation requirements for IPE in silo fashion (Interprofessional Education Collaborative Expert Panel, 2011; Interprofessional Education Collaborative, 2016). This means that the IPE Steering Committee was challenged to develop a course that met the unique IPE needs for all 7 programs. In this process, the IPE Steering Committee was challenged to learn each profession's accreditation guidelines in detail to ensure the course developed would meet the needs of all.

Table 1. Accreditation Guidelines

Professional School	Accrediting Body	Focus of Standards
Dentistry	Commission on Dental Accreditation of ADA	Students should have educational experiences in which they coordinate patient care within the health care system relevant to dentistry.
Emergency Medical Services	Commission on Accreditation of Allied Health Education Programs (CAAHEP)	The program should ensure educational interaction of physicians with students.
Medicine	Liaison Committee on Medical Education (LCME)	The program should prepare medical students to function collaboratively on health care teams that include health professionals from other disciplines to provide coordinated services to patients.
Medical Residents/ Fellows	Accreditation Council for Graduate Medical Education (ACGME)	Residents/fellows should participate as team members in real or simulated interprofessional clinical site.
Nursing – Graduate and Undergraduate	Commission on Collegiate Nursing Education (CCNE)	The curriculum and instructional processes of the program should reflect educational theory, interprofessional collaboration research and current standards of practice.
Occupational Therapy	Accreditation Council for Occupational Therapy Education (ACOTE) of AOTA	The student should be able to communicate, coordinate and work interprofessionally with those who provide services in order to clarify each member's responsibility in executing components of an intervention plan.
Pharmacy	Accreditation Council for Pharmacy Education (ACPE)	The curriculum should prepare all students to provide entry-level, patient centered care in a variety of practice settings as a contributing member of an interprofessional team.
Physical Therapy	Commission on Accreditation in Physical Therapy Education (CAPTE)	The didactic and clinical curriculum should include interprofessional education directed toward the development of interprofessional competencies including values/ethics, communication, professional roles and responsibilities and teamwork.

Furthermore, interprofessional education has been identified as resource heavy though it does not generate revenue for an institution (Reeves, Perrier, Goldman, Freeth, & Zwarestein, 2013). The development and implementation of IPE is further complicated by the infusion of distance learning which has become more commonplace in higher education (Kena, et al., 2015). At Creighton, these factors triangulated, presenting multiple challenges for the IPE Steering Committee charged with developing and implementing the IPE course. In this section, the authors will focus on the challenges of developing and implementing IPE 400 Introduction to Collaborative Care.

Throughout the development of the introductory IPE course, the IPE Steering Committee faced many challenges directly related to a lack of infrastructure for interprofessional education. This is consistant with the literature on the subject which clearly identifies that the establishment of an IPE infrastructure is a challenge across many academic institutions (Ho, Jarvis-Selinger, Borduras, Frank, Hail, Handfield-Jones, Ferdinands, 2008; Gilbert, 2005; Carlise, Cooper & Watkins, 2004). Specifically in the experience described here, the lack of infrastructure presented challenges in accessing the resources necessary to successfully design and implement the IPE 400 course. This challenge was confounded by a lack of understanding of interprofessional collaboration among faculty, staff and adminstrators, and systemic barriers to implementing an interprofessional course.

The IPE activities at Creighton have traditionally been an add-on to normal faculty workload. These activities were fueled by the passion of a few individuals acting as champions for IPE. None of the health science programs involved had faculty with designated assignment to develop and implement IPE. As a consequence, only one member of the entire IPE Steering Committee was relieved of some current duties to assist in the development of the IPE 400 course. The rest of the team took on the course development activities in addition to current workload. The IPE Steering Committee's experience was again similar to others in that time to design and implement IPE, in itself, has been identified as a significant barrier to successful implementation (Kroboth, et al., 2007).

Furthermore, the structure of the university is not currently set up to allow significant collaborations among the multiple health sciences schools and colleges. The health sciences programs are divided into multiple schools and colleges each with its own leadership, curriculum, and resources. At its beginnings, the IPE Steering Committee found IPE to exist in almost a "no man's land." Resources and structures to support each health sciences program were not shared. For example, each health science school has unique resources for instructional design and technical support. The committee struggled to identify where support for the design and implementation, as well as technical support for IPE 400 could be centered. The committee was informed by staff in multiple departments that no assistance could be provided because the course was designated as IPE. The lack of ownership of IPE initiatives further complicated the issues of faculty workload and forced the faculty members to take on duties outside their expertise to establish the course.

During this same time, significant leadership changes occurred in the university administration and among those assigned to lead IPE. With each leadership change, the team was forced to re-educate leaders on the importance of IPE. It was noted each leader holds a unique perspective on the implementation and support for IPE. These leadership changes also impacted the communication of the development of the IPE course which caused some internal conflict upon rollout of the course.

Several challenges encountered required negotiation to reconcile resources to support IPE within the University. For example, the committee found great differences in the manner in which each educational program handles credit hours, approval of courses, tracking for accreditation and even course scheduling.

Originally, the IPE Steering Committee proposed a 3-credit hour course. In the negotiations to ensure each profession participated, this was reduced to.5 credits.

To offer flexibility to each profession's program, the Committee allowed each program to determine how the course would be offered. In this process, some professions chose to have the course as a stand-alone for the.5 credit and others chose to embed the course into another. Tuition also arose as an issue. In some programs, the addition of a course or credits makes no impact on tuition costs as students pay a lump sum of tuition but in other programs students pay by credit hour. In the tuition scenario, there was concern that students paying extra for the IPE course may feel punished and therefore, demotivated to take the required course. The IPE Committee was challenged to work with each profession to identify strategies around tuition barriers for each stakeholder group.

The IPE Steering Committee also allowed each profession to determine when the course would be implemented in their curriculum. Although this offered flexibility to the programs, it presented challenges when bringing the course to the Registrar. The course had to be categorized correctly and differently for each profession. This challenge was then followed by the issue of students registering for the course and taking it at different times. Each professional program had different start and stop dates and unique implementation timelines due to their individual curricula. As with the example of technological support to design the course, the issues of course credits and how each profession would implement the course required members of the IPE Steering Committee to step out of their scope working directly with the University Registrar to meet the needs of everyone.

In addition to negotiating the final content and time commitment for the course, the course proposal had to be approved by the curriculum committee from each profession. This means the course was presented to seven curriculum committees, one for each profession's department. Without a clear structure for interprofessional course approval, the course implementation timeline was impacted, taking months to approve due to the existing course review processes. The IPE Steering Committee members spent significant amounts of time presenting and explaining the intent of the course to many stakeholders. Although this was an important step for acceptence, it slowed down the process and further exhausted the already burdened IPE Steering Committee members.

A widely recognized challenge in the implementation of IPE is the number of both professions and students that need to be involved in IPE (Cameron, et al., 2009). The IPE Steering Committee at Creighton faced this same challenge of educating approximately 900 students per year across 7 professions, as previously mentioned. In three of the programs, hybrid education with distance learners presented a further challenge. It was imperative to ensure all students, whether campus or distance, receive IPE. The IPE Steering Committee was well aware of the challenges of IPE in an online format including its limitations in allowing students to apply interprofessional concepts (Luke, et al., 2009). However, due to resources and the number of students, the IPE Steering Committee was forced to keep an open mind in its pedagogical approaches for IPE.

Despite a long history of online education courses at Creighton, this experience did not include familiarity with developing a self-paced course nor one intended to meet the needs of the large numbers of students; not to mention a course for students across the health professions programs. Lastly, IPE Steering Committee Members had voluntarily taken on the additional workload of developing the course, but the ongoing need for faculty to manage a course of this magnitude presented another difficulty. These aspects presented significant trials for the Committee to overcome.

In summary, the Interprofessional Education Steering Committee faced many challenges throughout the development and implementation of IPE 400 Introduction to Collaborative Care. Many of these resulted from the structure of the education of health professions students which does not inherently support collaboration. Challenges were often unpredictable and were met along the way in attempting to plan, approve and implement the IPE 400 course. The authors suspect these challenges resonate with many others who are attempting or have been successful in implementing IPE initiatives. However, in this process, the Interprofessional Education Steering Committee was able to discern many solutions and recommendations for future implementation of IPE initiatives.

SOLUTIONS AND RECOMMENDATIONS

Despite all the challenges faced in the development and implementation of the introductory IPE 400 course, the IPE Steering Committee was able to identify solutions to many of the challenges. It often took creative problem solving and significant innovation along with grit and tenacity to maintain the momentum. Yet, research supports an openness and willingness to tackle such challenges is what leads to high performing teams and enhanced collaboration (Friedman & Bernell, 2006). The Committee team of individuals from diverse health care backgrounds and levels of experience were strengths further ensuring the successful implementation of the IPE course.

The need for leaders who champion such efforts has been highly supported in the literature for successful IPE (Barker, Bosco, & Oandasan, 2005). In addition, IPE champions and leaders need to be able to promote organizational change and maintain "a strong belief in the importance of IPE and a commitment to carrying it through" (Farnsworth, Peterson, Neill, Neill, & Lawson, 2015; Fook, D'Avray, Norrie, Psoinos, Lamb & Ross, 2013, p. 286).

The difficulties cited were all resolved by collaborative work and negotiation that would be unique to the University's structure. The authors have identified four core areas where the Committee was able to categorize the solutions to the challenges encountered. These include:

1. Creation of infrastructure to support interprofessional education and collaborative practice;
2. Faculty champions who continue to promote interprofessional education;
3. An ongoing dedication of the Interprofessional Steering Committee members and other faculty who have displayed a willingness to collaborate and evolve; and
4. The innovation to develop a course which provides a foundation of interprofessional knowledge for all health sciences students whether they are campus or distance based. Each of these solutions will be discussed in dctail in this section.

Creation of Infrastructure

The development of IPE 400 Introduction to Collaborative Care was a grassroots effort of a group of dedicated health sciences faculty. Ideally and widely supported in the literature, academic institutions should have an IPE infrastructure in place with faculty assigned to IPE with offloading of other teaching responsibilities to develop such a course (Bridges, Davidson, Odegard, Maki, & Tomkowiak, 2011; Blue, Mitcham, Smith, Raymond & Greenberg, 2010). Administrative support with a budget and assigned staff is also highlighted as important (Bridges, et al., 2011). In the current infrastructure of our university, at the time of the IPE 400 course approval, the curriculum committee of each profession had to review and approve the course. The length of this process impressed on the IPE Steering Committee the need to develop a group to approve IPE courses and activities. This group would include representatives from the respective disciplines to ensure an expedited process for review and approval of IPE in future efforts. In the final proposal to the administration, the Committee recommended the need for an IPE Curriculum Committee as part of the future infrastructure to support IPE. The suggested committee could fast track and approve IPE courses and activities as well as provide recommendations on the best assessment tools for faculty to evaluate student learning. Additionally, there should be resources delegated for staff support for technology, student recruitment, and data reporting. The proposal highlighted exemplars from other institutions acting as leaders in IPE and was shared with administrators.

Although the authors feel an infrastructure is important for success and recommend it for other institutions, the IPE Steering Committee did not have such a structure in place at the time of the IPE 400 course development and implementation. In order to make the course a reality, the IPE Steering Committee had to begin by advocating for resources. One faculty member on the Committee was given a courseload reduction by her School's administration and was charged with leading the design of the course. The project was also assigned an instructional designer with expertise in the university's learning management system. These two assets should be noted as a best practice in ensuring that the institution puts resources behind such large-scale IPE initiatives. Time and expertise of supportive faculty and staff are critical to the success of such an endeavor.

The IPE Steering Committee supported the lead instructor by developing and approving the content for the course. The lead instructor worked closely with the instructional designer to solve problems encountered in making the learning activities self-paced within the learning management system. All of the members of the team had to be innovative to develop robust pedagogical approaches to ensure the students have an optimal learning experience. Though not ideal, in reality, institutions may not be in the situation to develop an infrastructure prior to implementing IPE. The importance of advocating for resources to get started is crucial, as was found in the authors' situation. Although these minimal resources are not what is recommended in the literature, the successful design and implementation of our course relied on the next recommendation for the ultimate success which is the need for faculty champions.

Champions

Although IPE is a strategic initiative for the institution, multiple personnel changes in administrative leadership during the Interprofessional Education Steering Committee's work stalled approval of financial resources to fully support an IPE infrastructure and curriculum. Truly, the individual faculty members from across the health professions making up the IPE Steering Committee acted as champions for the development and implementation of the IPE 400 course despite the challenges.

Champions have been identified as individuals in support of designing and implementing IPE (Kelley & Aston, 2011). They have been recognized as necessary to ensure interprofessionalism occurs (Travaglia, Nuges, Greenfield, Westbrook & Braithwaite, 2011). The role of the IPE champion includes faculty members "from each discipline willing to commit the time needed for planning and execution of IPE courses and activities" (Kroboth, et al., 2007, p. 5). These champions spread the message of the importance and value of IPE, challenge current systems that prevent IPE and develop innovative strategies to ensure IPE is possible. Without faculty champions, a course like IPE 400 Introduction to Collaborative Care would never happen.

Beyond the IPE Steering Committee, several administrators acted as champions pushing higher administration and encouraging the faculty champions on the Committee to keep moving forward. Accomplishments were celebrated and recognized by the Committee as progress and praise was provided by these champion administrators. Members of the Committee were recognized for their work by some administrators. After all, "it has been estimated that planning for a course or activity that is purposefully interprofessional may take as much as three times the amount of time of traditional course planning" (Kroboth, et al., 2007, p. 7). IPE 400 was no exception. Recognition of the efforts of the IPE Steering Committee disseminated to the university staff and faculty from the University Provost was important. Without administrative champions and support, wide scale IPE is not possible and this exemplar is no exception (Ho, et al., 2008).

Champions are also individuals who remain committed to a cause despite many odds (Barker, Bosco & Oadasan, 2005). In the exemplar presented here, faculty representatives from each health science program served on the IPE Steering Committee for more than three years. There was little turnover in membership; yet, new champions were recognized by the IPE Steering Committee and brought forward. During its tenure, the IPE Steering Committee met on a monthly, or even more frequent basis, as needed to conduct its activities. In addition to the IPE 400 course development, the IPE Steering Committee conducted an IPE inventory of curricular offerings and developed a logic model and budget for a future IPE infrastructure and curriculum. During this time, there was also discussion of an opportunity to construct an IPE building on campus. Although this did not come to fruition, the IPE Steering Committee was tasked with providing support to this initiative as well. All of these activities occurred in addition to the development and implementation of IPE 400 Introduction to Collaborative Care. Several of these faculty representatives also served on their department's curriculum or assessment committees and were able to act as a liaison between the IPE Steering Committee and their school's committees regarding IPE initiatives.

These champions have to constantly speak the message of the importance and value of IPE. They must continue to push forward despite distractions to the original charge and still maintain their current workload. As with any change, some individuals are resistant and this factor challenged the Committee members to face a willingness to evolve, another solution to address ongoing challenges.

Willingness to Evolve

The reality is that interprofessional collaboration, at any level, requires willingness (Oandasan & Reeves, 2005). Individuals and teams have to negotiate and compromise to reach outcomes and be successful. In preparation for the course development, there was significant time spent within the IPE Steering Committee meetings discussing and negotiating credit hours, IPE activities, and best options to offer an IPE course for all students. The literature on IPE clearly identifies that factors such as time, scheduling and curricula present challenges in implementing IPE (Carlisle, Cooper & Watkins, 2004). Openly discussing the factors that impede IPE helped the committee members to learn what obstacles each program faced regarding tight student schedules, curricular overload, and specific accreditation standards. Through the committee discussions, it was determined that each program should maintain autonomy as to when their students would complete the IPE 400 course. Essentially, the IPE Steering Committee wanted to be viewed as a resource for IPE on campus providing support to each profession's department, rather than a dictator of policy. This flexibility was intended to promote acceptance and ensure that- the implementation of the IPE 400 course was valued.

As the IPE Steering Committee explored implementation of the IPE 400 Introduction to Collaborative Care course, it became clear that a creative and open approach would be important especially in the initial offering of the course. In some circles, the implementation of the course was not viewed as a resource to address upcoming disciplinary accreditation guidelines for IPE. Instead, some saw it as imposing curriculum. This required the faculty champions on the IPE Steering Committee to think and talk openly about how to meet the needs and concerns of all involved. For example, as previously stated, during the process of course development, the course was cut from 3 credits to.5 credits. The IPE Steering Committee had to work through compromises to ensure participation by each health professions programs. Although opinions varied on the required credits, it was decided it was more important for all seven disciplines to participate and compromise on content rather than to exclude any profession.

Ultimately, the course was comprised of 5 lessons including:

Lesson 1: What is IPE and Interprofessional Collaborative Care?
Lesson 2: Defining the Members of the Health Care Team.
Lesson 3: What is a team?
Lesson 4: Working in a Health Care Team.
Lesson 5: Interprofessional Collaborative Practice in Action at Creighton.

Willingness and openness to change and compromise were critical to the design of the course and innovation was required for implementing the course.

Innovation

In addition to willingness, the Interprofessional Education Steering Committee had to be innovative to meet the needs of diverse health professions programs and the large number of students. Innovation and creativity have always been values of interprofessional collaboration (Hammick, Freeth, Koppel, Reeves & Barr, 2007). As cited, IPE tends to be underresourced and undervalued. These factors force champions to be creative and innovative for interprofessionalism's inception and advancement (Mast, Rahman, Schatzman, Bridges, & Horsley, 2015). From the beginning, innovation was critical to ensure that the IPE 400 course would be successful for both campus and distance learners. It had to fit into multiple curricula across multiple timelines. This led the IPE Steering Committee to determine an introductory online, self-paced course was the best option.

At the time of the course development, no courses at Creighton University had been implemented as self-paced courses. Historically, there had not been an online course with enrollment of all health sciences students across the seven professions. Both of these challenges forced the faculty and the instructional designer to work very closely and engage in creative problem solving to design a course that was both rigorous and easily navigated. The IPE Steering Committee also wanted the course to be interactive with application of the course materials. All of the IPE Steering Committee members felt if the course was too passive, it would send an inherent message that interprofessionalism is not of value. The IPE Steering Committee members spent a significant amount of time in the development of the level of complexity of the course activities to ensure learning occurred. As educators, no one wanted the course to be viewed as a waste of time by students or other faculty members. Therefore, each lesson required students to review a pre-recorded lecture, readings or videos, and participate in a learning activity.

One strategy that was used to ensure the course provided rich pedagogical experiences was the use of branched learning activities. Branched learning is viewed as a rigorous method for online learning to challenge students to develop critical thinking skills (Wiecha & Barrie, 2002; Datta, 2012). This approach has been used in online simulation as a successful learning approach (Al-Dahir, Bryant, Kennedy, & Robinson, 2014). The IPE 400 course contains two branched learning activities. The first branched learning activity involves the viewing of a video case of a patient with a spinal cord injury. Students then are asked to identify which team members they feel would address certain health issues for the patient. The intent of the activity is to ensure students do not just passively define the roles of health care providers on the health care team, but to analyze and determine which provider is appropriate to handle certain aspects of the case scenario. In the second branched learning activity, students analyzed a case and then engaged in a clinical reasoning activity on how to best handle the case. The intent of these branched learning activities is to promote clinical reasoning and a chance for application of course content.

To address the issue of the number of students, the course was designed for the student to progress through locked activities that had to be completed successfully so they could proceed. Each lesson and learning activity was structured in a progressive order so that students were required to complete each learning activity in a specific order. In some lessons, students were provided word codes within the branched learning activities that had to be used to move to the next lesson. This required the students to thoroughly read and review materials in order to advance to the next lesson. Building the course in this locked method was a new activity for the faculty and the instructional designer. Many discussions and meetings took place to ensure this element of the course was structured correctly.

At the completion of the course, students earn the Collaborative Care Badge. The badge demonstrates to students that the course has been successfully completed. This badge can be printed and placed in a portfolio. At the end of the semester, the instructors reviewed who had completed the badge and students were assigned a grade of satisfactory for completion or unsatisfactory for an incomplete course.

Prior to full implementation of the course, a pilot of a draft of the course was conducted. Students, faculty and staff at the institution were invited to complete the course and provide feedback through a survey. Based on this feedback, minor modifications were completed prior to the course implementation. Overall, the pilot feedback was very positive and yielded needs for only minor changes to the course.

The IPE Steering Committee recognized the need for technical support during course implementation due to the large scope of the course. The members of the IPE Steering Committee advocated for and were assigned a technical support person to assist if students had any technical issues with the course. This person's contact information was placed in the course for students if assistance was needed. Amazingly, only one student contacted the technical assistance staff person in the first semester of implementation and their concern was determined to be user error. As with any innovative and new pedagogy, it is im-

Figure 1. Collaborative Care Badge

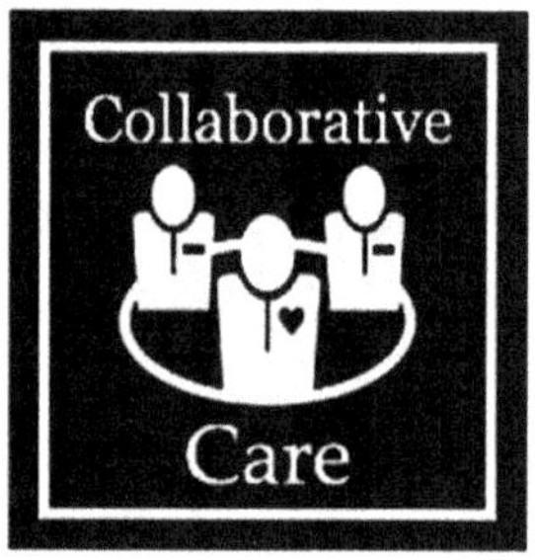

Collaborative Care

Thank you for your participation in Creighton University's Introduction to Collaborative Care course. You now have foundational knowledge of interprofessional collaboration. You will use this information both during interprofessional learning experiences as part of your health sciences education at Creighton University and also in clinical practice. This badge represents your completion of this course. You can print a copy for your records.

Requirements for completion:

To receive this badge the participant must successfully complete all five lessons within IPE 400 Introduction to Collaborative Care. Students receive a Satisfactory for the course upon completion.

portant to trial and test, seek feedback and get support if aspects go wrong. All of these processes were keys to successful implemention of IPE 400.

Assessment is an important step when implementing a new and innovative pedagogy. The IPE Steering Committee felt it was important to assess student learning on IPE and also their experience in the course. Both aspects ensure a positive learning experience for students and empower educators to make changes as needed for ongoing learning. To that end, a voluntary end of course survey was added to the course as a forum for students to provide feedback both on content and the experience of the course. At the time of this submission, 849 students had completed the course with more set to take it in an upcoming semester. Out of the 849 students, 548 completed the end of course survey leading to a response rate of 65%. Of the 548 respondents, 96% reported that instructions in the course were clear and easy to follow. Overall, 89% reported that the course enhanced their knowledge of interprofessional collaborative care. In future iterations of the course, the end of course evaluation will be required. The Team Skills Scale, a valid and reliable interprofessional education assessment tool, was included as a pre-post-test in the course (Grymonpre, et al., 2010). Data from the tool are in the stages of being analyzed to determine how the course impacts perceptions of teamwork.

Although many challenges were faced in the design and implementation of IPE 400, it is clear that the successful implementation of the course relied on multiple factors. The authors feel that implementing IPE requires identifying and addressing challenges. A summary of these challenges and the solutions to overcome them is summarized in Figure 2.

FUTURE RESEARCH DIRECTIONS

The tenets of quality health care delivery coupled with specialized accrediting bodies' standards for interprofessional education are changing the way educators in the health professions think about curriculum design, implementation and assessment (Zoreck & Raehl, 2013). Multiple options for content delivery and learning experiences provide a wide array of opportunities to develop best practices that will lead to the achievement of expected graduate outcomes. The current economic challenges in higher

Figure 2. Summary of Challenges and Solutions

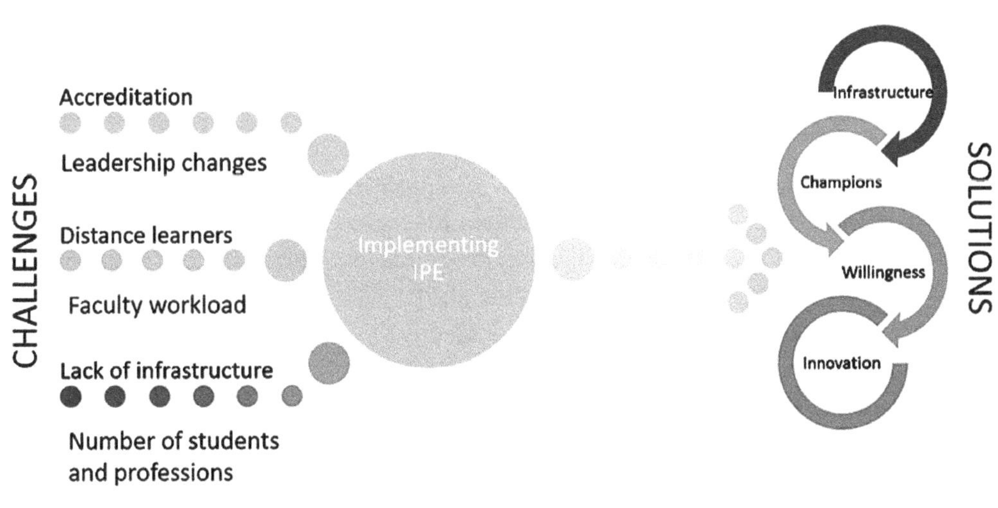

education and healthcare require that these best practices be both efficient and effective for faculty and students aligning with the Triple Aim (Berwick, Nolan, & Whittington, 2008). The Triple Aim addresses improving the patient experience of care and the health of populations along with reducing the cost of health care. It triangulates with the initiatives discussed in this book chapter.

The emphasis on interprofessional education to prepare health care professionals to participate in collaborative care led to the development of an introductory course to teach foundational concepts to students across the health professions. Student performance outcomes from the course as well as student satisfaction with the course content and delivery method are being assessed as students in the first cohort complete the course. Longer term assessment will focus on the following key dimensions:

- Did the course prepare students to engage in further interprofessional coursework and learning experiences including simulated and authentic healthcare delivery?
- Are students prepared to engage in interprofessional collaborative care throughout their education? It will be important to gauge the perceptions of the students, clinical teachers/preceptors as well as patients.
- Are graduates of the health professions programs prepared to meet the demands of the workplace?

Evaluation of the IPE model described in this chapter needs to extend beyond the student/graduate outcomes. This model has potential effects on the discipline-specific curricula of the seven health sciences programs and the faculty in these programs, both those directly involved in the IPE initiative as well as those who are not. Resource factors including cost, time, space and personnel warrant consideration with respect to the effectiveness and efficiency of the initiative. It poses the question: Is this model sustainable?

Programmatic accreditation standards related to IPE and collaborative care vary across the health professions. The authors wonder: Does this model of IPE allow for the diversity of experiences needed by each program? In addition, does the model lead to the outcomes set forth by the Institute of Medicine (2015) and the Interprofessional Education Collaborative (Interprofessional Education Collaborative Expert Panel, 2011) designed to meet the needs of society?

Future research focused on IPE models will provide evidence for needed changes and enhancements. Rich descriptions of diverse models will allow academic institutions to explore and replicate best practices as they look to offer quality and diverse IPE.

CONCLUSION

Development of the IPE 400 Introduction to Collaborative Care course grew from a necessity to address the movement of health care toward a model of interprofessional collaborative practice. The desire and need to change health care delivery in the United States has led, over time, to the establishment of accreditation standards for health care education programs to prepare students to fit into this model (Interprofessional Education Collaborative Expert Panel, 2011). Health professions educators have been faced with the daunting task of finding efficient and effective means to meet the demands of these new requirements (Reeves, Perrier, Goldman, Freeth, & Zwarnstein, 2013).

At Creighton University, this required the coordination and involvement of seven separate programs all currently trying to fulfill the requirements specific to each discipline. The challenges encountered grew from the diversity of these programs, the isolation of the traditional educational models and the intense requisite curriculum content of each profession. Essentially, implementing interprofessional education is a culture change and culture change is never easy (Pecukonis, Doyle & Bliss, 2007). In addition, the institutional structure of the University lacked pathways for the bridging between the various schools and colleges that is critical for these challenges to be addressed. The ways of thinking and traditional policies had to be challenged for the IPE 400 course implementation to be a success.

The IPE Steering Committee was charged with divining an approach to solving these challenges. The development of this self-paced online introductory course was to establish a baseline of knowledge of the concepts and scope of interprofessional collaboration. The course became a requirement for students in all health sciences programs in the University in 2015. The innovative nature is displayed in a course that is flexible enough to fit into the curriculum of each discipline at varying times and educational levels, as a stand-alone course or embedded in another course, with minimal demands on already busy faculty.

The solutions to the many problems encountered were summarized in four categories: 1. Infrastructure to manage this course and, ultimately, the more advanced experiences that the students will need to reach our goal of educating collaboration ready graduates. 2. Champions within each program that can effectively act as a liaison between their programs and IPE planning. 3. Willingness to evolve the programs to encompass the concepts of interprofessional collaboration. 4. Innovation necessary to address the complex nature of the difficulties.

The implementation of this course has been successfully realized. The students appear to have had no significant problems with access and navigation of the course. Results from the end of course survey were favorable in regards to the ease of completion the course and the perceived enhancement of the student's knowledge of interprofessional collaborative care. This implementation has accomplished the goal of providing foundational knowledge to a multitude of diverse learners and preparing them to continue on in further experiences to become collaboration ready. The success of the course in meeting the needs of the students as they engage in more advanced interprofessional experiences in their education and, ultimately, in the workplace will be further assessed over time.

REFERENCES

Al-Dahir, S., Bryant, K., Kennedy, K. B., & Robinson, D. S. (2014). Online virtual-patient cases versus traditional problem-based learning in advanced pharmacy practice experiences. *American Journal of Pharmaceutical Education*, *78*(4), 1–8. doi:10.5688/ajpe78476 PMID:24850938

Association of American Medical Colleges. (2016). *Notable trends and five future forces*. AAMC.

Barker, K. K., Bosco, C., & Oandasan, I. F. (2005). Factors in implementing interprofessional education and collaborative practice initiatives: Findings from key informant interviews. *Journal of Interprofessional Care, 19*(sup1), 166-176.

Berwick, D. M., Nolan, T. W., & Whittington, J. (2008). The triple aim: Care, health, and cost. *Health Affairs*, *27*(3), 759–769. doi:10.1377/hlthaff.27.3.759 PMID:18474969

Blue, A. V., Mitcham, M., Smith, T., Raymond, J., & Greenberg, R. (2010). Changing the future of health professions: Embedding interprofessional education within an academic health center. *Academic Medicine*, *85*(8), 1290–1295. doi:10.1097/ACM.0b013e3181e53e07 PMID:20671454

Bower, B. L. (2016). *Distance education: Facing the faculty challenge*. Retrieved from http://www.westga.edu/distance/ojdla/summer42/bower42.html

Bridges, D. R., Davidson, R. A., Odegard, P. S., Maki, I. V., & Tomkowiak, J. (2011). Interprofessional collaboration: Three best practice models of interprofessional education. *Medical Education Online*, *16*(0), 1–10. doi:10.3402/meo.v16i0.6035 PMID:21519399

Cameron, A., Rennie, S., DiProspero, L., Langlois, S., Wagner, S., Potvin, M., & Reeves, S. et al. (2009). An introduction to teamwork findings from an evaluation of an interprofessional education experience for 1,000 first-year health science students. *Journal of Allied Health*, *38*(4), 220–226. PMID:20011821

Carlisle, C., Cooper, H., & Watkins, C. (2004). Do none of you talk to each other?: The challenges facing the implementation of interprofessional education. *Medical Teacher*, *26*(6), 545–552. doi:10.1080/61421590410001711616 PMID:15763834

Datta, C. (2012). The rise of E-learning and opportunities for Indian family physicians. *Journal of Family Medicine and Primary Care*, *1*(1), 7–9. doi:10.4103/2249-4863.94441 PMID:24478993

Farnsworth, T. J., Peterson, T., Neill, K., Neill, M., & Lawson, J. (2015). Understanding the Structural, Human Resource, Political, and Symbolic Dimensions of Implementing and Sustaining Interprofessional Education. *Journal of Allied Health*, *44*(3), 152–157. PMID:26342612

Fook, J., dAvray, L., Norrie, C., Psoinos, M., Lamb, B., & Ross, F. (2013). Taking the long view: Exploring the development of interprofessional education. *Journal of Interprofessional Care*, *27*(4), 286–291. doi:10.3109/13561820.2012.759911 PMID:23659644

Gilbert, J. H. (2005). Interprofessional learning and higher education structural barriers. *Journal of Interprofessional Care, 19*(sup1), 87-106.

Gilbert, J. H., Yan, J., & Hoffman, S. J. (2010). A WHO report: Framework for action on interprofessional education and collaborative practice. *Journal of Allied Health*, *39*(Supplement 1), 196–197. PMID:21174039

Grymonpre, R., van Ineveld, C., Nelson, M., Jensen, F., De Jaeger, A., Sullivan, T., & Booth, A. et al. (2010). See it – do it – learn it: Learning interprofessional collaboration in the clinical context. *Journal of Research in Interprofessional Practice and Education*, *1*(2), 127–144.

Hammick, M., Freeth, D., Koppel, I., Reeves, S., & Barr, H. (2007). A best evidence systematic review of interprofessional education: BEME Guide no. 9. *Medical Teacher*, *29*(8), 735–751. doi:10.1080/01421590701682576 PMID:18236271

Ho, K., Jarvis-Selinger, S., Borduas, F., Frank, B., Hall, P., Handfield-Jones, R., & Ferdinands, L. et al. (2008). Making interprofessional education work: The strategic roles of the academy. *Academic Medicine*, *83*(10), 934–940. doi:10.1097/ACM.0b013e3181850a75 PMID:18820523

Institute of Medicine. (2015). *Measuring the impact of Interprofessional Education (IPE) on collaborative practice and patient outcomes*. Retrieved from http://nationalacademies.org/hmd/reports/2015/impact-of-ipe.aspx#sthash.nrPQl0Ah.dpuf

Interprofessional Education Collaborative. (2016). *Core competencies for interprofessional collaborative practice: 2016 update*. Washington, DC: Interprofessional Education Collaborative.

Interprofessional Education Collaborative Expert Panel. (2011). *Core competencies for interprofessional collaborative practice: Report of an expert panel*. Washington, DC: Interprofessional Education Collaborative.

Kelley, A., & Aston, L. (2011). An evaluation of using champions to enhance inter-professional learning in the practice setting. *Nurse Education in Practice*, *11*(1), 36–40. doi:10.1016/j.nepr.2010.06.003 PMID:20630804

Kena, G., Musu-Gillette, L., Robinson, J., Wang, X., Rathbun, A., Zhang, J.,... Dunlop Velez, E. (2015). The condition of education 2015 (NCES 2015-144). Washington, DC: U.S. Department of Education, National Center for Education Statistics. Retrieved from http://nces.ed.gov/pubsearch

Kroboth, P., Crismon, L. M., Daniels, C., Hogue, M., Reed, L., Johnson, L., & Maine, L. L. et al. (2007). Getting to solutions in interprofessional education: Report of the 2006-2007 professional affairs committee. *American Journal of Pharmaceutical Education*, *71*(19), 1–8. PMID:17429501

Luke, R., Solomon, P., Baptiste, S., Hall, P., Orchard, C., Rukholm, E., & Carter, L. (2009). Online interprofessional health sciences education: From theory to practice. *The Journal of Continuing Education in the Health Professions*, *29*(3), 161–167. doi:10.1002/chp.20030 PMID:19728380

Mast, L. J., Rahman, A., Schatzman, B. I., Bridges, D., & Horsley, N. (2015). Innovations in continuing professional education: A model to impact interprofessional collaboration. *International Public Health Journal*, *7*(1), 65–77.

Morrison, J. L. (2000). *Challenges in implementing distance learning programs*. Retrieved from htttp://horizon.unc.edu/projects/resources/44items.html

Oandasan, I., & Reeves, S. (2005). Key elements for interprofessional education. Part 1: The learner, the educator and the learning context. *Journal of Interprofessional Care, 19*(sup1), 21-38.

Pecukonis, E., Doyle, O., & Bliss, D. L. (2008). Reducing barriers to interprofessional training: Promoting interprofessional cultural competence. *Journal of Interprofessional Care*, *22*(4), 417–428. doi:10.1080/13561820802190442 PMID:18800282

Reeves, S., Perrier, L., Goldman, J., Freeth, D., & Zwarenstein, M. (2013). Interprofessional education: Effects on professional practice. *Cochrane Database of Systematic Reviews*, (3): 1–21. doi:10.1002/14651858.CD002213.pub3 PMID:23543515

Travaglia, J. F., Nugus, P., Greenfield, D., Westbrook, J., & Braithwaite, J. (2011). Contested innovation: The diffusion of interprofessionalism across a health system. *International Journal for Quality in Health Care*, *23*(6), 629–636. doi:10.1093/intqhc/mzr064 PMID:22003045

Wiecha, J., & Barrie, N. (2002). Collaborative online learning: A new approach to distance CME. *Academic Medicine*, *77*(9), 928–929. doi:10.1097/00001888-200209000-00031 PMID:12228097

Zorek, J., & Raehl, C. (2013). Interprofessional education accreditation standards in the USA: A comparative analysis. *Journal of Interprofessional Care*, *27*(2), 123–130. doi:10.3109/13561820.2012.718295 PMID:22950791

KEY TERMS AND DEFINITIONS

Champions: Individuals who support and carry an initiative forward.

Core Competencies for Interprofessional Collaborative Practice: A collection of competencies for interprofessional education and collaborative practice.

Distance Learning: Learning that occurs away from the primary educational site.

Innovative Pedagogy: Pedagogy that offers an alternative learning experience Accreditation standards: discipline-specific requirements for education.

Interprofessional Collaborative Practice: Involves the deliberative interaction of two or more different health care professionals.

Online Education: Learning that occurs in an online environment.

Self-Paced Course: A course, usually online, that learners do at their own pace.

Chapter 11
Informal Learning in Medical Education

Misa Mi
Oakland University William Beaumont School of Medicine, USA

ABSTRACT

A great deal of valuable learning—informal learning—takes place within medicine's informal and hidden curriculum. It is this kind of informal learning that brings about more diverse and personal learning gains. Informal learning contributes to individuals' continuing professional development, personal mastery, and capacity building. Recognition of informal learning can be the key to the development of a strong lifelong learning orientation for learners as they go through the process of developing and forming their professional identity. Expanded insights into the informal learning process will contribute to the design and development of strategies, methods, and informal learning spaces that promote a broader spectrum of human learning within formal medical education settings. It is hoped that discussion on informal learning will also stimulate interest in investigating the impact of informal learning on learners across the spectrum of medical education.

INTRODUCTION

Physicians are expected to pursue a lifelong discipline of continuous learning and professional development throughout the lifespan of their career. Lifelong learning has been regarded as a vital skill for any physician committed to providing current, safe, and high-quality medical care to individual patients (Schrock & Cydulka, 2006). Lifelong learning is considered as an indicator of professionalism. Accreditation bodies for educational programs require lifelong learning goals integrated into medical education curricula across the spectrum of medical education (Accreditation Council for Graduate Medical Education, 2002; Liaison Committee on Medical Education, 2016). Previous research establishes the link between past academic performance and a lifelong learning orientation (Hojat, Veloski, & Gonnella, 2009) and between the orientation and future academic achievement (Schrock & Cydulka, 2006).

Lifelong learning occurs in both formal and informal learning opportunities afforded by the workplace (Nisbet, Lincoln, & Dunn, 2013) or in the medical school educational environment. Learning involves

DOI: 10.4018/978-1-5225-2098-6.ch011

Copyright © 2017, IGI Global. Copying or distributing in print or electronic forms without written permission of IGI Global is prohibited.

both formal and informal learning processes that overlap as well as interact (Peeters et al., 2014). Learning is also a reflexive process. Learning facilitates a process which enables the learner to reflect on his/her life and learning environment (Medel-Anonuevo, Ohsako, & Mauch). In the educational arena, recommendations for promoting lifelong learning or active learning have been primarily focused on fostering and facilitating participation in formal learning.

Informal learning contributes to individuals' continuing professional development, personal mastery, and capacity building. As informal learning can complement and supplement formal learning in reaching learning goals and objectives, it would likely foster the development of individual lifelong learning skills and attitude. Students who are trained for careers in the fast changing health care system need to master more than just clinical skills; they should develop skills necessary for becoming master adaptive learners—"expert, self-directed, self-regulated and lifelong workplace learners"(American Medical Association, 2015).

Engaging in informal learning may pique learners' interest or curiosity, lead them to enroll in a formal education program to expand what they have informally learned before. Learners in a formal learning program upon completion of their learning experience may decide to continue learning informally by self-directed learning (Peeters et al., 2014). When learners are encouraged to reflect on their self-directed learning and recognize that their informal learning is an additional and tangible way of continuous learning, they will identify connections between formal and informal learning activities. As a result, the recognition could facilitate their lifelong learning which becomes more concrete (Livingstone, 1999).

Recognizing informal learning and creating a culture for the organizational learning that embraces informal learning will likely develop an enabling condition for developing master or expert lifelong learners who engage in continuing professional development and professional socialization. The Liaison Committee on Medical Education (LCME) requires that the medical curriculum in a medical school include "self-directed learning experiences and time for independent study to allow medical students to develop the skills of lifelong learning" (Liaison Committee on Medical Education, 2016). Furthermore, the recognition of informal learning can be the key to the development of a strong lifelong learning orientation for students as they go through the process of developing and forming their professional identity. The recognition encourages them to appreciate more their own learning capacities, identify their personal learning preferences, recognize the connections between diverse learning activities, and better understand the use of informal learning as a lifelong endeavor (Werquin, 2010).

How do medical educators leverage informal learning opportunities and develop strategies to promote a continual learning mode for lifelong learning? There is still a lack of understanding of and insight in informal learning in medical education. Similarly, there is little discussion about informal learning that occurs between students (Ozolins, Hall, & Peterson, 2008) and between students and faculty. Education research has been predominately focused on formal learning--the intentional, preprogrammed, and structured part of learning.

This chapter will define informal learning in relation to lifelong learning; address multifarious aspects of informal learning and its associations with various factors; discuss approaches to supporting informal learning; and offer recommendations for medical education and research with respect to informal learning. Expanded insights into the informal learning process will contribute to the design and development of strategies, methods, and informal learning spaces that promote a broader spectrum of human learning within formal medical education settings. It is hoped that the knowledge of informal learning will stimulate interest in investigating the impact of informal learning on learners in the medical school educational environment.

BACKGROUND

Differentiating Between Formal and Informal Learning

Formal learning takes place within formal education settings or through training programs in institutions and organizations; it has learning objectives and is professionally planned or institutionally organized. It ultimately leads to recognized diploma, certificate, or qualifications. In the formal learning process, learners have an explicit learning goal to gain knowledge, skills, and/or competences; they intentionally participate in formal learning and thus, are conscious of their learning during learning activities (Peeters et al., 2014). However, a great deal of valuable learning—informal learning--also takes place in everyday life (Werquin, 2010). Informal learning is considered as a "very normal, very natural human activity." People just don't seem to be aware of their learning. Being so invisible, it is usually taken for granted (Tough, 2002). Livingstone (1999) defines informal learning as

Any activity involving the pursuit of understanding, knowledge or skill which occurs outside the curricula of educational institutions, or the courses or workshops offered by educational or social agencies.... Informal learning is undertaken on one's own, either individually or collectively, without either externally imposed criteria or the presence of an institutionally authorized instructor. (Livingstone, p. 51)

Informal learning is also regarded as learning by experience or just as experience. It is predominantly unstructured and experiential. It has no set objective in terms of learning outcomes; it is never organized nor intentional from the learner's standpoints (The Organisation for Economic Co-operation and Development, 2010). Informal learning is driven by one's choices, preferences, and intentions (Marsick & Volpe, 1999). It permeates through one's own routines and daily work. It occurs "just in time" or spontaneously within the context of real work, as we face a challenge, dilemma, problem, or unanticipated need. Since it cannot be planned or preprogrammed, it will not necessarily lead to predetermined outcomes (Marsick & Volpe, 1999), but it can sustain and complement formal learning and "lead to participation in formal education and the other way around" (Peeters et al., 2014, p. 183).

Informal learning is a complex and multifarious concept; it is central to any form of learning that takes place at work or in other spheres of life. It is characteristically collaborative and co-participatory, usually leading to context-specific forms of knowledge and skills (Swanwick, 2005). In the informal learning process, learning is implicit because it can result in acquisition of knowledge independently of conscious attempts to learn and without explicit knowledge about what was taught (Reber, 1993).

Types of Informal Learning

Informal learning has been defined and classified in different ways. Schugurensky proposed a taxonomy of informal learning in three forms/types: self-directed learning, incidental learning and socialization (Table 1) (Schugurensky, 2000).

On a continuum of informal learning, incidental learning is somewhere between directed learning and socialization. As the extent of intention, reflection, awareness, and accessibility increases, the focus moves from the unconscious forms of informal learning to self-directed learning. Although learning through socialization is unintentional and unconscious, it can be made explicit or overt through a process

Table 1. Taxonomy of informal learning

Types	Description
Self-directed learning	• Learning initiated by individuals (alone or as part of a group) without the assistance of an educator • May involve preset goals. • A resource person may be present. • Intentional: the individual wants to learn something outside the formal, structured learning experience. • Conscious: the individual is aware that she or he is learning something.
Incidental	• Learning experiences that occur when the learner did not have any previous intention of learning something out of the experience, but after the experience, she or he becomes aware that some learning has taken place • Unstructured, embedded in daily life
Socialization	• Tacit learning • Internalization of values, attitudes, behaviors, skills, etc., that occur during one's everyday life • Unstructured, embedded in daily life • Unintentional: No priori intention of acquiring them • Unconscious: Unaware of the learning that occurs

of retrospective recognition that is internally generated or externally led, immediately after the learning experience or many years after it. The internally generated retrospective recognition is likely triggered through an inductive process of learners' self-reflection on or in action in the learning environment or reflective practice in the workplace. Debriefing after the fact may prompt the externally led retrospective recognition. The retrospective recognition has another added benefit for learners to develop an inductive mindset and reflective skills (Schugurensky, 2000).

The typology for informal learning describes the nature of and three levels of intention for informal learning: implicit, reactive, and deliberative (Eraut, 2004). Implicit learning is defined as the process of acquiring knowledge without conscious attempts to learn and explicit knowledge about what was learned (Authur, 1993). Reactive learning is intentional and occurs in the middle of the action. It can result from observation of effects of action; taking notice of ideas, opinions, and impressions; asking questions; and brief near-spontaneous reflection on past experience, events, or incidents. In contrast, deliberate learning has a definite learning goal with time set aside for acquiring new knowledge. Deliberate learning activities include discussion and review of past actions, communications, events, and experiences; engagement in decision making, problem solving, and planned informal learning.

Another type of learning is referred to as non-formal learning. "Such learning may occur at the initiative of the individual but also happens as a by-product of more organized activities, whether or not the activities themselves have learning objectives" (The Organisation for Economic Co-operation and Development, 2010). This type of learning may or may not be intentional. It is usually organized in some way, even if it is loosely organized. For example, non-formal learning activities arranged by an educational institution, a public library, or a community center are examples of such activities without formal credits granted in such non-formal learning situations (Ainsworth & Eaton, 2010). Given that the non-formal learning is a concept on which there is the least consensus, the chapter will be focused on informal learning.

In medical education, the educational or learning environment is widely used as an overarching concept that embraces different types of curricula. Hafferty (1998) conceptualized the multiple dimensional nature of the medicine's educational milieu as being subject to three interrelated spheres of influences:

The stated, intended, and formally offered and endorsed curriculum; an unscripted, predominantly ad hoc, and highly interpersonal form of teaching and learning that takes place among and between faculty and students (informal curriculum); and a set of influences that function at the level of organizational structure and culture (the hidden curriculum). (p. 404)

Informal learning is related to the informal and hidden curriculum (Marsick, Watkins, Callahan, & Volpe, 2009). The informal curriculum, usually student driven, involves all activities initiated by students to address their individual learning needs such as passing examinations. Medical students indicated that the informal curriculum helped them pass the exams (e.g., via past student notes), and they perceived the informal curriculum as important to enable them to be and think like doctors. However, learning from both the informal and formal curriculum could increase students' workload, and the cumulative effort from students who felt the urge to attend to both the informal, student driven curriculum and formal curriculum could contribute to a sense of feeling overwhelmed (Peeters et al., 2014). In the hidden curriculum, students can learn from faculty's unintentional behaviors, beliefs, and attitude, and from implicit social and cultural rules. Learning by informal ways in the hidden curriculum qualitatively and quantitatively plays a more important role, and is more highly valued, than formal methods (van Mook et al., 2010).

Both, the informal and hidden curriculum, constitute part of the learning environment in medicine and to a great extent, contribute to the informal learning process and outcomes. Recognizing the latent and implicit side of medical education would help educators get a better understanding of and appreciation for how much of what students come to know is grounded in learning activities and interactions that take place outside of the formally defined learning environments (Hafferty, 1998). The understanding of the influence of informal learning or the informal curriculum can help raise awareness of any possible conflict in learning expectations from the individual student and the education program (formal curriculum).

Development of Informal Learning

Learners can use a variety of sources for informal learning such as patient encounters, the Internet, social media, schools, colleagues, students of upper classes, friends, and relatives. Informal learning can occur at any age, individually or as a group, and in any space (e.g., school, workplace, elevator, corridor, cafeteria, student lounge, library). Informal learning can contribute to learners' knowledge base, expand and strengthen their skills and values, or lead them to challenge their assumptions and values, or radically change their existing prior knowledge and approaches. Informal learning can also reinforce the learning acquired in formal education (Schugurensky, 2000). It can also contradict the learning acquired in formal ways (Schugurensky, 2000), in part because it is often idiosyncratic, influenced by chance, and happens in a haphazard fashion (Marsick & Volpe, 1999).

Given the importance of informal learning in improving one's capacity, an organization or institution needs to cultivate a learning culture or environment that rewards curiosity and experimentation and supports individuals in identifying a goal for learning but leaves the learning process to individuals because the learning process is not determined by the organization. A variety of activities can be deliberately and purposefully designed to foster informal learning at the workplace. These activities include teaming, meetings, peer interaction/communication, networking, supervision, mentoring, coaching, shift change, cross training, exploration, on-the-job training, documentation, execution of one's job, site visits, etc.

(Center for Workforce Development, 1998). In his research, Eraut (2004) identified 5 types of work activity that regularly gave rise to learning:

- Participation in group activities;
- Working alongside others;
- Tackling challenging tasks;
- Problem solving;
- Working with clients.

Working with patients in a healthcare setting is part of learners' daily routines. All these activities help facilitate a process of acquisition (learning) rather than transmission of information (Swanwick, 2005).

FACTORS ASSOCIATED WITH INFORMAL LEARNING

Informal Learning in the Learning Environment

Various factors at the individual/personal, group, institutional, community, and society levels interact to constitute the overall educational environment (Miller, 1978). Research conducted by Gruppen and Stansfield (in press) reveals a much greater impact of personal-level factors—components of the learning environment--on how medical students perceive the medical school educational environment than institution-level factors. Learners' attitude toward lifelong learning and their inclination for informal learning as part of personal-level factors or learner variables may exert a certain impact on learners' perceptions of the educational environment. Informal learning that takes place at the individual, group, and institutional levels is indispensable to the process by which learners develop into expert professionals and assimilate into a particular culture of a profession. Much of how the process operates or can be enhanced goes unrecognized in medical education. Paying attention to different dimensions of the environment may enrich learning experiences and enhance the learning process that would in turn facilitate the progression from a novice to an expert in medical practice.

The learning process involves many things/activities that learners do informally outside the formal curriculum to aid their learning and to grasp the process of becoming a doctor (Ozolins et al., 2008). These activities can affect learners' perceptions of the learning environment. Interventions and strategies at the learner or personal levels in the learning environment should be designed to support formal learning that encourages students to engage in more self-directed informal learning. Effective interventions should support for informal learning as well.

Examples of interventional cfforts include encouraging retrospective recognition--learner reflection on different types of learning to help them become conscious of any unintentional learning process. The reflection has potential for advancing informal learning to additive learning and transformative learning. Additive learning refers to addition of knowledge and improvement of skills and values; transformative learning indicates learning experiences that lead learners to challenge their assumptions and values and to change their existing prior knowledge and approaches (e.g., learning strategies) (Schugurensky, 2000). Given the complexity of the definition and dynamics of the learning environment, future research is warranted to investigate how interactions among learners and of learners with faculty or individual differences (both in characters and in behavior) can lead to different experiences and perceptions of the learning environment (Gruppen & Stansfield, in press).

Informal Learning in the Workplace Environment

Informal learning constitutes the most important way of acquiring and developing the skills and competencies required at work (Boud & Garrick, 1999; Skule, Stuart, & Nyen, 2002). Work- or performance-based learning has taken center stage in the training and ongoing professional development of the medical workforce. Informal learning plays an important role in professional development of the workforce and has been identified as a major component of graduate medical education (Swanwick, 2005) and continuing medical education (CME). Engagement in clinical practice on a daily basis affords a condition or environment that serves as a precursor to informal learning. Without engagement, learning may be superficial or nonexistent.

Previous research on the impact of formal learning opportunities (e.g., CME workshops, didactic sessions) in the medical education literature reveals a limited impact of such formal training on changing physician practice (Bloom, 2005), physician behaviors, or health care outcomes (Davis et al., 1999; Davis, Thomson, Oxman, & Haynes, 1995). Physicians' clinical practice is influenced by many forces or factors, including their professional aspirations, curiosity, desire for new or enhanced competence, pressures from patients and colleagues, pressure from the healthcare institution in which they worked, and the social and cultural milieu of their practice settings. Among these factors, personal factors were reported to be associated with larger and more complex changes, while professional and social forces with smaller and simpler changes (Fox & Bennett, 1998). One personal factor can be related to physicians' lifelong, self-directed learning evolving around patient care problems, a changing practice environment, or new competencies required to practice medicine differently, effectively, or efficiently.

In self-directed learning, the focus is on the individual; however, physicians are also engaged in informal learning from their work with patients, other healthcare professionals, or in consultation with colleagues. Informal learning is the most pervasive type of learning in the workplace. The observation that it is not teaching or training but learning has resulted in a shift in perspective: the goal of education is to facilitate learning (Fox & Bennett, 1998). Therefore, organizations need to purposefully provide a working environment that makes time and space for learning and promotes and encourages opportunities for continual informal learning (Marsick & Volpe, 1999). These opportunities are developed to suit individual learning styles and meet different learning needs and to enable learners to pull information and knowledge at any place and at any time when they need it, so they can gain certain control of their own learning. Therefore, it is important to understand the natural patterns of physicians' learning in their daily practice so that their learning can be facilitated through opportunities provided for self-assessment, acquisition of knowledge and skills, and reflection on clinical performance.

Informal Learning through Interprofessional Learning and Practice

Informal learning is social and linked to learning of others. Learning, thinking and knowing are relations among people in activity (Lave & Wenger, 1991). In Marsick's point of view, relations are a key to building informal learning communities (2009). The social relations developed in such communities provide a fertile ground for informal learning and enriched personal experiences. Most workplace learning occurs on the job rather than off the job (Eraut, 2004). In a clinical setting, learning by personal experiences and informal ways quantitatively plays a more important, and more valued role (van Mook et al., 2010).

Interprofessional education is introduced to health education programs to develop health professions students' awareness and understanding of the value and impact of roles, skills and expertise of other health professions and to prepare them to communicate and work effectively with interprofessional patient care teams in future practice. In the interprofessional workplace, health professionals are engaged in informal interprofessional learning through their every day work practice. They learn from their interactions with patients, colleagues and situations to further develop their knowledge and skills and apply them to patient care (Nisbet et al., 2013). The clinical practice setting affords interprofessional learning experiences through implicit, reactive, and deliberate activities as Eraut described in the typology of informal learning (Eraut, 2004). Examples of these activities include reading of medical record notes, discussion of issues with patients and other patient care team members, reflection on optimal patient care through debriefing after team-based patient grand rounds, discussion and evaluation of past action and care plan implementation experiences, and interprofessional collaboration and consultation and decision making.

Informal learning activities as part of everyday practice, however, are rarely considered learning activities by participants (Eraut, 2004), due to their serendipitous, implicit nature (Freeth, Hammick, Reeves, Koppel, & Barr, 2008). Freeth and colleagues suggest that some of the informal learning activities should be moved towards the more visible spectrum of planned interprofessional education (2008). Eraut provides 4 practical justifications for making the informal learning explicit: 1) improving the quality of individual or team performance through feedback on performance; 2) communicating tacit knowledge to others; 3) increasing accountability for one's actions; and 4) constructing tools to further assist in decision-making and reasoning (2000).

Benefits of informal workplace interprofessional learning are difficult to quantify; however, the learning provides alternative cost-effective ways leading to potential benefits such as less time spent away from the workplace on structured formal learning programs, reduced patient care costs (e.g. hospital bed days), improved patient safety, reduced duplication of services, engaged and motivated staff, increased job satisfaction, and enhanced relevance and application of learning (Nisbet et al., 2013). These potential beneficial outcomes warrant organizational/institutional efforts in designing jobs, work practices, workflow, work schedules, and work relationships in ways for health care professionals to interact with one another within and beyond their professional boundary; seek responses to challenges that they have identified; and collaboratively and collectively solve patient care problems (Marsick & Volpe, 1999).

Informal Learning Mediated by Technologies

Mobile technologies and online social media are ubiquitous among medical students, residents, and practicing physicians. Learning no longer occurs in a formal setting as in a brick and mortar building; it can take place at any time and any place either in a physical environment or the virtual world.

Only formal learning acquired in accredited institutions with verifiable grades and transcripts used to be considered credible. Informal learning was discounted or assumed to be of less value or merely an addition to a *proper education* (Ainsworth & Eaton, 2010). As the society makes strikes in the 21st century, e-learning or mobile learning is taking place anywhere and anytime. Learning is not solely confined to one's workplace or formal learning environment anymore thanks to the connectedness enabled by mobile technologies (mobile devices such as mobile phones, iPad, and wearable watches). Mobile devices play a role in revolutionizing learning due to their portability, mobility, light weight, connectedness. Since lifelong learning is required as part of health education programs and professional practice, informal learning via mobile devices and the Internet should be credited with adding value to one's fund of knowledge and repertoire of skill sets in one's pursuit of lifelong learning.

The web and social media have enormous potential for informal learning. It has become one of key ways for people to obtain information, whether the information is good or bad, credible or unreliable. The web fits very well into informal learning. People do not have to go to or sit in class for learning to take place; they can engage in learning anywhere and at anytime and in any way of their choice. With the proliferation and ubiquitous existence of mobile devices, internet-based learning is much easier and more convenient and thus, has infiltrated people's personal and professional life. Even if students sit in a classroom, they can step in and out between the physical environment and virtual world. In their virtual world, they may engage in learning-related activities, looking for answers, searching for background knowledge, or practicing online board exam questions. They also engage in non-learning related activities such as online shopping, watching sports games, or chatting with a friend or peer.

Millennium learners grow up with the Internet, and their own existence and learning environment are excessively influenced by their access to the Internet and social media. In response to student behaviors in class, medical educators and administrators react by setting up and mandating attendance policies or professionalism guidelines for social media use to ensure expected learning outcomes and professional behaviors. Allen Tough's landmark study on adult learning described and documented self-directed learning that is widespread and occurs as part of adults' everyday life. His study uncovered the 20/80 percent split between institutionally organized learning and informal learning: 73% of all adult learning planned by the learner herself or himself (the learner decides what to learn and how to learn); 3% with a friend, co-worker, or family member; 4% with a peer group getting together to learn something without using any kind of professional assistance (Tough, 2002; Tough, 1979). As more research evidence surfaces and becomes available on what the web and social media are doing to learning across the spectrum of medical education, it is prudent that medical educators make evidence-based educational decisions. It is known that medical students do not tolerate the one-size-fits-all educational model any more (Triola, 2016, April). By harnessing the Internet and social media to create diverse opportunities to encourage omnipresent informal learning in the digital age, the spectrum of learning would be cultivated in support of individualized learning paths, and learning will take on an intrinsic worth for each student with different learning needs and goals and unique characteristics.

Informal Learning in Communities of Practice

Most informal learning is tacit and accomplished through social modeling (Marsick & Volpe, 1999). Interactions among learners have a great impact on the educational environment (Gruppen, Rytting, & Marti, in press), because thinking and learning are both situated in both physical and social contexts and learners not only interact with each other, but with the learning environment (Orsmond & Zvauya, 2015). To promote learning at the workplace, medical educators need to provide a breadth of access to opportunities for learning. "The workplace is responsible for shaping both unintentional and intentional learning activities through its participatory practice" (Swanwick, 2005). Lave and Wenger's research discovers that the foremost and more fundamental educational process in action was learning rather teaching in apprenticeships (1991). "The learning process is very much shaped by the environment in which the learner finds himself/herself" (Medel-Anonuevo et al., 2001). Lave and Wenger developed the concept of community of practice to describe a model of learning based on social interaction and collaboration among peers (1991). It is within the interaction, collaboration and participation that practice, meaning, identity, and community emerge and evolve, all of which interact to constitute context (Wenger, 1998). The context or social milieu facilitates engaged participation, relationship building, and communal resources sharing.

Given the nature of the contextualized learning that occurs in a community of practice, members in the community become socialized and enculturated in a profession by participating in the community. They begin to make meanings of what works for their shared goal or experience and gain tacit knowledge or skills in their practice or chosen specialty. Learning communities are burgeoning in medical schools as an effort to stimulate and support learner-learner interactions and to improve the learning environment. They influenced learning inside and outside of the overt curriculum (Orsmond & Zvauya, 2015) and were associated with more positive perceptions of the learning environment (Smith et al., 2016). They are also a viable approach to supporting lifelong learning and informal learning through members' participation in group activities and working alongside others. Communities of practice support the social-cultural dimension of informal learning, which is collaborative and participatory and perceived to be important for professional identity formation. Medical educators need to leverage communities of practice by designing structures for supporting meaningful learner communities for social, human-to-human interaction. The interaction allows "newcomers" (e.g., underclassmen, novices) and "old-timers" (e.g., upperclassmen, experts) to interactively engage in group activities, collaborative and collective learning, shared problem solving, and completion of given tasks (Barab, Warren, Del-Valle, & Fang, 2006).

Informal Learning by Evidence-Based Practice

Evidence-based medicine (EBM) was introduced as an approach to the practice of medicine to improve the quality of patient care over two decades ago. The approach signifies a paradigm shift from the traditional medical practice. EBM is defined as "the conscientious, explicit, and judicious use of current best evidence in making decisions about the care of individual patients" (Sackett, Rosenberg, Gray, Haynes, & Richardson, 1996). In making decisions about caring for individual patients, the approach calls for the integration of the best available, current, valid, and relevant evidence with clinicians' knowledge and expertise and patients' preferences, values, and needs. EBM is a process of lifelong, self-directed learning in which caring for patients creates a need for acquisition of new knowledge about diagnosis, prognosis, treatment, and other health care related issues (Bhandari et al., 2003; Burneo, Jenkins, & Bussiere, 2006). Evidence-based practice involves steps in action and calls for a new set of skills: asking a focused clinical question derived from a patient care problem; acquiring the evidence; appraising the evidence critically and determining its applicability; applying the evidence by integrating it with clinical expertise and the patient's preferences; and assessing the clinician's performance with the patient (Sackett, Straus, Richardson, & Rosenberg, 2000; Schardt, 2001).

Based on EBM principles, the EBM process always starts and ends with the patient. A patient care problem or clinical need during a patient encounter offers a challenge or a problem to be resolved; the problem serves as a trigger or internal or external stimulus for learning within a given context of patient care. The learning can be viewed as the informal and incidental learning that Marsick and Watkins describe as the heart of adult learning (Marsick & Watkins, 2001); the learning is relevant to clinical practice in the patient care context.

It should be pointed out that practicing EBM is not acquired instantly but developed over time (Liu & Stewart, 2007). It represents an approach to lifelong learning in which the patient encounters cue the acquisition of knowledge (Green, 2000). The EBM approach is the continuity of learning and transfer process, and it is a cyclic process likened to the learning cycle of informal and incidental learning described by Marsick and Watkins (2001). The cycle in a patient care setting would start with a patient problem that presents a new challenge. To make sense of the challenge, various contextual factors need to be interpreted. These factors might involve the patient unique circumstance, the clinical decision-making process, willingness and motivation to learn, availability of appropriate resources, and a given clinical practice environment.

Interpretation of the context leads to choices about alternative actions for the health care professional (Marsick & Watkins, 2001). These choices are guided by clinical judgment and expertise and by a search for the current best available evidence to inform clinical decision-making. Once a solution is identified, and an action is taken, patient outcomes are assessed to determine if the outcomes match the intended results or consequences. The step of judging patient care outcomes and reflection on action enable the learner to draw lessons learned; and it also leads to a new understanding and frame that the learner would resort to when encountering a new patient problem. The step brings back full circle to the beginning of the learning cycle. The learning cycle of informal and incidental learning processes is well aligned with the cyclic process of evidence-based practice. The process can become a natural extension of whom the learners are and how they approach knowledge. Incorporating EBM principles or the cyclic process of evidence-based practice into education programs across the spectrum of medical education would foster a culture of evidence-based practice that supports informal learning and development of problem-solving, self-directed, lifelong learning skills.

SOLUTIONS AND RECOMMENDATIONS

Leveraging Social Media to Promote Informal Learning

Social media such as Facebook and Twitter is enjoying immense popularity among students of the millennium generation due to its attributes of openness, collaboration, and user-generated content (Cain & Fox, 2009). It affords additional advantages of informality, mobility, and less rigid time and physical constraints. Facebook can serve as a tool to promote social learning and contribute to the informal learning environment. It allows users to share content online and engage in interaction and discussion. A course or program director or instructor can use Facebook as a feasible platform for exposing students to diverse ideas, thoughts, and perspectives shared by influential external experts and thought leaders who are already active on Facebook. When using Facebook as an informal approach to exposing student to content not covered in a structured course core content, several strategies can be taken to enhance the informal learning environment (Cain & Fox, 2009).

Any educator who considers using Facebook should be cautioned against making the use of Facebook or other social networking technologies as a course requirement because students resent such a requirement to use these applications for educational purposes. The use of social networking tools can be innovative and creative in supporting active learning, problem-solving, or team building; however, the requirement for students to participate in manufactured or mediated social media groups may create a potential 'creepy treehouse' effect. Learners may view it as "infringement on the sanctity of their peer groups or perceive faculty members as intruders in their private online spaces" (Young, 2008). In contrast to the more structured, traditional forms of online-based discussion that is likely graded and requires student participation, the informal approach to learning by means of a Facebook group page should be optional for students.

When creating a Facebook group page as an informal learning strategy to enable an informal learning environment, learners should not be required to join Facebook, view the Facebook group page or make a specific number and/or type of posts to a Facebook group page. The Facebook group page could be used to expose learners to practitioners, external guest experts, and thought leaders, who share perspectives and thoughts as 'outsiders' to expand learners' knowledge of topics not included in class or pertaining to topics in the course syllabus. Content for posts should not be pre-selected, nor regularly scheduled.

Educator Role Change to Facilitate Informal Learning

It is not uncommon that in undergraduate medical education, there is too much to teach in the content packed curriculum and too little time for students to learn and reflect on learning. Medical educators have the tendency to over-control: they make all choices for learners; set all course and session objectives in their teaching; tell learners exactly what to learn and how to learn; and determine how to evaluate learning against stated objectives. Learners are forced to follow all that is taught or told. Regardless of preset objectives, good intention of educators, and expectations of learners, educators face the challenge of teaching classes with a low student attendance rate or teaching students distracted by social media activities. Adult learners have a desire to determine what to learn, how to learn, and set their own learning pace. If the instructional goal in medical education is to get learners to learn and ultimately, bring about patient-oriented clinical outcomes, medical educators need to free learners up so that they can learn more and learn more enthusiastically. By doing that, learners may actually accomplish more learning by being freer.

Recruitment and Development of Faculty to Promote Informal Learning

Informal learning also takes place in the informal curriculum through personal interactions with faculty, mostly in a personalized and unstructured way. When each class session in the formal curriculum ends, faculty may continue to interact with students beyond the formal classroom setting, nurture the community life, remain responsive to student inquiries through informal teaching, and address students' needs. These faculty exhibit their commitment to students and display attitudes that are indispensable to the development of professionalism and active citizens (Peeters et al., 2014).

When addressing the impact of the informal and hidden curriculum on student learning and the relationship with the learning environment, the practice of recruiting teachers for faculty positions should not overlook those attitudes and competencies necessary for professional and community life. Teachers who show high levels of these competencies will increase the odds that students will model these competencies and help shape their character building.

Faculty who come into contact and interact with students constitute part of the informal and hidden curriculum in a medical school. Support for informal learning and its integration with formal learning necessitates faculty development efforts in developing their skills and expertise in using tools, information technologies, and social media so that they can communicate and interact with students in different learning spaces efficiently and effectively. In addition, faculty need training to expand their knowledge of the taxonomy or spectrum of human learning and the impact of the informal and hidden curriculum because what they do and say overtly may influence learners beyond the formal curriculum.

Any component of the curriculum may contribute to part of the learning environment that makes an impression on learners. It is necessary to develop faculty in such a way that will empower them to embrace the role of both teacher and lifelong learner (Triola, 2016). Students can take the cue from faculty through their role modeling and mentoring as lifelong learners. The understanding of the concept and impact of the informal learning or the informal curriculum underlying the learning environment allows medical educators and administrators to better address and assess the importance of role models in the learning that takes place in the learning environment (Hafferty, 1998).

Another important aspect of faculty development is to encourage collaboration between faculty and learners. In collaborating with learners, faculty can involve students in setting up their learning goals, mapping learning content, shaping the design of learning management systems, developing technology-enhanced learning spaces, and charting their longitudinal progression from medical student to practicing physician. Students' partaking in these activities helps them grow into intrinsically motivated, self-directed learners who choose to learn, integrate learning with application problems, and achieve learner-driven learning goals in classroom or clinical practice settings.

Decision-Making Informed by Big Data Analysis

A variety of big data exist in various formats and come from different sources in institutional or organizational settings. Vast volumes of big data may be derived from websites (e.g., institutional websites, Internet, Intranet), learning management systems, online learning resources, and usage of the Internet and social media. E-learning data and data from assessment of learning processes and outcomes at each level or milestone of learners' progression can also be tracked, integrated, and analyzed in aggregate at multiple points for improving learning outcomes. The big data captured and analyzed can provide insights that likely lead to better data-driven decisions on developing and innovating curricula, optimizing learning processes and outcomes, and improving the learning environment (Triola & Pusic, 2012).

Triola and Pusic suggest that institutions should work collaboratively to establish a multiple institutional data network to prospectively collect data over time on leaners from multiple educational/training programs and professional settings. The data can be analyzed for information to answer specific questions on types of learning at each educational/training program setting. The data may be also compared for the relative impact of educational variations in curricula and training programs (Triola & Pusic, 2012). The information derived from data analysis may provide insights into the impact of potential personal and institutional factors of the medical school educational environment on informal learning. As a result, data-driven and informed decision-making on interventions to improve the environment can be practiced and shared across institutions to enhance students' informal learning and make it additive and transformative to their educational experiences.

FUTURE RESEARCH DIRECTIONS

Recognition of Informal Learning

Educators tend to be oblivious to informal learning. They even do not notice their own informal learning. It would be empowering, helpful, and supportive to encourage learners to look at their own learning (Tough, 2002) because of its additive and transformative nature in the learning process. If learners may not be fully aware of their own fund of knowledge or its potential value, they are unable to put all their learning to full or better use. It is important for educators to recognize non-formal and informal learning outcomes to make learners' fund of knowledge from informal learning more visible and more valuable to their learning goals and outcomes. Both educators' recognition and learners' self-awareness of informal learning outcomes give informal learning value for further formal learning (Werquin, 2010).

Recognition of informal learning outcomes provides validation of competences resulted from informal learning that can potentially lead to exemption from certain coursework requirements or parts of a formal study/educational program (Werquin, 2010). The approach may let students complete formal education more quickly and efficiently and reduce their medical education debt since they may opt out for certain courses for which they have already mastered and assessed for the required course content. Allowing for fast track through their formal medical education program by making the most of their non-formal and informal learning would likely increase the supply of physicians in primary care careers (e.g., family medicine); it would also motive learners to engage in self-directed learning in their academic career.

Recognition of non-formal and informal learning for the purpose of shortening study trajectories necessitates a well-developed mechanism for identification, assessment, and documentation that is tested and retested and validated. The mechanism involves many issues such as the type of guidance provided for learners, self-assessment tools for learners to evaluate their own learning, and sources and types of feedback for learners. The mechanism also takes into consideration an information/data system to track, store, and analyze data on learning progression and outcomes, and faculty's responsibility for facilitating and monitoring student learning, and student affairs personnel's strategies in counseling and career guidance.

Evaluation of Informal Learning

Most of what is learned in medical school takes place within medicine's informal and hidden curriculum rather than with formal course offerings (Hafferty, 1998). It is this kind of informal learning that brings about more diverse and personal learning gains. "To some degree the science of medicine is associated with the formal curriculum, and the art of medicine associated with the informal and hidden curriculum" (Ozolins et al., 2008, p. 610). The art of medicine may be perceived as so-called 'soft skills' that are often learned rather than taught (Holford & van der Veen, 2003). Both science and art of medicine are integral to the processes of becoming a doctor.

Recognition of informal learning outcomes requires valid methods to assess the outcomes. Traditional assessment in the formal curriculum, however, was perceived to be inadequate because a large proportion of student learning that takes place was not captured and assessed. There was clearly an imbalance between the assessment that was attributed to the formal and informal curriculum (Ozolins et al., 2008). Instruments used for the traditional assessment are more than just assessment tools used to evaluate learning; they serve as "vehicles for conveying what is and is not important within the organization (Hafferty, 1998, p. 405). These tools are awash with messages reinforcing what should be valued and how medical education should be structured and delivered. However, much of what students come to know about the nature, art, and practice of medicine occurs at an implicit level beyond the formal curriculum. Evaluation methods that excessively depend on multiple–choice questions to measure learning outcomes against pre-stated, measurable, objectives in a course render conflicts between the formal curriculum and informal and hidden curriculum. Since this type of evaluation conveys to learners the message about what is important and what is not important, they would focus their learning on what would be tested on examinations at the expense of learning the 'soft skills' -- the art of medicine, which is important for providing humanistic healthcare.

In the era of the "staggering ascendance of science and technology, along with current healthcare economics" (The Arnold P. Gold Foundation, 2013), it is becoming more critical to inculcate in learners a strong lifelong learning orientation in a rich learning environment that values and promotes informal learning. Learners' personal experience or informal learning process during their academic career is of vital importance to the formation of their medical professional identity and establishment of their clinical credibility. Thus, medical educators face the question on how traditional evaluation can be reformed to capture, monitor, and recognize the informal learning processes and outcomes. Tools to assess informal learning are lacking or seriously underdeveloped. Indicators traditionally used to measure formal learning outcomes in education or training (e.g., attendance rates, contact or training hours, change in knowledge and skill, level of qualification) are inadequate for assessing informal learning. Given the lack of indicators to measure informal learning, Skule proposes that assessment for informal learning should focus on factors or learning conditions that are most conducive to learning at the workplace or in the learning environment (2004).

There is relatively little research attention to informal learning across the spectrum of medical education; few evaluation methods are available to measure informal learning in medical education. Future investigative efforts are much needed to glean empirical evidence on the nature and processes of informal learning in medical education and to develop standardized and psychometrically sound instruments to validate, recognize, and measure informal learning or the informal curriculum in medical education programs.

CONCLUSION

The chapter offers an overview of informal learning within the context of medical education. Insights in and attention to informal learning in the learning environment may offer medical schools an additional way of guiding student learning directly or indirectly. An increased emphasis on self-directed learning strategies and acknowledgement of the value of informal learning may eventually benefit students in terms of their formal and informal learning processes. Much remains to be learned about various factors or dimensions of the learning environment. These factors will contribute to the understanding, advancement, and assessment of informal learning processes and outcomes that will have an impact on the development of lifelong learning oriented physicians.

REFERENCES

Accreditation Council for Graduate Medical Education. (2002). *ACGME Core Competencies*. Retrieved May 1, 2016, from http://www.ecfmg.org/echo/acgme-core-competencies.html

Ainsworth, H. L., & Eaton, S. E. (2010). *Formal, non-formal and informal learning in the sciences*. Retrieved May 1, 2016, from http://files.eric.ed.gov/fulltext/ED511414.pdf

American Medical Association. (2015). *Accelerating change in medical education with visionary partners and bold innovations*. Retrieved April 22, 2016, from http://www.ama-assn.org/ama/pub/about-ama/strategic-focus/accelerating-change-in-medical-education/innovations.page-envisioning-expand

Authur. (1993). *Implicit learning and tacit knowledge: An essay on the cognitive unconscious*. Norwood, NJ: Oxford University Press.

Barab, S., Warren, S. J., Del-Valle, R., & Fang, F. (2006). Coming to terms with communities of practice: A definition and operational criteria. In J. A. Pershing (Ed.), *Handbook of human performance technology: Principles, practices, and potential* (3rd ed.; pp. 640–664). San Francisco, CA: Pfeiffer.

Bhandari, M., Montori, V., Devereaux, P. J., Dosanjh, S., Sprague, S., & Guyatt, G. H. (2003). Challenges to the practice of evidence-based medicine during residents surgical training: A qualitative study using grounded theory. *Academic Medicine*, *78*(11), 1183–1190. doi:10.1097/00001888-200311000-00022 PMID:14604884

Bloom, B. S. (2005). Effects of continuing medical education on improving physician clinical care and patient health: A review of systematic reviews. *International Journal of Technology Assessment in Health Care*, *21*(3), 380–385. doi:10.1017/S026646230505049X PMID:16110718

Boud, D., & Garrick, J. (1999). *Understanding learning at work*. London: Routledge.

Burneo, J. G., Jenkins, M. E., & Bussiere, M. (2006). Evaluating a formal evidence-based clinical practice curriculum in a neurology residency program. *Journal of the Neurological Sciences*, *250*(1-2), 10–19. doi:10.1016/j.jns.2006.06.013 PMID:16859711

Cain, J., & Fox, B. I. (2009). Web 2.0 and pharmacy education. *American Journal of Pharmaceutical Education*, *73*(7), 120. doi:10.5688/aj7307120 PMID:19960079

Center for Workforce Development. (1998). *The teaching firm: Where productive work and learning converge. Report on research findings and implications*. Newton, MA: Education Development Center, Inc.

Davis, D., O'Brien, M. A., Freemantle, N., Wolf, F. M., Mazmanian, P., & Taylor-Vaisey, A. (1999). Impact of formal continuing medical education: Do conferences, workshops, rounds, and other traditional continuing education activities change physician behavior or health care outcomes? *Journal of the American Medical Association*, *282*(9), 867–874. doi:10.1001/jama.282.9.867 PMID:10478694

Davis, D. A., Thomson, M. A., Oxman, A. D., & Haynes, R. B. (1995). Changing physician performance. A systematic review of the effect of continuing medical education strategies. *Journal of the American Medical Association*, *274*(9), 700–705. doi:10.1001/jama.1995.03530090032018 PMID:7650822

Eraut, M. (2000). Non-formal learning and tacit knowledge in professional work. *The British Journal of Educational Psychology*, *70*(Pt 1), 113–136. doi:10.1348/000709900158001 PMID:10765570

Eraut, M. (2004). Informal learning in the workplace. *Studies in Continuing Education*, *26*(2), 247–273. doi:10.1080/158037042000225245

Fox, R. D., & Bennett, N. L. (1998). Continuing medical education: Learning and change: Implications for continuing medical education. *British Medical JournalJ*, *316*(7129), 466–468. doi:10.1136/bmj.316.7129.466 PMID:9492684

Freeth, D., Hammick, M., Reeves, S., Koppel, I., & Barr, H. (2008). *Effective interprofessional education: development, delivery, and evaluation*. Oxford, UK: Wiley-Blackwell.

Green, M. L. (2000). Evidence-based medicine training in internal medicine residency programs: A national survey. *Journal of General Internal Medicine*, *15*(2), 129–133. doi:10.1046/j.1525-1497.2000.03119.x PMID:10672117

Gruppen, L., Rytting, M., & Marti, K. (in press). *The educational environment.* Academic Press.

Gruppen, L. D., & Stansfield, R. B. (in press). *Personal and institutional components of the medical school education environment*. Academic Press.

Hafferty, F. W. (1998). Beyond curriculum reform: Confronting medicine's hidden curriculum. *Academic Medicine*, *73*(4), 403–407. doi:10.1097/00001888-199804000-00013 PMID:9580717

Hojat, M., Veloski, J. J., & Gonnella, J. S. (2009). Measurement and correlates of physicians' lifelong learning. *Academic Medicine*, *84*(8), 1066–1074. doi:10.1097/ACM.0b013e3181acf25f PMID:19638773

Holford, J., & van der Veen, R. (2003). *Lifelong learning, governance and active citizenship in Europe*. Guildford: ETGACE.

Lave, J., & Wenger, E. (1991). *Situated Learning: Legitimate Peripheral Participation*. Cambridge, UK: Cambridge University Press. doi:10.1017/CBO9780511815355

Liaison Committee on Medical Education. (2016). *Functions and Structure of a Medical School: Standards for Accreditation of Medical Education Programs Leading to the MD Degree*. Retrieved March 15, 2016, from http://lcme.org/publications/

Liu, J. C., & Stewart, M. G. (2007). Teaching evidence-based medicine in otolaryngology. *Otolaryngologic Clinics of North America*, *40*(6), 1261–1274. doi:10.1016/j.otc.2007.07.006 PMID:18021839

Livingstone, D. (1999). Exploring the iceberg of adult learning: Findings of the first Canadian survey of informal learning practices. *Canadian Journal for the Study of Adult Education*, *13*(2), 49–72.

Marsick, V. J. (2009). Toward a unifying framework to support informal learning theory, research and practice. *Journal of Workplace Learning*, *21*(4), 265–275. doi:10.1108/13665620910954184

Marsick, V. J., & Volpe, M. (1999). The nature and need for informal learning. *Advances in Developing Human Resources*, *1*(3), 1–9. doi:10.1177/152342239900100302

Marsick, V. J., Watkins, K., Callahan, M., & Volpe, M. (2009). Informal and incidental learning in the workplace. In M. C. Smith & DeFrates-Densch (Eds.), Handbook of research on adult learning and development (pp. 570-599). New York, NY: Routledge.

Marsick, V. J., & Watkins, K. E. (2001). Informal and incidental learning. *New Directions for Adult and Continuing Education*, *89*(89), 25–34. doi:10.1002/ace.5

Medel-Anonuevo, C., Ohsako, T., & Mauch, W. (2001). *Revisiting lifelong learning for the 21st century*. UNESCO Institute for Education. Retrieved March 1, 2016, from http://www.unesco.org/education/uie/pdf/revisitingLLL.pdf

Miller, J. (1978). *Living Systems*. New York, NY: McGraw-Hill.

Nisbet, G., Lincoln, M., & Dunn, S. (2013). Informal interprofessional learning: An untapped opportunity for learning and change within the workplace. *Journal of Interprofessional Care*, *27*(6), 469–475. doi: 10.3109/13561820.2013.805735 PMID:23789898

Orsmond, P., & Zvauya, R. (2015). Community of learners: Charting learning in first year graduate entry medical students during problem-based learning (PBL) study. *Advances in Health Sciences Education: Theory and Practice*, *20*(2), 479–497. doi:10.1007/s10459-014-9542-4 PMID:25118861

Ozolins, I., Hall, H., & Peterson, R. (2008). The student voice: Recognising the hidden and informal curriculum in medicine. *Medical Teacher*, *30*(6), 606–611. doi:10.1080/01421590801949933 PMID:18608968

Peeters, J., Backer, F. D., Buffel, T., Kindekens, A., Struyven, K., Zhu, C., & Lombaerts, K. (2014). Adult learners' informal learning experiences in formal education setting. *Journal of Adult Development*, *21*(3), 181–192. doi:10.1007/s10804-014-9190-1

Reber, A. (1993). *Implicit Learning and Tacit Knowledge*. Oxford, UK: Oxford University Press.

Sackett, D. L., Rosenberg, W. M., Gray, J. A., Haynes, R. B., & Richardson, W. S. (1996). Evidence based medicine: What it is and what it isn't. *British Medical Journal*, *312*(7023), 71–72. doi:10.1136/bmj.312.7023.71 PMID:8555924

Sackett, D. L., Straus, S. E., Richardson, W. S., & Rosenberg, W. (2000). *Evidence-based medicine: How to practice and teach EBM* (2nd ed.). New York, NY: Churchill Livingstone.

Schardt, C. (2001). Evidence-based medicine and the hospital librarian. *Journal of Hospital Librarianship*, *1*(2), 1–14. doi:10.1300/J186v01n02_01

Schrock, J. W., & Cydulka, R. K. (2006). Lifelong learning. *Emergency Medicine Clinics of North America*, *24*(3), 785–795. doi:10.1016/j.emc.2006.05.012 PMID:16877143

Schugurensky, D. (2000). *The forms of informal learning: Towards a conceptualization of the field*. Centre for the Study of Education and Work.

Skule, S. (2004). Learning conditions at work: A framework to understand and assess informal learning in the workplace. *International Journal of Training and Development*, *8*(1), 8–20. doi:10.1111/j.1360-3736.2004.00192.x

Skule, S., Stuart, M., & Nyen, T. (2002). International briefing 12: Training and development in Norway. *International Journal of Training and Development*, *6*(4), 263–276. doi:10.1111/1468-2419.00164

Smith, S. D., Dunham, L., Dekhtyar, M., Dinh, A., Lanken, P. N., Moynahan, K. F., & Skochelak, S. E. et al. (2016). Medical Student Perceptions of the Learning Environment: Learning Communities Are Associated With a More Positive Learning Environment in a Multi-Institutional Medical School Study. *Academic Medical Documentation*. doi:10.1097/ACM.0000000000001214

Swanwick, T. (2005). Informal learning in postgraduate medical education: From cognitivism to culturism. *Medical Education*, *39*(8), 859–865. doi:10.1111/j.1365-2929.2005.02224.x PMID:16048629

The Arnold P. Gold Foundation. (2013). *About us: Overview*. Retrieved May 1, 2016, from http://humanism-in-medicine.org/about-us/

The Organisation for Economic Co-operation and Development. (2010). *Recognition of Non-formal and Informal Learning*. Retrieved April 29, 2016, from http://www.oecd.org/edu/skills-beyond-school/recognitionofnon-formalandinformallearning-home.htm

Tough, A. M. (2002). *The iceberg of informal adult learning*. NALL Working Paper, 49. Retrieved May 2, 2016, from http://nall.oise.utoronto.ca/res/49AllenTough.pdf

Tough, A. M. (1979). *The adult's learning projects: A fresh approach to theory and practice in adult learning* (2nd ed.). Austin, TX: Learning Concepts.

Triola, M. M. (2016). *Eduational innovation in a continuously learning health care system.* Keynote address delivered at the conference of the Central Group on Educational Affair, Ypsilanti, MI.

Triola, M. M., & Pusic, M. V. (2012). The education data warehouse: A transformative tool for health education research. *Journal of Gradudate Medical Education*, *4*(1), 113–115. doi:10.4300/JGME-D-11-00312.1 PMID:23451320

van Mook, W. N., de Grave, W. S., Gorter, S. L., Muijtjens, A. M., Zwaveling, J. H., Schuwirth, L. W., & van der Vleuten, C. P. (2010). Fellows' in intensive care medicine views on professionalism and how they learn it. *Intensive Care Medicine*, *36*(2), 296–303. doi:10.1007/s00134-009-1644-8 PMID:19771410

Wenger, E. (1998). *Communities of practice: Learning, meaning, and identify*. New York, NY: Cambridge University Press. doi:10.1017/CBO9780511803932

Werquin, P. (2010). *Recognizing non-formal and informal learning: Outcomes, Policies and Practices.* Retrieved April 25, 2016, from http://www.eucen.eu/sites/default/files/OECD_RNFIFL2010_Werquin.pdf

Young, J. R. (2008). When professors create social networks for classes, some students see a 'Creepy Treehouse'. *The Chronical of Higher Education*. Retrieved April 1, from http://chronicle.com/blogs/wiredcampus/when-professors-create-social-networks-for-classes-some-students-see-a-creepy-treehouse/4176

KEY TERMS AND DEFINITIONS

Big Data: An extremely large volume of data sets, structured or unstructured, that may be searched, captured, analyzed, curated, and stored to reveal patterns, trends, and associations, especially relating to human behaviors and interactions, to enable and inform better decisions on important issues.

Communities of Practice: Formed by groups of people who engage in collective, collaborative learning and share a concern, an interest, or passion for something that they do or learn how to do it better. Learning resulted from communal activities may or may not be intentional.

Evidence-Based Medicine: A paradigm of practicing medicine by integrating the best available current clinical research evidence with clinical expertise and patient circumstances, preferences, and biology.

Formal Learning: Learning that takes place within formal education settings or through formal training programs in institutions/organizations; it is structured, professionally planned, institutionally organized, with preset learning objectives and expected outcomes and anticipated, recognized diploma, certification, or qualifications.

Interprofessional Education and Practice: Learning and experiential or practical experiences resulted when learners from diverse health professions or educational programs are engaged in or participate in collaborative and collective learning and health care practice.

Learning Environment: Diverse physical locations, context, or culture in which students learn; qualities and characteristics of a learning environment are determined by a wide variety of factors; school policies, governance structures, and other features may also be considered elements of a "learning environment."

Lifelong Learning: The ongoing, voluntary, self-directed, self-motivated pursuit of learning for either personal or professional reasons throughout one's lifetime.

Medical Education: A continuum of education involving undergraduate medical education of an initial four year education program leading to a doctor of medicine degree (MD); graduate medical education of newly graduated MDs entering into a residency program for three to seven years or more of professional training in a medical specialty and additional training in a fellowship program (one to three years) for those who want to become highly specialized in a subspecialty; and continuing medical education of physicians who must complete yearly coursework and receive a certain number of continuing medical education (CME) credits per year to ensure their knowledge and skills remain current after they obtain a license to practice medicine following their residency or fellowship training.

Social Media: Computer-mediated tools that allow people to create, share, contribute, or exchange information, ideas, knowledge, and multimedia materials in virtual communities and networks. The term is often used interchangeably with web 2.0 or emerging technologies.

Chapter 12
Virtual Patients in Health Professions Education

A. J. Kleinheksel
Shadow Health, Inc., USA

ABSTRACT

The field of health professions continues to struggle with the impact of increasing practitioner and educator shortages. Health professions education is also faced with the issues of limited clinical placements and an increasing demand for online education. To address these issues, health professions educators have increasingly turned to simulations to provide experiential learning in safe, controlled environments. One of the newest simulation technology innovations to emerge is that of virtual patient simulations. This chapter reviews the context in which virtual patients have emerged, the range of virtual patient technologies available, and the ways in which health professions educators currently use virtual patient simulations.

INTRODUCTION

Healthcare in America is at a crossroads. As the population of the United States ages, more healthcare providers are needed, yet these same aging citizens are retiring from their healthcare careers. As a result, there are significant and imminent shortages in many fields of the health professions (Kreitzer, Kligler, & Meeker, 2009). The Bureau of Labor Statistics (2013) has identified registered nurses, licensed practical and licensed vocational nurses, home health aids, and nursing assistants as being among the occupations with the largest projected number of job openings due to growth and replacement needs. Nearly one-third of current registered nurses will reach retirement age within the coming decade (Health Resources and Services Administration, 2013). Family physicians and general internists are also facing similar shortages due to the increasing and aging population (Colwill, Cultice, & Kruse, 2008; Salsberg & Grover, 2006). However, to exacerbate the issue, there are shortages of health professions educators as well, and educational institutions cannot meet the demand of those applying to their programs (Dutile, Wright, & Beauchesne, 2011; Mancuso-Murphy, 2007; Salsberg & Grover, 2006). Another issue faced by health professions educators is the limited availability of clinical placements for their students (Hall, 2006;

DOI: 10.4018/978-1-5225-2098-6.ch012

Copyright © 2017, IGI Global. Copying or distributing in print or electronic forms without written permission of IGI Global is prohibited.

Kassam, Kwong, & Collins, 2013). In addition, these challenges in health professions education must be addressed within the context of an increasing demand for nontraditional educational programs, as health professions education is experiencing the fastest growing online enrollments of any field (Lytle, 2011).

Though health professions education programs struggle with high demand and limited resources in changing educational environments, they must still teach the knowledge, skills, and attitudes necessary to produce competent and safe professionals. To help meet the demand for the comprehensive education necessary to educate these health professionals, health professions educators have turned to simulations as a way to provide some portion of the experience in clinical environments necessary to develop safe and effective procedural, communication, and clinical reasoning skills (Aggarwal et al., 2010; Forsberg, Georg, Ziegert, & Fors, 2011; Guise, Chambers, Conradi, Kavia, & Välimäki, 2012; Schmidt, Goldhaber-Fiebert, Ho, & McDonald, 2013; Wilt & King, 2012). Although task trainers, roleplaying, standardized patients, and high-fidelity manikins have been used in the health professions for decades, a more recent development in healthcare simulations is that of virtual patients (Cendan & Lok, 2012; Cook, Erwin, & Triola, 2010; Rosen, 2008). The objective of this chapter is to document the emergence of virtual patient simulation in health professions education, and to define the range of technologies within this category of clinical simulation.

BACKGROUND

Medical errors are a significant cause of patient harm and morbidity in health care today (E. J. Lewis, Baernholdt, & Hamric, 2013). In the education of health professionals, faculty of all disciplines seek to teach their students the diagnostic reasoning and communication skills, and to foster the teamwork and self-confidence needed to provide safe and effective care in order to prevent these errors (Consorti, Mancuso, Nocioni, & Piccolo, 2012; Cook et al., 2010). Simulation is an established and effective method of providing a safe, risk-free environment where students can practice new skills and apply new knowledge without posing a threat to actual patients (Nehring & Lashley, 2009). There is strong evidence that the use of simulation can meet identified learning objectives and increase self-reported measures of engagement, satisfaction, and self-confidence (Arnold, Johnson, Tucker, Chesak, & Dierkhising, 2011; Cook et al., 2010; Howard, Englert, Kameg, & Perozzi, 2011). Existing literature also identifies simulation as an effective educational strategy for the achievement of patient safety learning outcomes (Blum & Parcells, 2012; Cook et al., 2012; Thornock, 2013). Simulation has been identified by anesthesiology researchers as a successful strategy for improving patient safety, decreasing patient morbidity, identifying latent errors, and facilitating improvements to process (Aebersold & Tschannen, 2013; Shear, Greenberg, & Tokarczyk, 2013). While it is difficult to pinpoint simulation as the cause of decreased medical errors, Durham and Alden (2008) described patient safety as a complex concept that includes not only the prevention of medical errors, but also the development of critical thinking and decision-making, effective communication, and the promotion of teamwork, all of which have been identified as outcomes achieved through the use of simulations (Aggarwal et al., 2010; Stanley & Latimer, 2011; Stevens et al., 2006; Stroup, 2014; Sweigart, Burden, Carlton, & Fillwalk, 2014).

Medical education began using human patient simulation at the turn of 20th century (Bradley, 2006). The subsequent introductions of mathematical descriptions of pathophysiology and the development of virtual worlds further advanced the uses of simulations in health professions education, and the environments in which they are conducted (Rosen, 2008). However, the use of manikins, standardized patients, and virtual simulations have only gained wide acceptance in health professions education since the turn of the 21st century (Bradley, 2006; Rosen, 2008). The United States military was instrumental in the broader adoption of simulation technology in medicine, and accounted for 80% of all modeling and simulation work prior to 1990 (Rosen, 2008). Currently, the field of medical simulation provides a variety of modalities through which to teach healthcare professionals (Cook et al., 2012). From task trainers to standardize patient actors to patient avatars, simulation allows for the development and reinforcement of clinical reasoning and psychomotor skills (Bradley, 2006; Forsberg et al., 2011; Nehring & Lashley, 2009; Rosen, 2008). The safe, risk-free environments that simulations provide are of significant value in the education of an ever-increasing number of students in health professions education, particularly due to the persistent shortage of health professions educators (Hayden, Smily, Raij, Kardong-Edgren, & Jeffries, 2014; Kassam et al., 2013; Mancuso-Murphy, 2007).

VIRTUAL PATIENT SIMULATION

One of the most recent modalities to be applied in the field of health professions simulation is that of virtual patients. The use of virtual patients in health professions education has been applied to a wide range of disciplines, including medical, pharmacy, clinical therapy, dental, and nursing education (Benedict & Schonder, 2011; Huang, Reynolds, & Candler, 2007; Kenny, Parsons, Gratch, Leuski, & Rizzo, 2007; Kiegaldie & White, 2006; Stevens et al., 2006). The critical literature review conducted by Cook and Triola (2009) proposed that virtual patients are a cost-effective, satisfying and effective method of simulation. However, virtual patients do have limitations, the most conspicuous of which is their deficiency in assessing the psychomotor domain; virtual patients have been shown to be better suited to the assessment of the cognitive and affective domains within the simulation environment. As a result, in many cases the learning objective of a virtual patient simulation is to teach, reinforce, and/or assess clinical reasoning skills. Cook and Triola (2009) have gone as far as to assert that the development of clinical reasoning is in fact the only valid learning objective for a virtual patient simulation, as non-analytical thinking will mature an individual healthcare provider's practice and lead to safer, more effective patient care decisions. The use of virtual patient simulations for the development of clinical reasoning is most often evident when virtual patients are used in a conjunction with self-reflection activities, as virtual patient simulations have been shown to facilitate a critical level of reflection, which is a crucial component to the development of clinical reasoning (Kleinheksel, 2014). However, though virtual patients are uniquely positioned to facilitate the development of clinical reasoning, Cook and Triola also noted that the assessment of virtual patient simulations often employs only an algorithmic approach to evaluation, which scores a student on the completeness of information they elicited rather than evaluating their clinical reasoning abilities. Prior research on virtual patient simulations have included qualitative, quasi-experimental controlled, and comparative designs, all of which found no significant difference between identified learning outcomes and learner satisfaction when compared to other methods of simulation (Consorti et al., 2012; Cook et al., 2010). Virtual patient simulations have also been shown to demonstrate large positive effect sizes for knowledge, clinical reasoning, and other skills when compared with no intervention (Consorti et al., 2012; Cook et al., 2010).

Virtual patient simulations offer several distinct benefits when compared to other types of manikin and standardized patient simulations, many of which stem from the flexibility offered within a virtual patient's implementation (Consorti et al., 2012; Dutile et al., 2011). Unlike high-fidelity simulations, virtual patients do not require the substantial initial financial investment by an institution, the clinical lab space on campus, or the dedicated technical staff to run a computer-operated manikin, which is a particular advantage for online and blended programs, as well as smaller programs with limited space available (McKeon, Norris, Cardell, & Britt, 2009). Virtual patients also do not require the investment of resources that are necessary to train a standardized patient actor, nor are they restricted by the space and scheduling limitations of examining a standardized patient (Kiegaldie & White, 2006; Stevens et al., 2006; Triola et al., 2006). The objective nature of a virtual patient simulation also differs from a standardized patient actor, who may grow tired of repeated simulations and deviate from the prescribed dialogue, or who could introduce explicit or implicit bias into their assessment of a student.

Virtual patient simulations have been used to replace some portion of clinical hours for those programs that have limited access to clinical placements, such as rural institutions, and to replace lab hours for advanced students in online programs spread over a large geographic area (Hayden et al., 2014). Virtual patients allow for the exposure of students to specific cases that may not be easily simulated through a manikin or standardized patient actor, including at-risk populations such as children with developmental disabilities (Sanders et al., 2008), adults with post traumatic stress disorder (Kenny, Parsons, Gratch, & Rizzo, 2008), and patients with a mental illness (Foster et al., 2014; Guise et al., 2012). A significant benefit of virtual patients is their asynchronous computer-based delivery, which is especially beneficial for distance education, working professional, and other nontraditional students who have competing commitments of their time and location. An asynchronous virtual patient simulation can be used by a working student who is taking a break on their shift at work, or by a nontraditional student who does their assignments late at night while their children are sleeping. Virtual patients are appealing to faculty due to their consistency, as they provide an objective and replicable experience to each student that can be used as a standardized assessment, or as a common point of reference in the classroom. This consistency of experience also can allow students to conduct the same virtual patient simulation multiple times, facilitating self-remediation of their previous performance deficiencies. Another explicit value to faculty is the transparency of student performance provided by virtual patient simulations. A virtual patient records every question asked, action taken, and decision made by a student, allowing faculty to identify deficiencies in knowledge or skills more precisely (Kelley, 2015).

While virtual patient simulations offer many benefits, they are cost-prohibitive to develop internally, with estimated costs ranging from $10,000 to $50,000, plus the cost of maintenance (Cendan & Lok, 2012; Cook & Triola, 2009; Huang et al., 2007). As a result, many health professions programs adopt one or more of the commercially developed virtual patient simulation applications available. Virtual patient software is currently available for purchase from educational technology and publishing companies such as Shadow Health (The Digital Clinical Experience), Wolters Kluwer (vSim) and i-Human Patients. Faculty may select a particular virtual patient simulation based on their perceived needs and the ways in which the available features of a simulation align with those needs. This has resulted in the emergence of virtual patients as a profitable commercial market within health professions education, one that is projected to reach $508.7 million in 2019 (Meticulous Research, 2014).

Virtual Patient Technologies

The technology described in prior virtual patient research has varied widely. Though many studies have used the same term of "virtual patient" to describe their simulations, several earlier studies, including those by Stevens, et al. (2006) and Kenny, Parsons, Gratch, Leuski, and Rizzo (2007), described the use of more dynamic and responsive tools that would have been better differentiated as a patient avatar or virtual character simulation as was done by Filichia, et al. (2011). Other studies have described a robotic full-scale manikin simulation as a virtual patient (Cendan & Lok, 2012; Cooper & Taqueti, 2004).

Though any simulation technology can be categorized by fidelity, the term high-fidelity simulation typically refers to a dynamic full-body manikin, which may be stationary, computer-operated, or operated by a technician. This type of simulation is conducted in a lab or other dedicated space, and often requires a trained specialist to facilitate their use. Other terms used to describe this type of simulation technology are patient simulator, human patient simulator, or full-scale simulator. Though less common, computer-operated high-fidelity manikin simulations have also been called virtual patients or electronic patients (Arnold et al., 2011; Cendan & Lok, 2012; Cook & Triola, 2009; Cooper & Taqueti, 2004; Nehring & Lashley, 2009).

Early screen-based virtual patients fall within the category of computer-assisted instruction. These programs typically included patient cases, multimedia instructional materials, feedback delivery, or other computer-based educational simulation technologies. The characteristic that differentiates computer-assisted instruction from modern virtual patients and virtual simulation environments is the lack of learner input and interaction within computer-assisted instruction. Computer-assisted instruction is a term found most often in the field of education (Cook & Triola, 2009; Nehring & Lashley, 2009).

Computer-based, asynchronous, interactive clinical scenarios are most commonly considered to be a virtual patient simulation. These programs allow students to either follow the progression of a linear case, or affect the outcome by the choices they make (Cook & Triola, 2009). Learner input can be selected from existing options, typed, or spoken as they interview, examine, order tests, and diagnose the virtual patient. Some virtual patient applications allow instructors to develop their own scenarios and cases. There are both open-source and commercial virtual patient simulations available. The media employed in some virtual patients are two-dimensional images or pictures accompanied by text within a database of patient information and responses, while other virtual patients are three-dimensional characters that can move and respond to student input. Assessment is sometimes embedded within the software, yet often instructors must evaluate the success of a virtual patient simulation (Cook et al., 2010; Huang et al., 2007; Kiegaldie & White, 2006).

Interactive, synchronous, virtual learning environments used to conduct individual or team-based simulations online are called immersive virtual reality simulations. Recent literature has referred to the patients within these synchronous virtual clinical simulations as patient avatars (Miller & Jensen, 2014; Sweigart et al., 2014). These virtual reality simulations require the participation of people to control each avatar within the virtual environment. Typically, a faculty member will control the patient in the case for each student, similar to the way in which a standardized patient actor will repeat their performance for each student. Studies that have used immersive virtual reality simulations have often employed the Second Life virtual world (Nehring & Lashley, 2009; Stewart et al., 2010; Sweigart et al., 2014).

Though often categorized as a virtual patient in research studies, the most recent development in virtual patient technology is that of the virtual character simulation, also called a virtual standardized patient, or digital standardized patient. A virtual character simulation is a virtual experience involving a more dynamic clinical simulation than a linear virtual patient case. Within the virtual environment, a virtual character is a three-dimensional, multimodal digital patient that can speak, move, and respond to learners using a conversation engine or other similar responsive input technology. This is the newest and least researched simulation technology in the field of virtual simulation (Consorti et al., 2012; Cook &

Triola, 2009; Cook et al., 2010; Stevens et al., 2006). A virtual human is similar to a virtual character, though it requires dedicated space and specialized hardware to create the mixed reality environment in which students can interact directly with the screen-based, often life-sized character through dynamic feedback systems that record a student's speech and movement (Johnsen, Raij, Stevens, Lind, & Lok, 2007).

Within the field of virtual clinical simulations, researchers and professionals have often used some of these terms interchangeably, or used one term to describe two very different technologies. The confusion stems from the overlapping nature of the terminology. The range of uses for each simulation technology can make it difficult to discern the meaning of a term within the literature. Though some research includes pictures or screen captures of the technology referenced, there are a number of published articles that do not include visual aids, and also do not adequately define the technology being studied. Health professions simulations instruction and research could benefit greatly from the standardization of simulation terminology. This author takes the position that the term standardized patient avatar should be adopted and defined as a computer-based, asynchronous, and interactive clinical simulation in which a student can conduct an interview through unprompted text or speech, and provide input or make choices in the examination or treatment of a simulated patient in a virtual environment. This definition builds upon the definition of a virtual patient proposed by Cook and Triola (2009), who defined virtual patient simulations as a "specific type of computer program that simulates real-life clinical scenarios; learners emulate the roles of health care providers to obtain a history, conduct a physical exam, and make diagnostic and therapeutic decisions." However, the term virtual patient has been used to describe such a wide range of technologies over the past decades it is difficult to immediately recognize the type of technology being employed. The term standardized patient avatar also builds upon the definition of a standardized patient, in which an actor is hired to perform the role of a predesigned patient, and then contributes to the evaluation of a student's communication and interview skills (Nehring & Lashley, 2009; Rosen, 2008). The definition of a standardized patient avatar serves to differentiate the use of the most immersive and engaging asynchronous virtual patient technologies currently available, and is both more inclusive of health professions students who may not make diagnostic or therapeutic decisions as part of their health care role or at that particular stage of their education, and more restrictive in the exclusion of synchronous computer programs, virtual reality, and high-fidelity simulations. This definition of a standardized patient avatar includes virtual characters, digital standardized patients, and virtual patient technologies that are delivered asynchronously and solely via personal computer without any additional hardware that is not standard with a typical laptop or desktop PC. This definition excludes synchronous immersive virtual reality simulations, linear patient cases and other computer-assisted instruction, and computer-operated manikin simulations, as well as virtual humans and virtual characters that require peripheral technology to interact with the simulation. The use of a more specific and restrictive definition can benefit the field of health professions education in two ways. First, the modern field of education now has a greater and more nuanced understanding of educational technologies. Not every clinical simulation technology that uses a computer is a virtual patient, and not every virtual learning environment is a virtual reality simulation. By acknowledging different computer-assisted technologies with more precise terminology, developers and users of standardized patient avatar technology can better understand the intent and unique benefits of this particular kind of clinical simulation. Second, because the asynchronous nature of standardized patient avatars contributes unique benefits and facilitates specific uses, the research conducted on standardized patient avatars can be more easily indexed and searched for, which will contribute to a clearer understanding of the technology for emerging scholars and research-based practitioners alike.

Virtual Patients in Medical Education

Although virtual patient technology has been in existence for decades, Huang, Reynolds, and Chandler (2007) found that only 24% of medical schools in the United States and Canada were incorporating virtual patient simulation technologies in their curriculum. However, significant research has been conducted on a range of virtual patient technologies demonstrating significant outcomes in medication education. Medical faculty, computer scientists, and educational technologists have researched virtual patients within medical education. Computer science research has been conducted on the input and feedback mechanisms of a virtual patient, including speech input, which requires natural language processing, behavior generation, speech generation, and animation output. This research has demonstrated significant outcomes, including in the training of psychiatry residents and novice psychotherapists in their interviewing of a patient with post traumatic stress disorder (Kenny, Parsons, & Rizzo, 2009; Kenny et al., 2008).

Virtual patients have proven to be particularly effective in development of patient interviewing and therapeutic communication skills (Cendan & Lok, 2012). This confirms earlier research, which suggested that the outcomes of virtual patient simulations were more successful when their structure was designed around a narrative rather than a problem to solve, but also that well-constructed virtual patients had the capability to affect emotional reactions within medical students (Bearman, Cesnik, & Liddell, 2001). Other more recent interdisciplinary research has been conducted to evaluate the efficacy of the virtual characters, including in the hand-off exchange between physicians, in anatomy education, and in the use of virtual character simulations as an assessment strategy for undergraduate medical students (Botezatu, Hult, Tessma, & Fors, 2010; Filichia et al., 2011; Tworek, Jamniczky, Jacob, Hallgrimsson, & Wright, 2013). Studies have also been conducted comparing virtual patients to other simulation technologies. Deladisma et al. (2007) found that, though to a lesser extent than they did with standardized patients, medical students expressed nonverbal communication and empathy in their virtual patient simulations.

Virtual Patients in Nursing Education

Studies on the application of virtual patient simulations in nursing education have addressed pre-licensure and graduate programs, as well as a range of nursing sub-disciplines from mental health to postgraduate critical care (Arnold et al., 2011; Forsberg et al., 2011; Guimond, Sole, & Salas, 2011; Guise et al., 2012; Kiegaldie & White, 2006; McKeon et al., 2009; Sanders et al., 2008; Walsh, 2011). Virtual patients in nursing education have been well received by students, who found them to be realistic and engaging, as well as a good opportunity to practice clinical skills (Forsberg et al., 2011). Apart from enjoying virtual patients, students also benefited from significant increases in both demonstrated mastery of content and perceived competency (R. A. Lewis, 2009; Sanders et al., 2008). The instructional benefits of virtual patient simulations most often cited in nursing education are the development of clinical reasoning skills, increased diagnostic knowledge, repeatable scenarios, asynchronous use, and improved confidence (Forsberg et al., 2011; Kiegaldie & White, 2006; R. A. Lewis, 2009; Mancuso-Murphy, 2007). The most recent research to emerge on virtual patients in nursing education found that nurses interacted with a screen-based, life-size virtual human surgeon in the same way they would with a real surgeon during a simulation in which the nurse had to speak up about a medical error when the surgeon was dismissive of their concern. This study concluded that simulation could help to train healthcare professionals to prepare for difficult interpersonal conflicts, which could prevent serious medical errors (Robb et al., 2015).

Virtual Patients in Dental Education

One other health profession that serves as an exemplar of the effective use virtual patient simulations is that of dental education. Virtual patient simulation delivered on a CD-ROM was used to increase student dentists' competency and confidence in their treatment of children with developmental disabilities. This study is noteworthy due to the diverse development team that designed the virtual patient case, which included pediatric dentistry faculty, educational specialists, an adult with a developmental disability, and parents of children with developmental disabilities. The case, which presented a 10-year-old child with Down syndrome and a toothache required students to make decisions on the appropriate interactions and procedures for the patient. The students reported satisfaction with the virtual patient experience, and demonstrated a significant change in knowledge as a result of the simulation (Kleinert et al., 2007). Dentistry faculty have also used virtual patient simulations to facilitate the practice of history taking. Students who used virtual patient simulations with free text input to interview their patient and review X-rays asked more relevant and thorough oral health history questions and spent more time on patient issues in their first real patient encounter than students who had only received traditional instruction. Researchers also found that students who engaged with the virtual patient demonstrated more empathy than their peers in the control group (Janda et al., 2004).

Curricular Integration of Virtual Patients

There is limited research on faculty's perceptions of virtual patients, however, the perceptions of simulation in general by faculty are largely positive. Though there are several studies on the barriers to adoption of new simulation modalities, the overwhelming majority of health professions faculty have used some type of simulation in their classroom (Sweigart et al., 2014). Nursing faculty experience the most significant resistance to simulation adoption with new or resource-intensive simulations, as role-playing and task trainers are widely accepted and established technologies in current nursing curriculum (Nehring & Lashley, 2009).

The most common positive perceptions of simulations among nursing faculty are achieving learning objectives and patient outcomes, providing meaningful feedback, facilitating self-reflection, improving clinical reasoning and critical thinking, providing unique clinical experiences that students would not otherwise experience, preparing students for professional practice, and flexibility of application (Akhtar-Danesh, Baxter, Valaitis, Stanyon, & Sproul, 2009; Conejo, 2010; Howard et al., 2011; Thornock, 2013). The modalities of high-fidelity and virtual patient simulations pose the most cited challenges in current research (Akhtar-Danesh et al., 2009; Howard et al., 2011). The most common dissatisfaction with the adoption of a new simulation modality is a perceived lack of support (e.g., facilitator, technical) and resources (e.g., time, space, financial) for integrating or facilitating the simulation technology (Akhtar-Danesh et al., 2009; Howard et al., 2011; Jansen, Berry, Brenner, Johnson, & Larson, 2010; Wilt & King, 2012). However, even when faculty are uncomfortable with new simulation technologies, there is a positive perception of the learning outcomes for students (Howard et al., 2011).

The intentional integration of a simulation modality into health professions curriculum is a critical component to its success. The lack of purposeful integration and unsystematic assignment of simulation activities can negatively affect learning outcomes (Clapper, 2011; Harder, 2009). Health professions faculty have considered the implementation of simulation a challenging and unfamiliar pedagogy, which can prevent intentional integration (de Hrussoczy-Wirth, 2010; Griffin-Sobel et al., 2010). For example, research has found that nursing faculty report a need for additional training in new technologies (Nguyen, Zierler, & Nguyen, 2011). Several studies have attempted to support faculty in the integration of simulation into their curriculum by creating faculty toolkits, using transdisciplinary teams, and providing faculty development programs (Griffin-Sobel, 2009; Griffin-Sobel et al., 2010; Webster, 2009). Because implementing simulation can be overwhelming for some faculty, literature-based integration methods have also been developed, which link scenarios with didactic information, prioritize debriefing, and provide opportunities for repetition (Jeffries, 2005; Kardong-Edgren, Starkweather, & Ward, 2008).

There is a wide range of ways in which virtual patient simulations might be integrated into health professions curricula (Cook & Triola, 2009). Due to the flexibility afforded by asynchronous computer-based simulations, faculty may use virtual patients to teach their students new content within the classroom; to provide an environment off-campus in which to allow their students to practice new skills and apply new knowledge; or as a summative assessment in order to evaluate the competency of their distance education students who do not have access to a standardized patient actor. In addition, although simulation has been shown to be an effective teaching strategy, simulation does change the dynamic of the student-teacher relationship. While conventional health professions education often relies on teacher-centric classroom strategies (e.g., lecture), simulation refocuses on the student, with the instructor serving as the facilitator (Jeffries, 2005; Murray, 2013). This refocus of attention is clearly apparent in virtual patient simulations, in which faculty are often not even present when a student is interacting with the virtual patient.

Five general categories of virtual patient simulation integration were identified in an exploratory factor analysis of virtual patient adoption and integration in nursing education by Kleinheksel (2015): *Hour replacement, Intensive integration, Leveling, Preparation,* and *Benchmarking*. The first category of integration behavior was that of *Hour replacement,* wherein faculty replaced clinical, practicum, or lab hours with ungraded time spent in virtual patient simulations. After the National Council of State Boards of Nursing found either no significant difference or a significant positive improvement between students in traditional clinical placements, and those students with either 25% or 50% of their clinical hours replaced with simulation (Hayden et al., 2014), and as more research explores the effectiveness and practical application of simulation technologies in nursing education, state boards of nursing and other health professions associations will likely continue to increase the amount of clinical hours eligible for replacement by simulation.

This is of particular importance because the replacement of clinical hours with virtual patient simulations also has the potential to help to alleviate the difficulty some programs experience in finding or funding clinical placements for their students. The category of *Intensive integration* was defined by a deep, time-intensive integration, in which faculty assigned the virtual patient simulations as a frequent, graded activity and created custom rubrics and worksheets to achieve learning outcomes not explicitly measured within the virtual patient program. These behaviors described an ability and desire by faculty to adapt the virtual patient to their unique goals, and an investment of the time required to engage in the grading of regularly assigned virtual patient simulations. Intensive integration addressed the difference between writing paper cases or designing standardized patient scenarios, in which faculty can address the exact clinical situation they feel is relevant to their curriculum and to the patient population their students will encounter, and the adoption of a commercially developed simulation program, which can be used as a regularly graded assignment, but may need modifications or adaptations to achieve a faculty's specific learning objectives.

The integration strategy of *Leveling* consisted of the use of virtual patients for the demonstration of complex concepts, the connection of content from other courses, or the summative assessment of proficiency. Faculty engaged in leveling behaviors the used the virtual patient program as illustration for the purpose of connecting concepts from other courses or content areas, a tool to introduce increasingly difficult principles, or as a summative assessment to establish proficiency at the end of the semester. The concept of demonstration is particularly well-suited to asynchronous virtual patient simulations, which can be assigned to students, and then used again either in the classroom or as a repeated assignment to exhibit or allow for the practice of more advanced techniques or skills. *Preparation* behavior was the integration strategy most often employed in the first semester of use of a virtual patient, or in situations in which the virtual patient was adopted due to administrative pressure, and consisted of the use of the virtual patient as a pass/fail activity assigned prior to classroom or lab hours in order to teach content, practice concepts, or to provide a common point of reference for an in-class discussion. This strategy included the assignment of the virtual patient before students attended lecture or lab activities as a way to introduce concepts, or to ensure students' readiness for expensive lab time.

Preparation is arguably the most basic integration strategy among the identified behaviors, due to the limited affect the virtual patient simulations have on the pedagogy of the course and the simple pass/fail assessment of student performance. While this category does leverage the objective nature of asynchronous virtual patients, students would gain greater benefits from the application of new skills and knowledge in a virtual patient simulation following a lecture or other content delivery. Students who are required to purchase their own license for virtual patient programs may also find less value in a virtual patient simulation when their effort is graded only as pass/fail if it is also given minimal academic weight in the course grade, or if faculty do not provide substantive feedback with their pass/fail assessment. *Benchmarking* described the use of the virtual patient as a formative assessment during the semester or to reinforce content after lecture. This integration strategy was employed by faculty who used the virtual patient to evaluate comprehension throughout the course of the semester (Kleinheksel, 2015).

As faculty adopt and integrate virtual patient simulations into their curriculum, intentional integration will facilitate greater satisfaction for both faculty and their students, and better learning outcomes. Virtual patients can be used as a supplementary activity, as a replacement for clinical hours, as an assessment tool, or as an environment in which to reinforce new knowledge and practice the application of skills. It is up to the faculty to evaluate the virtual patient technology and to assign the simulation to its most appropriate place within their curriculum.

CONCLUSION

Due to an increased need for safe and effective healthcare professionals, and fewer resources with which to train them, virtual patient simulations are likely to grow in number as they also grow in technological complexity. The use of virtual patient simulations has been shown to be an effective method to both supplement and replace existing clinical simulations and placements. Moving forward, in order to better differentiate the kinds of virtual patient technologies being described in research and in practice, the term standardized patient avatar should be used to describe the most dynamic and engaging of current virtual patients, which are computer-based, asynchronous, and interactive clinical simulations in which a student can provide input or make choices in the examination, interview, and treatment of a simulated patient in a virtual environment.

REFERENCES

Aebersold, M., & Tschannen, D. (2013). Simulation in nursing practice: The impact on patient care. *Online Journal of Issues in Nursing*, *18*(2), 83. PMID:23758424

Aggarwal, R., Soper, N., Ziv, A., Reznick, R., Mytton, O. T., Derbrew, M.,... Morimoto, T. (2010). Training and simulation for patient safety. *Quality & Safety in Health Care, 19*(4), i34-i43. doi:10.1136/qshc.2009.038562

Akhtar-Danesh, N., Baxter, P., Valaitis, R. K., Stanyon, W., & Sproul, S. (2009). Nurse faculty perceptions of simulation use in nursing education. *Western Journal of Nursing Research*, *31*(3), 312–329. doi:10.1177/0193945908328264 PMID:19176404

Arnold, J. J., Johnson, L. M., Tucker, S. J., Chesak, S. S., & Dierkhising, R. A. (2011). Comparison of three simulation-based teaching methodologies for emergency response. *Clinical Simulation in Nursing*, *9*(3), e85–e93. doi:10.1016/j.ecns.2011.09.004

Bearman, M., Cesnik, B., & Liddell, M. (2001). Random comparison of Virtual patient models in the context of teaching clinical communication skills. *Medical Education*, *35*(9), 824–832. doi:10.1046/j.1365-2923.2001.00999.x PMID:11555219

Benedict, N., & Schonder, K. (2011). Patient simulation software to augment an advanced pharmaceutics course. *American Journal of Pharmaceutical Education*, *75*(2), 1–9. doi:10.5688/ajpe75221 PMID:21519411

Blum, C. A., & Parcells, D. A. (2012). Relationship between high-fidelity simulation and patient safety in prelicensure nursing education: A comprehensive review. *The Journal of Nursing Education*, *51*(8), 429–U122. doi:10.3928/01484834-20120523-01 PMID:22624562

Botezatu, M., Hult, H., Tessma, M. K., & Fors, U. G. (2010). Virtual patient simulation for learning and assessment: Superior results in comparison with regular course exams. *Medical Teacher*, *32*(10), 845–850. doi:10.3109/01421591003695287 PMID:20854161

Bradley, P. (2006). The history of simulation in medical education and possible future directions. *Medical Education*, *40*(3), 254–262. doi:10.1111/j.1365-2929.2006.02394.x PMID:16483328

Bureau of Labor Statistics. (2013). *Occupations with the largest projected number of job openings due to growth and replacement needs, 2012 and projected 2022*. Retrieved from http://www.bls.gov/news.release/ecopro.t08.htm

Cendan, J., & Lok, B. (2012). The use of virtual patients in medical school curricula. *Advances in Physiology Education*, *36*(1), 48–53. doi:10.1152/advan.00054.2011 PMID:22383412

Clapper, T. C. (2011). Interference in learning: What curriculum developers need to know. *Clinical Simulation in Nursing*, *7*(3), e77–e80. doi:10.1016/j.ecns.2010.08.001

Colwill, J. M., Cultice, J. M., & Kruse, R. L. (2008). Will generalist physician supply meet demands of an increasing and aging population?. *Health Affairs (Project Hope)*, *27*(3), w232–w241. doi:10.1377/hlthaff.27.3.w232 PMID:18445642

Conejo, P. E. (2010). *Faculty and student perceptions of preparation for and implementation of high fidelity simulation experiences in associate degree nursing programs* (Ph.D. Dissertation). Available from ProQuest Dissertations & Theses Full Text. (305210649). Retrieved from http://search.proquest.com.lp.hscl.ufl.edu/docview/305210649?accountid=10920

Consorti, F., Mancuso, R., Nocioni, M., & Piccolo, A. (2012). Efficacy of virtual patients in medical education: A meta-analysis of randomized studies. *Computers & Education, 59*(3), 1001–1008. doi:10.1016/j.compedu.2012.04.017

Cook, D. A., & Triola, M. M. (2009). Virtual patients: A critical literature review and proposed next steps. *Medical Education, 43*(4), 303–311. doi:10.1111/j.1365-2923.2008.03286.x PMID:19335571

Cook, D. A., Brydges, R., Hamstra, S. J., Zendejas, B., Szostek, J. H., Wang, A. T., & Hatala, R. et al. (2012). Comparative effectiveness of technology-enhanced simulation versus other instructional methods. *Simulation in Healthcare, 7*(5), 308–320. doi:10.1097/SIH.0b013e3182614f95 PMID:23032751

Cook, D. A., Erwin, P. J., & Triola, M. M. (2010). Computerized virtual patients in health professions education: A systematic review and meta-analysis. *Academic Medicine, 85*(10), 1589–1602. doi:10.1097/ACM.0b013e3181edfe13 PMID:20703150

Cooper, J. B., & Taqueti, V. R. (2004). A brief history of the development of mannequin simulators for clinical education and training. *Quality & Safety in Health Care, 13*(Suppl 1), i11-i18. doi:13/suppl_1/i11

de Hrussoczy-Wirth, D. (2010). *Simulation in undergraduate nursing education curriculum: An integrated review of the literature (Unpublished Master of Nursing).* University of Victoria.

Deladisma, A. M., Cohen, M., Stevens, A., Wagner, P., Lok, B., Bernard, T., & Dickerson, R. et al. (2007). Do medical students respond empathetically to a virtual patient? *American Journal of Surgery, 193*(6), 756–760.

Durham, C. F., & Alden, K. R. (2008). Enhancing patient safety in nursing education through patient simulation. In R. G. Hughes (Ed.), *Patient safety and quality: An evidence-based handbook for nurses.* Rockville, MD: Agency for Healthcare Research and Quality.

Dutile, C., Wright, N., & Beauchesne, M. (2011). Virtual clinical education: Going the full distance in nursing education. *Newborn and Infant Nursing Reviews; NAINR, 11*(1), 43–48. doi:10.1053/j.nainr.2010.12.008

Filichia, L., Halan, S., Blackwelder, E., Rossen, B., Lok, B., Korndorffer, J., & Cendan, J. (2011). Description of web-enhanced virtual character simulation system to standardize patient hand-offs. *The Journal of Surgical Research, 166*(2), 176–181. doi:10.1016/j.jss.2010.04.052 PMID:20828726

Forsberg, E., Georg, C., Ziegert, K., & Fors, U. (2011). Virtual patients for assessment of clinical reasoning in nursing: A pilot study. *Nurse Education Today, 31*(8), 757–762. doi:10.1016/j.nedt.2010.11.015 PMID:21159412

Foster, A., Chaudhary, N., Murphy, J., Lok, B., Waller, J., & Buckley, P. F. (2014). The use of simulation to teach suicide risk assessment to health profession Trainees—Rationale, methodology, and a proof of concept demonstration with a virtual patient. *Academic Psychiatry*, 1–10. PMID:25026950

Griffin-Sobel, J. P. (2009). The ENTREE model for integrating technologically rich learning strategies in a school of nursing. *Clinical Simulation in Nursing*, *5*(2), e73–e78. doi:10.1016/j.ecns.2009.01.008

Griffin-Sobel, J. P., Acee, A., Sharoff, L., Cobus-Kuo, L., Woodstock-Wallace, A., & Dornbaum, M. (2010). A transdisciplinary approach to faculty development in nursing education technology. *Nursing Education Perspectives*, *31*(1), 41–43. doi:10.1043/1536-5026-31.1.41 PMID:20397480

Guimond, M. E., Sole, M. L., & Salas, E. (2011). Getting ready for simulation-based training: A checklist for nurse educators. *Nursing Education Perspectives*, *32*(3), 179–185. doi:10.5480/1536-5026-32.3.179 PMID:21834380

Guise, V., Chambers, M., Conradi, E., Kavia, S., & Välimäki, M. (2012). Development, implementation and initial evaluation of narrative virtual patients for use in vocational mental health nurse training. *Nurse Education Today*, *32*(6), 683–689. doi:10.1016/j.nedt.2011.09.004 PMID:22056146

Hall, W. A. (2006). Developing clinical placements in times of scarcity. *Nurse Education in Practice*, *6*(6), 319–325. doi:10.1016/j.nepr.2006.07.005 PMID:19040897

Harder, B. N. (2009). Evolution of simulation use in health care education. *Clinical Simulation in Nursing*, *5*(5), e169–e172. doi:10.1016/j.ecns.2009.04.092

Hayden, J. K., Smily, R. A., Raij, A., Kardong-Edgren, S., & Jeffries, P. R. (2014). The NCSBN national simulation study: A longitudinal, randomized, controlled Study Replacing clinical hours with simulation in Prelicensure nursing education. *Journal of Nursing Regulation*, *5*(2Supplement.).

Health Resources and Services Administration. (2013). *The U.S. nursing workforce: Trends in supply and education*. Rockville, MD: National Center for Health Workforce Analysis.

Howard, V. M., Englert, N., Kameg, K., & Perozzi, K. (2011). Integration of simulation across the undergraduate curriculum: Student and faculty perspectives. *Clinical Simulation in Nursing*, *7*(1), e1–e10. doi:10.1016/j.ecns.2009.10.004

Huang, G., Reynolds, R., & Candler, C. (2007). Virtual patient simulation at U.S. and canadian medical schools. *Academic Medicine*, *82*(5), 446–451. doi:10.1097/ACM.0b013e31803e8a0a PMID:17457063

Janda, M. S., Mattheos, N., Nattestad, A., Wagner, A., Nebel, D., Färbom, C., & Attström, R. et al. (2004). Simulation of patient encounters using a virtual patient in periodontology instruction of dental students: Design, usability, and learning effect in History-Taking skills. *European Journal of Dental Education*, *8*(3), 111–119. doi:10.1111/j.1600-0579.2004.00339.x PMID:15233775

Jansen, D. A., Berry, C., Brenner, G. H., Johnson, N., & Larson, G. (2010). A collaborative project to influence nursing faculty interest in simulation. *Clinical Simulation in Nursing, 6*(6), e223-e229. http://dx.doi.org.lp.hscl.ufl.edu/10.1016/j.ecns.2009.08.006

Jeffries, P. R. (2005). A framework for designing, implementing, and evaluating simulations used as teaching strategies in nursing. *Nursing Education Perspectives*, *26*(2), 96. PMID:15921126

Johnsen, K., Raij, A., Stevens, A., Lind, D. S., & Lok, B. (2007). The validity of a virtual human experience for interpersonal skills education. In *Proceedings of the SIGCHI Conference on Human Factors in Computing Systems*, (pp. 1049-1058). doi:10.1145/1240624.1240784

Kardong-Edgren, S. E., Starkweather, A. R., & Ward, L. D. (2008). The integration of simulation into a clinical foundations of nursing course: Student and faculty perspectives. *International Journal of Nursing Education Scholarship*, *5*(1), 1–16. doi:10.2202/1548-923X.1603 PMID:18673294

Kassam, R., Kwong, M., & Collins, J. (2013). Role-emergent model: An effective strategy to address clinical placement shortages. *The Internet Journal of Allied Health Sciences and Practice*, *11*(4).

Kelley, C. G. (2015). Using a virtual patient in an advanced assessment course.[doi]. *The Journal of Nursing Education*, *54*(4), 228–231. doi:10.3928/01484834-20150218-13 PMID:25692279

Kenny, P. G., Parsons, T. D., Gratch, J., & Rizzo, A. A. (2008). Evaluation of justina: A virtual patient with PTSD. In *Intelligent Virtual Agents,* (pp. 394-408). doi:10.1007/978-3-540-85483-8_40

Kenny, P. G., Parsons, T. D., & Rizzo, A. A. (2009). *Human computer interaction in virtual standardized patient systems. In Human-computer interaction. interacting in various application domains* (pp. 514–523). Springer. doi:10.1007/978-3-642-02583-9_56

Kenny, P. G., Parsons, T. D., Gratch, J., Leuski, A., & Rizzo, A. A. (2007). *Virtual patients for clinical therapist skills training*. Berlin: Springer Berlin Heidelberg; doi:10.1007/978-3-540-74997-4_19

Kiegaldie, D., & White, G. (2006). The virtual patient: Development, implementation and evaluation of an innovative computer simulation for postgraduate nursing students. *Journal of Educational Multimedia and Hypermedia*, *15*(1), 31–47.

Kleinert, H. L., Sanders, C., Mink, J., Nash, D., Johnson, J., Boyd, S., & Challman, S. (2007). Improving student dentist competencies and perception of difficulty in delivering care to children with developmental disabilities using a virtual patient module. *Journal of Dental Education, 71*(2), 279-286. doi:71/2/279

Kleinheksel, A. J. (2014). Transformative learning through virtual patient simulations: Predicting critical student reflections. *Clinical Simulation in Nursing*, *10*(6), e301–e308. doi:10.1016/j.ecns.2014.02.001

Kleinheksel, A. J. (2015). *Measuring the adoption and integration of virtual patient simulations in nursing education: An exploratory factor analysis (Unpublished PhD Dissertation)*. University of Florida.

Kreitzer, M. J., Kligler, B., & Meeker, W. C. (2009). Health professions education and integrative healthcare. *Explore (New York, N.Y.)*, *5*(4), 212–227. doi:10.1016/j.explore.2009.05.012 PMID:19608111

Lewis, E. J., Baernholdt, M., & Hamric, A. B. (2013). Nurses experience of medical errors: An integrative literature review. *Journal of Nursing Care Quality*, *28*(2), 153–161. doi:10.1097/NCQ.0b013e31827e05d1 PMID:23222195

Lewis, R. A. (2009). *The effect of virtual clinical gaming simulations on student learning outcomes in medical-surgical nursing education courses* (Ed.D. Dissertation). Available from ProQuest Dissertations & Theses Full Text. (305123049). Retrieved from http://search.proquest.com.lp.hscl.ufl.edu/docview/305123049?accountid=10920

Lytle, R. (2011, November 11). Study: Online education continues growth. *US News and World Report.* Retrieved from http://www.usnews.com/education/online-education/articles/2011/11/11/study-online-education-continues-growth

Mancuso-Murphy, J. (2007). Distance education in nursing: An integrated review of online nursing students' experiences with technology-delivered instruction. *The Journal of Nursing Education*, *46*(6), 252–260. PMID:17580737

McKeon, L. M., Norris, T., Cardell, B., & Britt, T. (2009). Developing patient-centered care competencies among prelicensure nursing students using simulation. *The Journal of Nursing Education*, *48*(12), 711–715. doi:10.3928/01484834-20091113-06 PMID:20000255

Meticulous Research. (2014). *Global virtual patient simulation market to reach $508.7 million by 2019* [Press Release]. Meticulous Research.

Miller, M., & Jensen, R. (2014). Avatars in nursing: An integrative review. *Nurse Educator*, *39*(1), 38–41. doi:10.1097/01.NNE.0000437367.03842.63 PMID:24300258

Murray, T. A. (2013). Innovations in nursing education: The state of the art. *Journal of Nursing Regulation*, *3*(4), 25–31. doi:10.1016/S2155-8256(15)30183-6

Nehring, W. M., & Lashley, F. R. (2009). Nursing simulation: A review of the past 40 years. *Simulation & Gaming*, *40*(4), 528–552. doi:10.1177/1046878109332282

Nguyen, D. N., Zierler, B., & Nguyen, H. Q. (2011). A survey of nursing faculty needs for training in use of new technologies for education and practice. *The Journal of Nursing Education*, *50*(4), 181–189. doi:10.3928/01484834-20101130-06 PMID:21117532

Robb, A., White, C., Cordar, A., Wendling, A., Lampotang, S., & Lok, B. (2015). A comparison of speaking up behavior during conflict with real and virtual humans. *Computers in Human Behavior*, *52*, 12–21. doi:10.1016/j.chb.2015.05.043

Rosen, K. R. (2008). The history of medical simulation. *Journal of Critical Care*, *23*(2), 157–166. doi:10.1016/j.jcrc.2007.12.004 PMID:18538206

Salsberg, E., & Grover, A. (2006). Physician workforce shortages: Implications and issues for academic health centers and policymakers. *Academic Medicine*, *81*(9), 782–787. doi:10.1097/00001888-200609000-00003 PMID:16936479

Sanders, C. L., Kleinert, H. L., Free, T., King, P., Slusher, I., & Boyd, S. (2008). Developmental disabilities: Improving competence in care using virtual patients. *The Journal of Nursing Education*, *47*(2), 66–73. doi:10.3928/01484834-20080201-05 PMID:18320957

Schmidt, E., Goldhaber-Fiebert, S. N., Ho, L. A., & McDonald, K. M. (2013). Simulation exercises as a patient safety strategy: A systematic review. *Annals of Internal Medicine*, *158*(5 Pt 2), 426–426. doi:10.7326/0003-4819-158-5-201303051-00010 PMID:23460100

Shear, T., Greenberg, S., & Tokarczyk, A. (2013). Does training with human patient simulation translate to improved patient safety and outcome? *Current Opinion in Anaesthesiology*, *26*(2), 159–163. doi:10.1097/ACO.0b013e32835dc0af PMID:23339975

Stanley, D., & Latimer, K. (2011). *'The ward': A simulation game for nursing students*. Academic Press. doi:10.1016/j.nepr.2010.05.010

Stevens, A., Hernandez, J., Johnsen, K., Dickerson, R., Raij, A., & Harrison, C. (2006). *The use of virtual patients to teach medical students history taking and communication skills.* Academic Press.

Stewart, S., Hansen, T. S., Pope, D., Schmidt, B., Thyes, J. G., Jambunathan, J., & Berthold, T. (2010). Developing a second life campus for online accelerated BSN students. *Computers, Informatics, Nursing, 28*(5), 253–258. doi:10.1097/01.NCN.0000388348.29174.9f PMID:20736721

Stroup, C. (2014). Simulation usage in nursing fundamentals: Integrative literature review. *Clinical Simulation in Nursing, 10*(3), e155-e164. http://dx.doi.org.lp.hscl.ufl.edu/10.1016/j.ecns.2013.10.004

Sweigart, L., Burden, M., Carlton, K. H., & Fillwalk, J. (2014). Virtual simulations across curriculum prepare nursing students for patient interviews. *Clinical Simulation in Nursing, 10*(3), e139-e145. http://dx.doi.org.lp.hscl.ufl.edu/10.1016/j.ecns.2013.10.003

Thornock, S. B. (2013). *Satisfaction of outcome achievement with web-enhanced teaching strategies in nursing education* (Ed.D. Dissertation). Available from ProQuest Dissertations & Theses Full Text. (1400228888). Retrieved from http://search.proquest.com.lp.hscl.ufl.edu/docview/1400228888?accountid=10920

Triola, M., Feldman, H., Kalet, A. L., Zabar, S., Kachur, E. K., Gillespie, C.,... Lipkin, M. (2006). *A randomized trial of teaching clinical skills using virtual and live standardized patients.* Academic Press. doi:10.1111/j.1525-1497.2006.00421.x

Tworek, J., Jamniczky, H., Jacob, C., Hallgrimsson, B., & Wright, B. (2013). The LINDSAY virtual human project: An immersive approach to anatomy and physiology. *Anatomical Sciences Education, 6*(1), 19–28. doi:10.1002/ase.1301 PMID:22791664

Walsh, M. (2011). *Narrative pedagogy and simulation: Future directions for nursing education.* Academic Press.

Webster, M. R. (2009). An innovative faculty toolkit: Simulation success. *Nurse Educator, 34*(4), 148–149. doi:10.1097/NNE.0b013e3181aabdf9 PMID:19574848

Wilt, K. E., & King, M. (2012). Time well spent: Integrating simulation into an accelerated 1-year BSN program. *Clinical Simulation in Nursing, 8*(3), e103-e107. http://dx.doi.org.lp.hscl.ufl.edu/10.1016/j.ecns.2010.10.002

KEY TERMS AND DEFINITIONS

Computer-Assisted Instruction: Patient cases, multimedia instructional materials, feedback delivery, or other computer-based educational simulation technologies. The characteristic that differentiates computer-assisted instruction from virtual patients and virtual simulation environments in the lack of learner input and interaction.

Fidelity: The concept of fidelity in medical simulations refers to the authenticity and accuracy of a tool or environment. Simulated patients and clinical settings are generally categorized into low-, moderate-, or high-fidelity categories.

High-Fidelity Simulation: Also called a human patient simulator or patient simulator, this term typically refers to a computer- or technician-operated, dynamic full-body manikin.

Immersive Virtual Reality Simulation: Also called a patient avatar simulation, immersive virtual reality simulations are interactive, synchronous virtual environments used to conduct individual or team-based simulations online. Studies on this type of simulation technology have often used the Second Life virtual world.

Simulation: The orchestration of a process or scenario for the purpose of teaching or reinforcing skills or knowledge in a low-risk environment. Clinical simulations can range from low-fidelity (e.g., case study or task trainer), to moderate fidelity (e.g., screen-based scenarios), to high-fidelity (e.g., dynamic, full-body manikin), where "fidelity" refers to the accuracy and realism of the system.

Standardized Patient Avatar: A computer-based, asynchronous, and interactive clinical simulation in which a student can conduct an interview through unprompted text or speech, and provide input or make choices in the examination or treatment of a simulated patient in a virtual environment.

Virtual Character Simulation: Also known as a virtual standardized patient, or digital standardized patient, a virtual character simulation is a virtual experience involving a dynamic, asynchronous, computer-based clinical simulation. Within a virtual environment, a virtual character is a three-dimensional, multimodal digital patient that can speak, move, and respond to learners using a conversation database or other similar responsive technology. Virtual character simulations may require peripheral hardware not typically included with a computer to represent tactile contact with part of a human body. Virtual humans are a virtual reality simulation with a virtual character.

Virtual Patient: Computer-based, asynchronous, interactive clinical scenarios that allow students to either follow the progression of a linear case, or to affect the outcome by the choices they make. Learner input can be spoken, typed, or selected from existing options as they interview, examine, order tests, and diagnose the virtual patient. Some virtual patient applications allow instructors to develop their own scenarios and cases. The media employed in some virtual patients are two-dimensional images accompanied by text within a database of patient information and responses, while others are three-dimensional characters that can move and respond to student input.

Chapter 13
Development and Evaluation of Neuroscience Computer-Based Modules for Medical Students:
Instructional Design Principles and Effectiveness

Kathryn L. Lovell
Michigan State University, USA

ABSTRACT

Interactive neuropathology computer-based teaching modules and other neuroscience computer-based resources were developed to provide individualized self-paced content information accompanied by images and self-assessment questions with feedback, along with problem-solving cases to facilitate application of neuroanatomy, neurology, and neuropathology concepts to patient cases. Initial implementation occurred in three curricula for second-year medical students. Evaluation of the modules was conducted using quantitative and qualitative methods to determine features of the modules that were important for students. This chapter will describe the instructional design principles that evaluation results identified as important and effective for student learning, and compare those to current principles for effective multimedia instructional design identified in a variety of research. Especially important principles applied in the neuroscience modules included cognitive load theory, retrieval practice and self-assessment, feedback, and learner control.

INTRODUCTION

Interactive computer-based teaching modules covering neuropathology content for second-year medical students were first developed by the author when interactive computer programs (e.g. Hypercard) and videodiscs with randomly accessible images became available (images from the second edition of Slice of Life videodisc, coordinated by Suzanne Stensaas, Ph.D., were utilized; most of the neuropathology images were provided by Margaret Z. Jones, M.D.). These factors were ideal for pathology content where

DOI: 10.4018/978-1-5225-2098-6.ch013

Copyright © 2017, IGI Global. Copying or distributing in print or electronic forms without written permission of IGI Global is prohibited.

gross and microscopic images are essential to the learning process. The goal of the modules was to provide individualized self-paced content information accompanied by images and self-testing questions with feedback, along with problem-solving cases to facilitate application of neuroanatomy, neurology, and neuropathology concepts to patient cases.

The development process included consideration of instructional design principles, production of initial topics (neoplastic disorders and cerebrovascular disorders), use-testing to determine student perceptions of technical and instructional effectiveness, and revisions based on student input. All images and diagrams were open source (Creative Commons or similar licensing). The interactive modules have been used continuously in the Colleges of Human Medicine and Osteopathic Medicine at Michigan State University since 1988, and repeated evaluations have demonstrated student support for the effectiveness of the instructional design principles. Periodic changes have been made based on changes in software and hardware, and access to additional images, and additional neuroscience units have been created for specific teaching goals.

The objectives of this chapter are to describe the development and structure of the neuropathology teaching modules and other units, including the instructional design principles utilized; to summarize results of evaluation of the modules by students; and to compare features of the modules with instructional design principles based on theories of learning and experimental evidence from other research.

BACKGROUND

Initial Structure and Implementation of Neuropathology Modules

Two neuropathology topics (neoplastic disorders and cerebrovascular disorders) were selected for initial module development and use-testing by students before additional topic modules were generated. The initial computer-based modules consisted of:

- Pre-test.
- Lesson utilizing text, diagrams and images (both normal and abnormal) with descriptions.
- Post-test (with immediate feedback for correct and incorrect answers).
- Clinical simulation emphasizing reinforcement of concepts in the lesson.
- Glossary.

A randomly accessible table of contents was available to permit learner control over lesson sequencing. The content of the units were based on paper modules with images provided in 35mm slide carousels developed previously by Dr. Margaret Z. Jones. Images in the modules were from the second edition of Slice of Life videodisc, coordinated by Suzanne Stensaas, Ph.D., University of Utah); most of the neuropathology images used were provided by Margaret Z. Jones, M.D., Michigan State University).

Hodgins & Lovell (1988) described the implementation of the initial two units in three curricular formats in the Colleges of Human Medicine and Osteopathic Medicine at Michigan State University (systems curriculum, discipline-based courses, problem-based independent study curriculum). The modules were designed to be usable by students in any order at any time, and could be used individually or in groups, and were required or optional for different sets of students. A log-in system and data tracking system recorded data during student use of the modules to determine the time spent in each component of each module.

The first formal evaluation of the two initial modules was described by Lovell et al. (1991). It should be noted that some of the evaluation related to using the new computer technology that was just beginning to be available in medical education. Students were given an evaluation form when the videodisc was checked out in the computer laboratory, and most students (over 80 for each module) completed the form. The evaluation form had three parts: Likert scale rating of effectiveness of different parts of the units; student preference for specific features of the units; and written comments. In addition, focus groups were organized to get feedback from students about hardware, utility of the modules to help students achieve levels of mastery, appropriateness of module content, organizational factors, motivational factors, and self-testing components within the module. Results indicated that students rated all aspects of the modules as very valuable in helping master the material, including content, images, diagrams, and review questions.

In addition, many of the open-ended comments emphasized the value and effectiveness of the interactive videodisc instructional modules in helping them master course content. About half of the students used the modules on a voluntary basis, even though the content was also covered in lectures and written course materials. Focus group session comment summaries included the following points: the modules were best suited for acquiring basic concepts and principles and practicing with case studies; the glossary and visual ability to compare normal and abnormal images were helpful; the organization was excellent and fit into the overall course; the reference points in each lesson were helpful. The self-evaluation components (post-test questions) were especially effective for students, and they suggested increasing the number of test questions.

After getting preliminary feedback on the two initial modules, additional modules were developed to encompass all of the neuropathology topics taught for second-year medical students, and further evaluation was conducted on effectiveness of specific features, to be discussed further in a different section of this chapter.

Cognitive Load Theory

Cognitive load theory describes learning effectiveness in terms of the capacity of working memory, which is limited. Working memory is divided into intrinsic, germane and extraneous loads and has a total that cannot be exceeded during the process of learning new material (Lau, 2014, Paas et al., 2010, Mayer, 2010, Mayer and Moreno 2010, Sweller 1994, and van Merrienboer and Sweller, 2010). Intrinsic load refers to the inherent difficulty of the material and typically cannot be altered by instructional interventions without altering the content to be learned (e.g. simplification). Extraneous load is imposed by instructional procedures, i.e. the attention paid towards the presentation of the material as compared to the intrinsic difficulty of the material itself. Germane load refers to the understanding of information through which to integrate the new knowledge into one's permanent memory, i.e. meaningful learning. Part of germane load involves connecting new information elements to existing frameworks in long-term memory. In cognitive load theory, intrinsic and extraneous cognitive loads are additive; if working memory is exceeded in a learning task, minimizing extraneous load can increase working memory capacity for germane load. Thus, reduction of extraneous cognitive load is a major goal of designing multimedia instructional materials in order to increase learning effectiveness.

Retrieval Practice (Testing Effect) and Self-Assessment

Karpicke and Blunt (2011) and Karpicke and Roediger (2008) demonstrated that a combination of study and tests is more effective than spending the same amount of time reviewing the material in some other way, such as rereading it. Rohrer and Pashler (2010) pointed out that surveys of college students show that most of them study almost entirely by rereading, with self-testing relatively rarely employed. In the author's experience this is also true for medical students, either because self-testing materials are not available or there is lack of awareness of the value of this approach. For many medical school pre-clinical courses, there is great variability in the availability of self-testing questions that are consistent with the objectives of the material to be tested over in a high-stakes course examination. Cognitive psychology research has demonstrated that repeated testing of information in any format produces superior retention compared to repeated study, a finding that is found across a wide variety of materials and experimental conditions (Larsen et al., 2008, Karpicke and Roediger, 2008, Karpicke and Blunt, 2011, Schmidmeier et al., 2011, Wood, 2009, and Rohrer and Pashler, 2010).

There are different types of tests that can be used to practice retrieval, including vocabulary tests, true-false statements, multiple-choice questions, short-answer questions, and essay or free recall questions. All are effective, but tests that require effortful retrieval of information, such as short-answer tests or free recall after reading a passage, or concept mapping, promote better retention and meaningful learning than tests based on recognition only such as multiple-choice tests. These results support the theory that retrieval practice enhances learning by retrieval-specific mechanisms that are more effective than episodes of repeated study.

According to Karpicke and Blunt (2011):

Not only does retrieval produce learning, but a retrieval event may actually represent a more powerful learning activity than an encoding event. This research suggests a conceptualization of mind and learning that is different from one in which encoding places knowledge in memory and retrieval simply accesses that stored knowledge. Because each act of retrieval changes memory, the act of reconstructing knowledge must be considered essential to the process of learning.

In the studies on retrieval practice, students also demonstrated inability to judge their own learning proficiency when they were asked to predict performance on an upcoming test. Karpicke and Blunt (2011) examined students metacognitive knowledge of the effectiveness of different types of learning activities (i.e. students predicted the percentage of information they would remember in 1 week). Students predicted that repeated studying would produce the best long-term retention on both factual and inference questions, and that practicing retrieval would produce the worst retention, even though the opposite was true. Thus students are not able to assess their level of competence or effectiveness of study strategies prior to an examination. This is also true for many medical students in the author's experience. An opportunity and encouragement for testing (or self-testing or self-assessment) is critical for students to assess their own level of knowledge and to most effectively learn and retain material.

Open Access and Creative Commons

One of the challenges in development of multimedia materials that will be open for all (open access) to use (through CD-ROM distribution or freely available on the Internet) is finding open access images or diagrams that illustrate the content, especially in the fields based on visual identification, such as anatomy, pathology and radiology. Carroll (2013) states that openness requires making the literature freely accessible under liberal terms that permit nearly all reuses so long as the author receives credit for the work when it's republished or adapted. Copyright owners seeking to grant permission to everyone have issued public licenses broadening the range of permitted uses, subject to certain conditions, e.g. attribution, use only for educational purposes, use only for non-profit endeavors. Creative Commons licenses (http://creativecommons.org/) are the most widely used for most educational materials, according to Carroll (2013). The Wikipedia community, for example, has adopted the Creative Commons Attribution ShareAlike license.

From 1985 to 2007, the Slice of Life Project (http://slice.utah.edu/sol/), based at the University of Utah, served as a nonprofit, cooperative venture creating and sharing educational materials using computers, multimedia, and new media in health care, health sciences, and medical education. Many people were instrumental in the Slice of Life Project, notably Dr. Suzanne S. Stensaas, who conceived of the videodisc and marshaled the cooperation and contributions of her colleagues, educators and research professionals in the health sciences and medical education. All of the images on the videodiscs could be used and adapted for non-profit educational purposes under a Creative Commons license.

The Health Education Assets Library (HEAL; http://library.med.utah.edu/heal/) was formed as a multi-institutional repository of multimedia learning objects for health sciences education. HEAL's vision was to create a premier national digital library for all levels of health sciences education by providing free and easy access to a large number of high-quality educational materials. This collection, which is no longer funded, still provides online access to many types of open source images, diagrams and videos.

More recently other initiatives have been developed with similar goals, at a variety of levels. For example, Open.Michigan (http://open.umich.edu/index.html) is a University of Michigan initiative that enables faculty, students, and others to share their educational resources and research with the global learning community. The Open Education Consortium (http://www.oeconsortium.org/) is a global network for open education. MedEdPORTAL (www.mededportal.org/), provided by the Association of American Medical Colleges, makes available stand-alone modules following a rigorous peer review process.

MAIN FOCUS OF THE CHAPTER

Evaluation Results for Neuropathology Modules

A series of evaluations by Lovell et al. (1991), Parkhurst et al. (1991), Lovell et al. (1993) and Lovell and Hodgins (2001) were conducted involving the neuropathology modules using videodisc images, and the CD-ROM version that included additional neuroscience practice applications and case studies. Results indicated that students found the units to be very effective in enhancing learning. The greatest assets of the units were in their visual impact, their ability to engage the learner as a participant rather than a passive listener (due to the interactive design), and self-assessment options. Several students noted that the units helped lengthen their attention span, and fostered problem solving rather than simple memorizing. When asked about specific features, students consistently mentioned the post-tests were especially useful, and the feedback explaining incorrect responses as well as reinforcing the rationale for the correct response, were relevant and extremely helpful.

Features of Neuropathology Modules that students considered very important included:

- High quality visual images that helped reinforce concepts.
- Flexibility in controlling location (easy navigation).
- Simultaneous display of both text and complete image or diagram.
- Indication of place in program (e.g. how many screens in remainder of section).
- Self-testing opportunities with explanations for right and wrong answers.
- Compatibility between the content and review questions.
- Flexibility in time allocation for completing the modules.
- Case studies to facilitate application of concepts to patient cases and attain higher level course objectives.

One objective in creating the modules was to accommodate different learner styles or characteristics. Students reported different patterns of use of the learner control options: pacing control, sequence control, content control, and whether to view the materials in groups or individually. The modules satisfied a variety of objectives including: as an advance organizer to acquire basic concepts; as a supplement to the lecture; for review; and for some students as a replacement for lecture.

Development of Neuroscience Resources for Specific Teaching Goals

After changes in the curricular structure for the Colleges of Human Medicine and Osteopathic Medicine, and based on changes in technology involving personal computers, further development occurred to build on the neuropathology teaching units, and to help students master areas that have been traditionally difficult and in which they have been observed to perform lower than expected on performance-based evaluations (Mavis et al., 1998).

Conversion of Neuropathology Modules to CD-ROM Format and Addition of Neuroanatomy Review Unit

The neuropathology modules were converted to a CD-ROM format, and a basic clinical neuroanatomy unit was added. Other units were developed to enhance problem-solving and integration of clinical and pathological concepts. Technical support and instructional design input was provided by Mark Hodgins. The CD-ROM was produced in the college facilities and distributed free of charge to students. Use was optional, but students were informed that the CD-ROM content covered the same material as the written neuropathology exams for the course, and that additional material for neuroanatomy review and problem-solving practice related to localization of lesions was available.

As part of the evaluation process after the CD-ROM was provided to students, Lovell and Hodgins (2001) showed that most students providing input (79% response rate for voluntary survey) used the CD-ROM. Response to the statement "The CD was effective in enhancing my understanding of the neuropathology objectives" was: Agree 13%, Strongly agree 85%. Response to the statement "The CD was effective in my review of neuroanatomy and localization of lesions" was: Agree 21%, Strongly agree 76%. Representative comments included the following: "The CD-ROM made studying less painful and learning easier;" "Questions had explanations and facilitated my learning greatly;" "I enjoyed having the pictures along with the readings. I also liked the fact that on the quiz questions answers were given as to why something was right or wrong;" "It helped my time management and assessment of learning." Since localization of lesions covered in neuroanatomy content is critical to diagnosis of a neurological disorder based on clinical presentation for a patient, the combination of units enhanced student understanding of the combined content.

Integration of Neuropathology and Patient Case Presentations

Another set of practice questions covering all neuropathology content with neuroanatomy reinforcement was developed after students performed more poorly than expected on an exam that included basic questions related to neuropathology images. This unit was designed to integrate a clinical scenario with the expected gross or microscopic pathology (clinic-pathological correlation), using 26 cases (Case A to Case Z). It was designed with short-answer questions with explanations rather than multiple-choice questions for several reasons: students would need to exert more effortful recall over a wider range of content, multiple concepts could be addressed more efficiently, and multiple-choice questions can be cumbersome to write.

An example of one scenario is "A 56-year-old man had been in good health. During an evening at home with his wife, he reported the sudden onset of a severe headache, and then lost consciousness. The patient died after several hours in the hospital. What is the diagnosis indicated by the history and brain section shown?" The image shows a coronal brain section with blood in the subarachnoid space and the lateral and third ventricles. Students can click a button "Show answer and explanation." The answer and explanation provided when a student clicks the button is: "The coronal section shows blood in the subarachnoid space, between the arachnoid and pia. Thus the diagnosis is subarachnoid hemorrhage. In this patient, a lumbar puncture would show bloody CSF. The most common cause of non-traumatic subarachnoid hemorrhage is ruptured saccular (berry) aneurysm. The history is also typical for ruptured saccular aneurysm, including sudden onset of headache ("worst headache of my life") and loss of consciousness ("Case History", n.d.).

This set of questions, designed to help students integrate pathology with features of a patient case, also included questions from multiple types of neuropathology disorders. The teaching modules were organized around topics (e.g. cerebrovascular disorders, neoplastic disorders, etc) and the post-test for each module included questions only on that topic. In contrast, the Neuropathology Case Examples (Cases A-Z) required students to think across topics, the process of interleaving. Rohrer & Pashler (2010) discuss interleaving as a process of combining testing or practice of different skills in a way that improves memory as compared to testing or practice blocked by type of skill. E.g. when baseball players practiced hitting three types of pitches that were either blocked or interleaved, interleaving improved performance on a subsequent test in which the batters did not know the type of pitch in advance. Blocked practice is important for initial learning, but provides students with a crutch that is unavailable during a cumulative exam, and in the real-world situations for which they are being trained. It is not surprising if they often struggle when asked to demonstrate a skill they have not previously practiced. More sets of practice problems utilizing interleaving across a number of topics can help students master the integration needed for comprehensive problem-solving related to patient cases.

Guided Problem-Solving Cases for Localization of Lesions

A set of 15 neuroanatomy problem-solving cases was developed to help students work through localization of lesions. These started with a patient scenario, e.g. "A 60-year-old man collapsed while at work. After he regained consciousness in the emergency room, neurological exam was performed with the following abnormalities noted: paralysis of the right arm and leg, dysarthria, deviation of the tongue to the left when protruded, loss of vibration, proprioception and discriminative touch sensation on the right side of the body (the face has normal sensation)." Relevant open-ended questions are asked and the student receives the answer and explanation when a button is clicked. These cases give students the opportunity to determine their answer before seeing the correct answer, and help with meaningful learning as well as self-assessment of their level of understanding ("Case History, n.d.).

Elements of Neuropathology Self-Instructional Modules and Neuroscience Units and Relation to Principles of Learning

The sections below focus on several features of the neuroscience self-instructional modules and discuss how they relate to instructional design principles to promote meaningful learning. These features can be viewed at http://learn.chm.msu.edu/neuropath/.

Self-Assessment and Feedback

As discussed in the Background section, retrieval practice markedly enhances learning and subsequent performance on a test. The Neuropathology Modules were designed with multiple-choice practice questions to facilitate student understanding of the content, and to facilitate their self-assessment of their ability to understand and apply the content. Some of the questions were at the recall level, and some required integration and application of concepts to a patient scenario. Some were intended to cover only chunks of material and some covered larger sets of material (interleaving). All were designed to enhance understanding through retrieval practice. Students consistently rated the practice questions in these modules as one of the most effective features and requested additional practice questions. Schmidmaier et al. (2011) found that in medical students learning clinical nephrology, repetitive testing promoted better recall than repetitive studying after 1 week; however after 6 months general recall was poor and no difference between the restudy and retest groups was observed.

Sets of cases for additional problem-solving were designed with open-ended questions, expecting students to retrieve an answer before clicking to get the answer and explanation. Rohrer and Pashler (2010) discuss the findings that tests that require effortful retrieval of information, such as short-answer questions, promote better retention than tests based on recognition only such as multiple-choice tests. Larsen et al. (2008) emphasize that production tests (e.g. short-answer, fill-in-the-blank) which require the test-taker to construct a response lead to better retention than recognition tests, presumably because production tests require more effortful retrieval of information from memory. The instructional design principles are consistent with students high rating of these in promoting understanding of the material.

The self-testing (multiple-choice questions and open-ended questions) in the modules all included feedback and explanations. Larsen et al. (2008) discuss the importance of feedback. Although testing improves retention in the absence of feedback, providing feedback enhances the benefits of testing by correcting errors and confirming correct responses. Also, the content of the feedback message is important, and should include the correct answer as well as other important information. The feedback for the modules was constructed to give the correct answer as well as give key information that students should focus on in answering similar questions.

The practice questions used as self-assessment also provide an opportunity for students to judge their own mastery of the content. Schumacher et al. (2013) states that most learners possess a limited ability to identify their knowledge gaps, and this was demonstrated in medical students by Schmidmaier et al. (2011). The limited ability of learners to assess and fill knowledge gaps plays out in study habits as well. Re-reading material is a common learning strategy but familiarity with information is often mistaken with knowing and understanding; thus individuals tend not to study what they perceive they already know, even if that perception is incorrect. Studies by Karpicke and Blunt (2011) also indicate that students are not able to accurately predict their performance on an exam. Thus it is important to provide students multiple opportunities to assess their own knowledge, both with respect to basic facts and to higher-level application of concepts.

Design of Content Presentation to Minimize Extraneous Processing in Cognitive Load

The Neuropathology Modules were designed to be straightforward concise descriptions of the key concepts in neuroscience and neuropathology content important for second-year medical students. Mayer (2008) discussed findings that students performed better on a problem-solving transfer test after receiving a concise lesson rather than an expanded lesson. According to the cognitive theory of multimedia learning, inserting extraneous material may cause learners to engage in extraneous processing – by using their processing capacity to attend to and process material that is not essential to building a mental model of the to-be-learned system. Learners given an expanded lesson may have less cognitive capacity for processing the essential material and therefore may be less likely to build a learning outcome that can be used to generate useful answers on a transfer test.

Efforts were made to write learning objectives and put key concepts in bold font to draw attention to these points. Also key features of images were represented in a caption of the image, with arrows, to emphasize the important terminology and put it in perspective. Mayer (2008) discussed the instructional design concept of signaling - the process of highlighting the essential material in the lesson. People learn better from a multimedia lesson when essential words are highlighted. Signaling can help guide the learner's attention toward the essential material.

When images were added to screen pages, the images were placed next to the text describing the concept displayed in the image, with the caption also visible on the same page. Mayer (2008) discussed the principle of spatial contiguity, i.e. that people learn better when corresponding words and pictures are presented near rather than far from each other on the page or screen.

Recommendations to manage cognitive load by Van Merrienboer and Sweller (2010) included replacing multiple sources of information, distributed either in space or time, with one integrated source of information. The Neuropathology Modules contained all of the neuropathology content taught for second-year medical students in our curriculum, and thus provided an integrated source of information to manage cognitive load and enhance learning.

Learner Control

The navigation of Neuropathology Modules in all forms (videodisc units, CD-ROM and Internet) was designed to be as flexible and straightforward as possible, and provide learner control over all elements, including the questions (which could be skipped if desired). Users could complete one or more units at a sitting, or could complete part of a unit, and the units were self-paced. This not only facilitated student variation in type of use, but also facilitated implementation of the module in various types of curricula, and for use as both initial learning modules, and for review in clerkships or residency. Learner control and flexible navigation were highly rated by students and fulfilled several goals of instructional design.

Clark and Mayer (2011) discuss learner control and navigation from several perspectives. For example, they recommend giving experienced learners more control. There are more significant differences between effectiveness of courses with learner or program control where learners have lower levels of prior knowledge and some evidence to suggest that some agency at higher levels has a positive effect. Plus there are the benefits in terms of reducing dropout and increasing engagement through agency. Pacing control generally means that learners spend more time on tasks but that more is learned and transferred better to real life situations. It is important that users can easily keep track of where they are and find other elements of the program. Clark and Mayer (2011) indicate that clear navigation leads to better retention of information. In the neuropathology and neuroscience modules, the clear flexible navigation was commended by students and the learner control of pacing in the modules enhanced engagement through agency and made it possible for students to effectively utilize the material at any level – initial learning, review within the course, review for board exams, review in clerkships or residency.

Learner control also can accommodate different learning approaches and styles of individual students. Friedlander et al. (2011) discuss individual learning and point out that individuals have various types of intelligence and show differences in the types of learning that they employ best. The flexible navigation with learning control also permits adaptability in curriculum implementation to meet variable curriculum objectives. I.e., the topics can be used in any order and at any time in the medical school curriculum to fit school and user needs in the context of blended and online learning formats. The structure of the current modules, which can be used either online or downloaded to a local device also permits student flexibility to use the modules in any location, even if an internet connection is not available.

SOLUTIONS AND RECOMMENDATIONS

The following are a few selected recommendations for the design of multimedia teaching materials that the author considers important based on student input and on results of cognitive psychology studies of learning principles.

- **Enhance knowledge of Evidence-Based Learning Strategies by Medical Education Faculty and Content Developers, in order to Promote the Application of Evidence-Based Instructional Design Principles:** Many of the faculty presentations in medical schools do not follow these principles, although there has been improvement in the last few years. Levinson (2010) wrote: "The majority of medical school lectures or grand rounds presentations run contrary to best practices in instructional design, often consisting of Power-Point slides with redundant text, 'death by bullet points' and – where graphics are used at all – trivial, seductive augmentation that probably reduces learning." One of the reasons is that, according to Levinson (2010), "institutions underfund quality curriculum content development, evaluation and improvement." Increasing the use of strategies that have been demonstrated to be effective in medical education, as developed by educators that know something about the topic, the audience and how people learn, would result in more efficient and effective learning by medical students and promote problem-solving and retention for application in clinical settings (Friedlander et al., 2011, Rohrer and Pashler, 2010, Mayer, 2008, Levinson, 2010, and Schumacher et al 2013).

- **Intentionally Utilize the Testing Effect (Retrieval Practice) to Help Students Learn:** Multiple practice tests of various formats (e.g. multiple-choice and short-answer questions) with feedback should be integrated into teaching materials or made easily available to students. This enhancement would help students learn and retain the content. While not as effective as short-answer or recall questions, the use of representative multiple-choice questions would also help students manage the multiple-choice question format of high-stakes testing, including many medical school course exams and licensing exams. Larsen et al. (2008) discussed studies indicating that feedback is crucial to learning from tests, and whenever possible feedback should include both answers and explanations to promote student understanding of the reason for errors. This was emphasized by Levinson (2010) who stated: "At the macro level of curriculum and programme design, one would like to see the integration of more opportunities for deliberate and mixed practice with expert feedback."
- **Enhance Availability of Multimedia Materials Using High Quality Open Source Images, Diagrams and Animations that could be used Without Copyright Issues:** One challenge the author and colleagues have encountered while developing multimedia teaching modules was finding enough appropriate high-quality digital materials. There are currently several sources of these images, but a developer has to search in many venues to find what is available and has limited options if no source is found. The availability of multiple diagrams, animations, images, videos to provide enhancement of concepts, multidisciplinary integration, and application to patient cases would enhance the effectiveness of medical education materials.

FUTURE RESEARCH DIRECTIONS

Cook et al. (2008) reported a meta-analysis of internet-based learning interventions in the health professions, with the conclusion that Internet-based learning is associated with large positive effects compared with no intervention, and recommended that future research should directly compare different Internet-based interventions. There are a variety of directions for such research and the discussion below focuses on only a few of these.

It has been well established that applying the principles of multimedia instructional design, retrieval practice, and cognitive load theory result in impressive effects on retention in non-health professions learners. It is expected that these effects will also apply to medical students. However, there has been little replication or extension of the findings in medical education settings. Future research should investigate which elements of instructional design are most effective for different types of content in medical education. This is important in order to plan development of multimedia materials that are highly effective but also consider the cost of design and production. For example, Ruiz et al. (2009) conducted a critical literature review related to animations and state: "Medical educators have used animations in a variety of computer-assisted learning applications, but few comparative studies have been published and the evidence is inconclusive. Research outside medical education shows conflicting results for studies comparing animations with static images. This may reflect differences in cognitive load induced by animation, or differences in the type of motion being illustrated. The benefits of animations may also vary according to learner characteristics such as prior knowledge and spatial ability. Features of animation that appear to facilitate learning include permitting learner control over the animation's pace, allowing learners to interact with animations and splitting the animation activity into small chunks."

More recent studies by Daly et al. (2016), Berney et al. (2015), Hoyek et al. (2014), and Keedy et al. (2011) have compared effectiveness of static versus animated images, and found no significant differences in student performance. Further research is needed to examine when and how more complex animated images or high-fidelity simulations can substantially enhance meaningful learning, and when static images, or other low-fidelity techniques, are just as, or more, effective, since production of multimedia instruction using more straightforward low-fidelity techniques is less costly and less time-intensive. Challenges in development of multimedia self-instructional materials include faculty and staff time, and it is important to distinguish the relative effectiveness of each type of instructional design for the intended purpose.

Research on effective support for different learning characteristics or learning styles is also important. Medical students need different degrees of assistance in integrating challenging concepts from different disciplines and in application of content to patient cases or interpretation of experimental findings. Interactive computer-based materials can provide options for those students who need specific types of assistance, e.g. a longer amount of time to cover the material, more opportunity to practice with explanations as part of the feedback, easily available resources to review previously learned concepts, and examples of the type of integration and application expected.

Another important direction is to enhance self-assessment for students to assist both with understanding of concepts and application of concepts to patient cases or interpretation of data. Students are not good at judging their own competence, and both low-fidelity computer instructional programs with self-testing options and high-fidelity simulations are needed to a greater extent. Research should focus on when simpler low-fidelity approaches are sufficient to enhance student identification of their own learning needs or practice, and when more expensive high-fidelity approaches are necessary.

CONCLUSION

Medical education will benefit from integration of current understanding of learning theory and evidence with educational strategies and curricular design. Important instructional design principles include cognitive load theory and importance of retrieval practice as part of the learning process. Medical students are adult learners with different backgrounds and abilities and learner characteristics. Self-paced interactive multimedia materials can substantially promote retention and understanding for students at a variety of levels of mastery. Self-instructional materials using appropriate instructional design principles should be available for students learning basic science material at the pre-clinical level, for students studying for board examinations, and for students in clerkships that are learning to apply material to diagnosis and treatment of patient problems. These can be available anyplace/anytime for the specific needs of each student and improve the efficiency and effectiveness of meaningful learning.

REFERENCES

Berney, S., Betrancourt, M., Molinari, G., & Hoyek, N. (2015). How spatial abilities and dynamic visualizations interplay when learning functional anatomy with 3D anatomical models. *Anatomical Sciences Education*, *8*(5), 452–462. doi:10.1002/ase.1524 PMID:25689057

Carroll, M. W. (2013). Creative Commons and the Openness of Open Access. *The New England Journal of Medicine*, *368*(9), 789–791. doi:10.1056/NEJMp1300040 PMID:23445090

Case History: Case B. (n.d.). Retrieved from: http://learn.chm.msu.edu/neuropath/content/neuropath_cases/neuropathology_cases/CaseB.html

Clark, R. C., & Mayer, R. E. (2011). *E-Learning and the science of instruction: Proven guidelines for consumers and designers of multimedia learning*. Chichester, UK: John Wiley and Sons Ltd. doi:10.1002/9781118255971

Cook, D. A., Levinson, A. J., Garside, S., Dupras, D. M., Erwin, P. J., & Montori, V. M. (2008). Internet-based learning in the health professions: A meta-analysis. *Journal of the American Medical Association*, *300*(10), 1181–1196. doi:10.1001/jama.300.10.1181 PMID:18780847

Daly, C. J., Bullock, J. M., Ma, M., & Aidulis, D. (2016). A comparison of animated versus static images in an instructional multimedia presentation. *Advances in Physiology Education*, *40*(2), 201–205. doi:10.1152/advan.00053.2015 PMID:27105738

Friedlander, M. J., Andrews, L., Armstrong, E. G., Aschenbrenner, C., Kass, J. S., Ogden, P., & Viggiano, T. R. et al. (2011). What can medical education learn from the neurobiology of learning? *Academic Medicine*, *86*(4), 415–420. doi:10.1097/ACM.0b013e31820dc197 PMID:21346504

Hodgins, M. W., & Lovell, K. L. (1988). CNS Neoplasms - Interactive videodisc instructional unit. *Bulletin of Pathology Education*, *13*, 89–90.

Hoyek, N., Collet, C., Di Rienzo, F., De Almeida, M., & Guillot, A. (2014). Effectiveness of three-dimensional digital animation in teaching human anatomy in an authentic classroom context. *Anatomical Sciences Education*, *7*(6), 430–437. doi:10.1002/ase.1446 PMID:24678034

Karpicke, J. D., & Blunt, J. R. (2011). Retrieval practice produces more learning than elaborative studying with concept mapping. *Science*, *331*(6018), 772–775. doi:10.1126/science.1199327 PMID:21252317

Karpicke, J. D., & Roediger, H. L. (2008). The critical importance of retrieval for learning. *Science*, *319*(5865), 966–968. doi:10.1126/science.1152408 PMID:18276894

Keedy, A. W., Durack, J. C., Sandhu, P., Chen, E. M., OSullivan, P. S., & Breiman, R. S. (2011). Comparison of traditional methods with 3D computer models in the instruction of hepatobiliary anatomy. *Anatomical Sciences Education*, *4*(2), 84–91. doi:10.1002/ase.212 PMID:21412990

Larsen, D. P., Butler, A. C., & Roediger, H. L. III. (2008). Test-enhanced learning in medical education. *Medical Education*, *42*(10), 959–966. doi:10.1111/j.1365-2923.2008.03124.x PMID:18823514

Lau, K. H. V. (2014). Computer-based teaching module design: Principles derived from learning theories. *Medical Education*, *48*(3), 247–254. doi:10.1111/medu.12357 PMID:24528459

Levinson, A. J. (2010). Where is evidence-based instructional design in medical education curriculum development? *Medical Education*, *44*(6), 536–537. doi:10.1111/j.1365-2923.2010.03715.x PMID:20604847

Lovell, K. L., Haf, J., & Hodgins, M. (1991). Development of neuropathology interactive videodisc instructional units. *Teaching and Learning in Medicine*, *3*(3), 156–158. doi:10.1080/10401339109539501

Lovell, K. L., & Hodgins, M. W. (2001). Implementation and evaluation of neuroscience technology resources for second-year medical students. In *Proceedings of Slice of Life/Computers in Health Care Annual Meeting*. Salt Lake City, UT: University of Utah.

Lovell, K. L., Parkhurst, P. E., Sprafka, S. A., Hodgins, M. W., & Bean, P. L. (1993). Quantitative and qualitative evaluation of interactive videodisc instructional modules in preclinical neuropathology education. *Teaching and Learning in Medicine*, *5*(1), 3–9. doi:10.1080/10401339309539579

Mavis, B. E., Lovell, K. L., & Ogle, K. S. (1998). Why Johnnie cant apply neuroscience: Testing alternative hypotheses using performance-based assessment. *Advances in Health Science Education*, *3*(3), 165–175. doi:10.1023/A:1009794026466 PMID:12386438

Mayer, R. E. (2008). Applying the science of learning: Evidence-based principles for the design of multimedia instruction. *The American Psychologist*, *63*(8), 760–769. doi:10.1037/0003-066X.63.8.760 PMID:19014238

Mayer, R. E. (2010). Applying the science of learning to medical education. *Medical Education*, *44*(6), 543–549. doi:10.1111/j.1365-2923.2010.03624.x PMID:20604850

Mayer, R. E., & Moreno, R. (2010). Nine ways to reduce cognitive load in multimedia learning. *Educational Psychologist*, *38*(1), 43–52. doi:10.1207/S15326985EP3801_6

Paas, F., Renkl, A., & Sweller, J. (2010). Cognitive load theory and instructional design: Recent developments. *Educational Psychologist*, *38*(1), 1–4. doi:10.1207/S15326985EP3801_1

Parkhurst, P. E., Lovell, K. L., Sprafka, S. A., Hodgins, M. W., & Bean, P. L. (1991). Evaluation of interactive videodisc instructional modules in preclinical neuropathology education. *Journal of Medical Education Technology*, *2*, 17–21.

Rohrer, D., & Pashler, H. (2010). Recent research on human learning challenges conventional instructional strategies. *Educational Researcher*, *39*(5), 406–412. doi:10.3102/0013189X10374770

Ruiz, J. G., Cook, D. A., & Levinson, A. J. (2009). Computer animations in medical education: A critical literature review. *Medical Education*, *43*(9), 838–846. doi:10.1111/j.1365-2923.2009.03429.x PMID:19709008

Schmidmaier, R., Ebersbach, R., Schiller, M., Hege, I., Holzer, M., & Fischer, M. R. (2011). Using electronic flashcards to promote learning in medical students: Retesting versus restudying. *Medical Education*, *45*(11), 1101–1110. doi:10.1111/j.1365-2923.2011.04043.x PMID:21988625

Schumacher, D. J., Englander, R., & Carraccio, C. (2013). Developing the master learner: Applying learning theory to the learner, the teacher, and the learning environment. *Academic Medicine*, *88*(11), 1–11. doi:10.1097/ACM.0b013e3182a6e8f8 PMID:24072107

Sweller, J. (1994). Cognitive load theory, learning difficulty, and instructional design. *Learning and Instruction*, *4*(4), 295–312. doi:10.1016/0959-4752(94)90003-5

Van Merrienboer, J. J. G., & Sweller, J. (2010). Cognitive load theory in health professional education: Design principles and strategies. *Medical Education*, *44*, 85–93. doi:10.1111/j.1365-2923.2009.03498.x PMID:20078759

Wood, T. (2009). Assessment not only drives learning, it may also help learning. *Medical Education*, *43*(1), 5–6. doi:10.1111/j.1365-2923.2008.03237.x PMID:19140992

KEY TERMS AND DEFINITIONS

Cognitive Load: Total amount of mental effort being used in working memory. Intrinsic cognitive load is the effort associated with a specific topic; extraneous cognitive load refers to the way information or tasks are presented to a learner; germane cognitive load refers to the work put into creating a permanent store of knowledge.

Computer-Based Teaching Module: Teaching format in which a multimedia program serves as a single source for learning.

Creative Commons: Organization promoting open access to Internet resources, and defining public licensing use for all types of copyrighted works.

Interleaving: Process of combining testing or practice of different skills in a way that improves memory as compared to testing or practice blocked by type of skill.

Learner Control: The process by which a user determines how to utilize different elements of a computer-based teaching module.

Meaningful Learning: A deep understanding of the material, which includes organization, integration and ability to apply the knowledge to new situations.

Multimedia Instruction: Presenting words and pictures (including images and diagrams) that are intended to promote learning.

Retrieval Practice: A process used as part of learning in which information must be recalled from memory; retrieval practice plays a critical role in consolidating learning.

Self-Assessment: The process of testing oneself to determine how much knowledge has been acquired or how well the knowledge can be applied.

Testing Effect: Evidence that students remember material better when they are tested over material than when they use repeated study but are not tested.

Chapter 14
Faculty Development for Clinical Educators:
A Competency Model for Continuous Improvement

Silvia Lizett Olivares Olivares
Tecnologico de Monterrey School of Medicine, Mexico

Martha Ruth Loyola Segura
Tecnologico de Monterrey School of Medicine, Mexico

Mildred Vanessa López Cabrera
Tecnológico de Monterrey School of Medicine, Mexico

Jorge Eugenio Valdez García
Tecnologico de Monterrey School of Medicine, Mexico

ABSTRACT

Since the Flexner report in the 20th century, teaching and learning process has evolved through: science learning, problem based learning, competency based learning and perspective learning. This evolution provides a consensus that educators need to develop competencies in their students to prepare them for an uncertain future. Competency refers not only to core knowledge or instrumental skills, but to inter-personal and systemic abilities required for lifelong learning. This transformation requires changes in both the educational model and faculty development programs. Previous research and proposals have defined important qualities and attributes; for clinical educators. The Faculty Development program presented here has been assessed with a mixed multiphase approach for continuous improvement process: 1) assessment of proposal, 2) assessment of implementation, 3) assessment of faculty experiences and 4) institutionalization of program. Results from this experience are presented, as well as other further challenges on this initiative.

INTRODUCTION

Since the Flexner report (1910) at the beginning of the 21st century, four phases of evolution of the teaching and learning process have been identified that demanded new roles and skills requirements for medical educators (Olivares, 2016). Medical students have participated for centuries with expert doctors on consultation, hospital patient rounds, and surgeries to learn from observation of the medical practice

DOI: 10.4018/978-1-5225-2098-6.ch014

Copyright © 2017, IGI Global. Copying or distributing in print or electronic forms without written permission of IGI Global is prohibited.

in situ (Graue-Wiechers, 2011). Passive learning among medical students should be questioned with the introduction of a variety of educational and pedagogical tools, such as multimedia, augmented reality, and simulation, available to provide a hands-on approach to medical education.

On the other hand, active participation of medical students should be properly addressed when attending actual patients. Accreditation agencies, governmental, and institutional regulations increasingly demand a formalization of the medical educator's roles and competencies to guarantee desired performance results (MacLeod, 2012). The general Medical Council (GMC), the UK's medical regulatory body, stated in its 2006 version of the document Good Medical Practice that all doctors should adopt the skills, attitudes and practices of a good teacher (Yeates, Stewart, & Barton, 2008). The quality and outcome of training could be legally challenged by trainees if they perceive failures in education delivery which could potentially lead to adverse outcomes for patients or health services (Rashid & Siriwardena, 2005). In this sense, clinician educators and institutions may be found responsible for an inappropriate supervision process and inadequate instruction.

Millennial students expect rewarding and challenging tasks from good instructors. From the students' perspective, the qualities of a good teacher have been the subject of considerable debate (Kiani, Umar, & Iqbal, 2014). A lack of understanding between teachers and learners can lead to a mismatch in expectations, frustration and reduced educational outcomes (Ross, 2014). In clinical teaching, teachers should consider factors such as physiological needs, learning goals, learning environment, teaching methods, and their professional behavior to create a positive environment for patients and learners (Omid & Haghani Fariba, 2016).

For these reasons, teaching in the clinical environment is a multifaceted endeavor that requires innovative approaches (Finn, Chiappa, Puig, & Hunt, 2011). Clinical teaching must be recognized as a complex learning situation influenced by the learning content, the setting and the actions and interactions of the participants (Nilson, Pennbrant, Pilhammar, & Wenestarm, 2010). University hospitals frequently expect clinicians, untrained in educational practice, to deliver teaching as an adjunct to increasingly high levels of patient service delivery (Konerman, Alpert, & Shashank, 2016). In many medical schools, educators still lack a structured career development pathway, and much education is delivered by researchers whose primary interest lies on scores for boards. Most junior faculty begin their careers with little formal training in education. For these reason, is imperative to design and implement faculty development programs which not only fulfill these stakeholders' expectations, but also which led to a satisfactory and rewarding task for the clinician educator himself/herself (MacLeod, 2012).

BACKGROUND

Khan and Chishti (2012) suggest that educators are required to become an inspirational guide to their students and to enable them to understand the mysteries of the world. They describe the importance of faculty development in the improvement of teachers' instructional methods, concepts and knowledge to ultimately positively affect the students' work. Olivares (2016) describes the evolution of the medical teacher since the beginning of the 20th century. The author describes four incremental phases of medical education which have required new roles and skills through time (Table 1).

Table 1. Learning approaches evolution in medical education (Olivares, 2016)

	Science Learning	Problem Based Learning	Competency Base Learning	Perspective Base Learning
Timeline in history	Beginning of XX century	Sixties	Seventies	Beginning of XXI century
Scope	Content	Context	Experimentation	Innovation
Teacher role	Lecturer	Tutor	Assessor	Mentor
Graduate expectations	Medical expert	Collaborator of a team	Professional on a health care system	Leader for systemic transformation

Science Learning

From a scientific perspective, the teacher has the knowledge, authority and status to deliver contents to students (Olivares, 2016). Since only some individuals have had formal education opportunities, the experienced professionals were the responsible to deliver science trough lectures. Written exams were the most common way to measure advance in learning. The required skills for faculty members on this academic approach were public speaking for specific disciplinary content, written examination design and grading.

Problem-Based Learning (PBL)

In order to engage and motivate students to learn, problem-based learning offered context and space for discussion and teamwork since its development in the 1960s. This format requires a tutor to facilitate knowledge. While there are several ways to implement PBL, the following are common steps:

1. Read the problem to identify prior knowledge and design learning goals.
2. Research and analyze new information that is hypothetically associated with the problem to build new semantic network to restructure knowledge.
3. Discuss alternatives on tutorial groups to discriminate options to define a solution.
4. Finally, explain inferences and course of action according to the presented solution.

This process requires assessment of student participation by a teacher in terms of preparation, argumentation and explanation applying observational rubrics. These additional interpersonal skills for teaching were ranked by Kiani, Umar and Iqbal (2014) as the most important skills required of a medical teacher.

Competency-Based Learning

Besides addressing patient health problems, clinicians in training must learn to relate to patients. They need to listen and understand, empathize and be aware of their own emotional responses and potential weakness (Ross, 2014). The term competency includes not only the core knowledge or the instrumental skills, but also other interpersonal and organizational abilities relevant to participate on an accredited health care institution. With this learning approach, teachers need to assume an evaluator role to examine their students' performance related to several competencies in a simulated environment.

Perspective-Based Learning

The teacher's role considering the perspectives approach is as mentor to guide the student to face a complex environment. Besides monitoring and debriefing the student on his or her performance as the health care institution is important to consider innovative strategies to improve processes, patient satisfaction and the society quality of life (Olivares, 2016).

This model requires teachers to design challenges for students to guide them to draw conclusions and answers to nonexistent situations. Since systemic thinking requires analysis based on multiple perspectives to generate empathy with the patient and the different variables of the environment it is necessary that the institution and its educational group provide students with educational experiences seek opportunities for the growing social demands. The challenges should train students in the ability to fully manage organizational processes through leadership, creativity, entrepreneurship, research, decision making and permanent quality care (Malcolm Baldrige National Quality Award, 2016). This training will allow them to perceive a holistic view of reality (Evans & Lindsay, 2014).

This incremental evolution for learning in medical education needs to be coupled with faculty member's preparation. Generally, physicians are well trained for diagnosis, prevention and treatment of diseases; PhDs have profound knowledge of their disciplines through research, but when they are hired to become faculty members, they have not received the proper training on pedagogical topics. Even when they may be experts on their discipline, they are rarely prepared for an educator's role (Harris, Krause, Parish and Smith, 2007). The growth of expectation on medical graduates as leaders, innovators and change agents is a challenge for medical schools. Clinical teachers are then responsible for helping their students and trainees to achieve this. The question is: how? (Ross, 2014).

CLINICAL EDUCATOR COMPETENCIES

In order to improve the educational vitality in teachers is important to include an adequate faculty development program to educate them on the required competences according to institutional policies and desired academic excellence (Wilkerson & Irby, 1998). The implementation process requires to be carefully executed to assure quality in the purposed results. According to Khan and Chishti (2012), the target of quality education can be achieved once the quality of teachers is enhanced. This includes credentials and competence for teachers since they are the primary agents for instructing quality education. The faculty development programs should continuously improve their results to achieve quality standards.

Several research studies have been conducted to define the profile of the clinician educator in terms of qualities, attributes, functions or competencies. Table 2 provides an overview of suggested clinical education competencies.

Duvivier, Van Dalen, Van Der Vleuten and Scherpbier (2009) developed a qualitative research to explore teachers' views on effective and desired teaching skills. A total of 10 teachers from a skills lab answered about desired qualities, competencies and strategies for undergraduate clinical skills teachers. Important qualities included: to be attracted to teaching, having sense of humor, respect students' limitations and to be responsible. The competences declared from this study were related to preparation of the teacher and educational background. Strategies for clinical learning included the use of reflective practice during physical examination skills or directly afterwards. Participants also emphasized to establish a wider perspective on the formulation of differential diagnosis and detection of an underlying pathology.

Table 2. Clinical educators' competencies suggested by different authors

Reference	Instructional Teaching	Assessment	Education in Clinical Settings	Other
Duvivier, Van Dalen, Vleuten, & Scherpbier (2009)	Preparation of the teacher/ educational background.		Reflective practice during and after physical examination skills	Passion for teaching/ Sense of humor
Atkinson, Ajjawi, & Cooling (2011)		Self-assessment	Coaching and feedback on clinical reasoning	
MacLeod (2012)	Design and planning of learning activities	Assessment and feedback to learners	Evidence based practice	Core values Management Leadership
Konerman, Alpert, & Shashank (2016)	Facilitation	Feedback Progress support	Revise rotations	Innovation Quality improvement
Kiani, Umar, & Iqbal (2014)	Knowledge of the subject Evidence based teaching	Exam oriented teaching		Ethical thinking Research Rapport with students
Nilson, Pennbrant, Pilhammar, & Wenestarm (2010)	Lecturing	Questions and answers	Piloting Prompting Suplementing Demonstrating Intervening	
Yeates, Stewart, & Barton (2008)	Preparation to teach Delivery of teaching		Teacher conduct as role model in clinic	Supporting activities
Rashid & Siriwardena (2005)	Individual teaching Professional development Learning plans Lecturing Curriculum planning	Formative and summative assessment	Reflective practice	Regulatory frameworks Research methods
Singh et al. (2013)	Instructional Time management Knowledge	Assessment		Personal qualities Interaction with colleagues Publications
Harris et al. (2007)	Teaching Curriculum development		Care management	Medical informatics Multiculturalism
Martínez-González et al. (2008)	Critical thinking promotion Medical knowledge Pedagogical skills	Assessment Self-directed learning	Mentor the student in the clinical practice	Bioethics education Motivation
Aguirre Huacuja et al. (2012)	Curriculum design Teaching strategies	Assessment design	Educational practice in several health care settings	Ethical and professional behavior promotion Educational research
Nogueira Sotolongo, Rivera Michelena and Blanco (2005)	Knowledge Pedagogical actions Communication skills	Assessment	Involvement of students on their learning	Educate on ethics and humanism Teamwork skills Use of information technology

Atkinson, Ajjqwi and Cooling (2011) relate the clinical reasoning literature to the general practice of family medicine context to provide clinical teachers with strategies to promote clinical reasoning. They define the developmental stages of clinical reasoning considering analytical and non-analytical methods as well as uncertain factors. Some strategies recommended for facilitating effective clinical reasoning include adequate exposure to cases, sufficient opportunity for reflection and coaching on reasoning in the context of cases from general practice. Clinical educators can teach trainees the importance of knowing when to get help trough metacognition and self-assessment processes.

MacLeod (2012) emphasized the importance to invest resources to assure quality of the training provided to medical students and trainees in health care settings. She recommends the framework developed by the Academy of Medical Educators (AoME) for training and development of the medical educator's workforce. This standard includes: core values; design and planning of learning activities; assessment and feedback to learners; educational research and evidence-based practice; educational management and leadership. The program may be defined considering *length* as years of experience of teaching in different contexts; the *breadth* as expanding to higher educational levels of disciplines and *depth* selecting research or improved knowledge on a specific area.

Konerman, Alpert and Shashank (2016) recognized that a successful academic clinician must also be a successful educator. The authors describe how at the National Heart and Lung Institute, Imperial College London (a department with approximately 75 full professors), it was set up as an education department in which salary full-time educators (clinical and nonclinical) to deliver medical teaching. This institute designed a formal curriculum for aspirants as clinician educators. The program includes a first section to lay the groundwork: create a culture, facilitation, feedback and motivation. A second part to take action: assessment, innovation, revise rotations and quality improvement. The last part is related to sustain the drive: progress support and celebration.

Kiani, Umar and Iqbal (2014) made a research to identify the most desired teaching skills for a medical teacher from the perspective of medical student according to variables presented on Figure 1. On teaching methodology they included exam oriented teaching and evidence-based teaching. Teaching skills considered were knowledge of the subject, rapport with students, enthusiasm and interaction with students. On commitment to grow the model includes ethical thinking and research.

Nilson, Pennbrant, Pilhammar and Wenestarm (2010) followed an ethnographic approach to look for meaning patterns, similarities and differences in how clinical teachers manage clinical teaching; There were identified these strategies: 1) Questions and answers, 2) Lecturing, 3) Piloting, 4) Prompting, 5) Suplementing, 6) Demonstrating and 7) Intervening as presented on Figure 2 according to the centerdeness and focus closer to the teacher or to the student.

Figure 1. Teaching skills for a medical teacher identified by medical students (Kiani, Umar, & Iqbal, 2014)

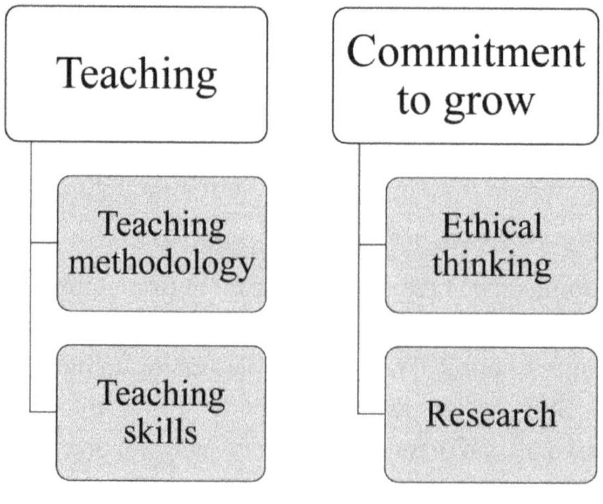

Figure 2. Pedagogical strategies used on clinical education (Nilson, Pennbrant, Pilhammar, & Wenestarm, 2010)

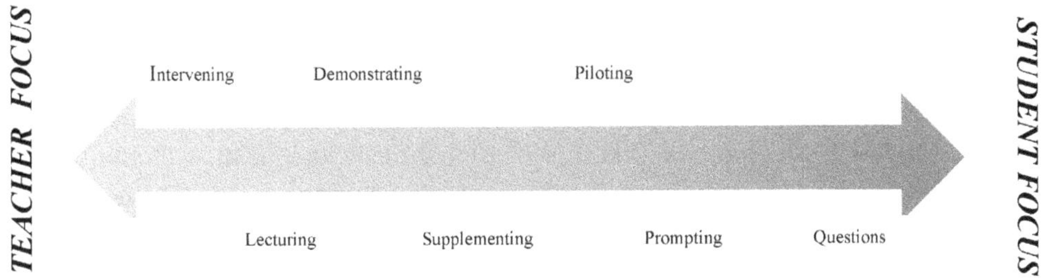

1. Questions and answers: clinical teachers ask questions to discuss and describe how to deal with medical problems.
2. Lecturing: this process focuses on an actual area of knowledge.
3. Piloting: by piloting the teachers prevent students from getting stuck in the management of a particular task. Thy use guiding questions, statements or signals to ensure that the student pays attention to focuses on specific content.
4. Prompting: This approach is useful in situations where the students appeared to need help in their assessment, problem solving or in communication with patients or nurses.
5. Supplementing: The strategy is characterized when teachers add complementary facts, or in some cases take over the students' communication.
6. Demonstrating: With this strategy the clinical teacher demonstrates how to act, assess, communicate, and perceive a problem.
7. Intervening: The teacher taking an authoritative role, interrupting the student and taking over the situation. In intervening, the clinical teacher focuses on getting the assignment completed.

Yeates, Stewart and Barton (2008) applied a Delphi technique to identify relevant skills attitudes and practices for clinical educators. The attributes which achieved ≥ 80% agreement at a basic level were:

1. Preparing to teach
   a. Identifies patients who are appropriate for student teaching
   b. Clearly communicates goals and outcomes
2. Deliver of teaching
   a. When appropriate, allows student to be involved with (rather than passively observe) clinical learning opportunities.
3. Teacher conduct
   a. Displays tolerance towards cultural issues and students beliefs without compromising institutional values
   b. Is an appropriate role model of clinical practice when teaching in a clinical environment
4. Supporting activities
   a. Knows who to contact if concerned about a student
   b. Promotes the necessity of gaining consent from patients to involve them in teaching

Singh et al. (2013) made a study to identify the qualities of the medical teacher from faculty perspective. They categorized in four domains these characteristics: classroom behaviour in instructional skills (communication, time management), interaction with students and colleagues (motivation, assessment, work well), personal qualities (puntual, unbiased, honest) and professional development (knowledge, publications, open to change). The top three desirable qualities of an effective teacher in their study were knowledge of subject, enthusiasm and communication skills.

According to Rashid & Siriwardena (2005) professional medical educators should be able to demonstrate skills and knowledge relating to: individual teaching, mentoring, continuing professional development (CPD), the use of learning plans, ability to demonstrate expertise in small groups teaching; lecturing, curriculum planning, reflective practice and educational research methods. The following is a draft curriculum for medical educators as a part of a master program.

1. Why become and educator in primary care?
2. Who are the learners?
3. The responsibilities of education and training
4. The regulatory frameworks and organization of training
5. Educational theory relevant to education/training in primary care
6. Appraisal and the educational plan
7. Assessment of learning needs, style and personally
8. E-learning
9. Formative and summative assessment
10. Assessing and addressing underperformance
11. Teaching communication skills
12. Developing a clinical audit ethos
13. Writing training reports
14. Approaches to small and large group learning
15. Multidisciplinary learning/interdisciplinary learning
16. Mentoring and reflective practice in teaching

Harris et al. (2007) determined categories of competencies according to the job description: leadership, administration, teaching, curriculum development, research, medical informatics and clinical practice. Considering the different roles in the health professionals' profile, a new design for a faculty development program was developed to address the complexity of teaching in an actual healthcare environment. They defined several competencies for a teacher-clinician role that combines medical family practice and teaching in the same setting. The required competencies for this profile included teaching, curriculum development, medical informatics, care management and multiculturalism as part of their academic skills.

Martínez-González et al. (2008) categorized the medical functions of a physician to healthcare practice, research, teaching, communication, administration and advocacy. The authors developed a list of 8 functions required for the medical teacher, which are related to pedagogical, interpersonal, managerial or bioethical perspectives:

1. Mentor the student in the clinical practice to identify healthcare problems.
2. Assess the student according to the graduate profile of his/her program.
3. Encourage the student to obtain new achievements.

4. Promote critical thinking among the students.
5. Stimulate the students' interests for medical knowledge, research and teaching.
6. Facilitate self-directed learning.
7. Develop bioethical behaviors in students.
8. Keep the teaching practice updated according to the new pedagogical trends

Aguirre Huacuja et al. (2012) also developed a competency model for medical teachers. They included six competencies in the model:

1. Curriculum design and development of the professional profile according to the institutional strategy and regulatory requisites.
2. Development of teaching strategies aligned to the institutional pedagogical model.
3. Efficient educational practice in several settings such as, hospitals, healthcare centers and science labs.
4. Development of ethical and professional behavior in students through education and example.
5. Design of reliable and valid assessment for learning results.
6. Commitment and participation in disciplinary or educational research.

Nogueira Sotolongo, Rivera Michelena and Blanco (2005) developed a list of basic competencies for medical teachers after applying a survey to family medicine doctors:

1. Knowledge expert on contacts.
2. Systemic focus on academic components: objectives, contents, methods, teaching techniques and assessment.
3. Organization, planning execution and control of pedagogical actions.
4. Design of academic objectives.
5. Involve students in their learning.
6. Educate students on ethics and humanism.
7. Use of information technology.
8. Teamwork skills.
9. Continuing development of academic skills.
10. Communication skills.

FACULTY DEVELOPMENT PROGRAMS FOR CLINICAL EDUCATORS

Several authors have recommended faculty development programs for clinical educators. According to Adamson et al. (2015), faculty development workshops and mentoring programs, can improve teaching skills and increase scholarly productivity. Training, mentoring, and support directed at medical education, appear as crucial for the success of clinician-educators as dedicated research experience is for physician-scientist. Through content analysis, Finn et al. (2011) found that the top five major areas that proved to be critical to effective clinical teaching were: question strategies, physical examination instruction, engagement of multiple learner's levels, learner-focused teaching, and teaching efficiency (time management). The CanMEDS role of Scholar promotes that medical trainees develop these types of competencies. The development of teaching skills in undergraduate medical students is therefore desirable, especially in view of the teaching obligations in residency programs (Marton, McCullough, & Ramnanan, 2014).

Ibrahim et al. (2015) found that clinical educators perceived that they faculty development program helped them on clinical skills, assessment of trainees, mentoring and teaching skills, but they still needed support on assessment of trainees (45.6%) curriculum development (45.6%), educational program evaluation (42.7%) and educational research (36.1%).

Boerbach, Lombarts, Keijzer, Heinerman and Arah (2012) found that 69% of residents considered that the teaching performance impacts the physician role and personal role of the clinical educator. Duvivier et al. (2009) found in their study that preparation of the teacher and educational background is relevant as clinical educator. According to the authors, new teachers should be provided with support, training and guidance to master these pedagogical techniques. Additionally their findings revealed that teachers value feedback form students and colleagues as it provides direction for improvement in both behavior and skills. The previous competency models showed several requirements for clinicians, so it was relevant to design a high quality faculty development program which may cover the most important characteristics to develop teaching, assessment, clinical education and other skills on faculty members for an adequate training to medical students.

PURPOSE OF THE STUDY

The School of Medicine at Tecnológico de Monterrey is a private university in Mexico that is highly interested in developing pedagogical skills among their faculty members. Since its founding in 1978, a student-centered educational approach has been implemented. The faculty members from basic science to medical science have been facilitators using problem-based learning and collaboration as teaching strategies. Faculty have participated in several courses regarding innovative pedagogical methods for higher education environments. Besides the benefits of the original training program offered by the university, the content was not customized for clinicians who do not educate in a traditional classroom.

The Development Program for Clinical Educators (DPCE) is a competency-based model which was designed to train faculty members to educate students in a medical context. The purpose of this study was to assess the quality of the DPCE according to the four moments established by Pérez Juste (2000). These four moments resemble to the fundamental quality management theory, which describes the importance of the continual improvement process, in which the evaluation represents the input to achieve superior performance standards (2006).

METHOD

A multiphase mixed method approach was conducted according to Creswell and Plano (2010). The mixed methods combine qualitative and quantitative instruments to inquire about a problem. According to the authors, a multiphase design is recommended to assess the impact of a long term project which will continue as a permanent program. In this case, the Development Program for Clinical Educators was introduced as a training program for every faculty member who participates in the School of Medicine.

The phases considered were the four assessment moments of Pérez Juste (2000). The author establishes that every training program must be assessed in four moments: 1) assessment of the proposal, 2) assessment of the implementation of the program, 3) assessment from faculty experiences and 4) institutionalization of the program, which is presented in Figure 3.

1. Assessment of the proposal. Considers the assessment of design taking into account purpose, function, methodology and relevance of the program prior to execution.
2. Assessment of the implementation of the program. Relates to information gathering to find improvement for the next implementation during the training program.
3. Assessment from faculty experiences. It is classified in positive and negative effects regarding the efficiency and effectiveness to achieve the objectives of the program after completion.
4. Institutionalization of program evaluation. Application of successive cycles of evaluation and continuous improvement to upgrade the program.

A qualitative approach was applied on proposal, implementation and institutionalization. A quantitative approach was selected for assessment from faculty experiences and institutionalization. In the following sections are presented detailed description of the inquiry and assessment process for continuous improvement on each moment.

Assessment of the Proposal

The model for the Development Program for Clinical Educators integrates six competences for faculty members on medical contexts: applying basic teaching skills; foster learning in the clinical setting; assessing and debriefing performance; managing healthcare educational technology; educating on bioethics and citizenship, and managing healthcare educational technology. Those six skills are represented in Figure 4.

The development program is based on the previously presented competency models (Table 2) as well as previous research on clinical educators and institutional policies. This qualitative approach, has been stated before by Taylor and Bogdan (1987) who recommend considering previous theories to validate its application. The assessment of this model was performed by the academic authorities of Tecnológico de Monterrey considering equivalence on the university program and requirements from

Figure 3. Phases of the study design

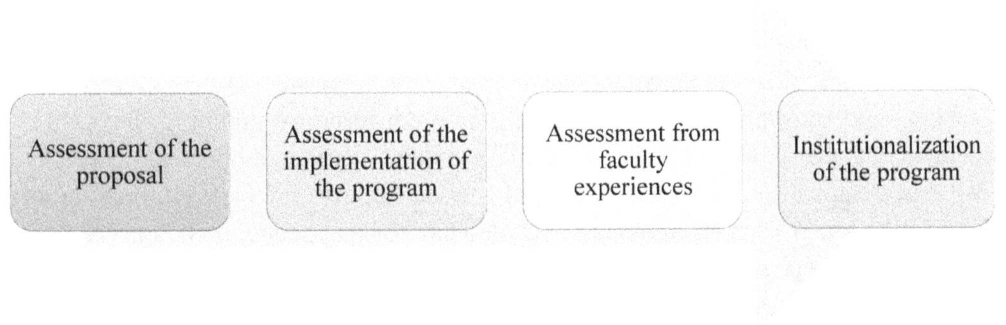

Figure 4. Competencies of the development program for clinical educator

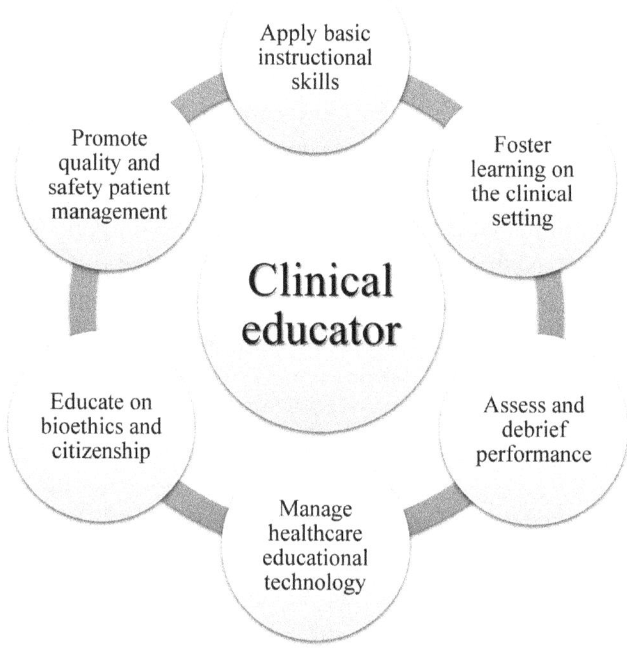

medical teachers. A comparison paired matrix was presented to them to demonstrate correspondence (Evans & Lindsay, 2014).

The purpose of the Development Program for Clinical Educators was to improve the faculty competencies in order to be applied to educational scenarios to enhance medical student's outcomes. The audience was primarily targeted to medical specialists who educate students in clinical settings such as: hospitals, emergency rooms, intensive care units, and consultation rooms amongst other scenarios. The pilot program considered two hour sessions during 18 weeks. After a review of purpose, content and targeted audience, a budget was assigned for a single group. This qualitative activity represented the first phase of the mixed method approach according to Creswell and Plano (2010). The following description introduces the content of the model on each competence.

Apply Basic Instructional Skills

Several authors declare that instructional development is part of the emergent core competencies needed by physicians who specialize in education. Harris et al. (2007) consider that faculty members should analyze teaching and learning styles of the students in order to prepare them for physical exams and patient interaction. Zabar et al. (2004) consider that a medical teacher should: ask learners to commit to diagnosis and treatment plans, request supporting evidence, give information, provide feedback on specific knowledge, check learning understanding on what was taught and, invite to generate questions. These behaviors encourage students to develop critical thinking and clinical reasoning on the acquired knowledge and experience. Critical thinking is a "purposeful reflective judgment that manifests itself in reasoned consideration of evidence, context, methods, standards and conceptualizations in deciding what to believe or what to do" (Facione, 1990).

Doukas, McCullough and Wear (2012) define critical thinking within the medical context as a skill set which enables the student to perform in a complex and uncertain environment where they must provide competent care. Its evidence is in the process that the student uses in the caring of the patient, where they must obtain data through observation, analyze by contrasting and identifying similarities with previous experience, and reflect for continuous improvement.

Ennis (1992) believes that there are four ways to teach critical thinking: general, infusion, immersion, and mixed. The general strategy refers to using specific courses or modules within a course to teach critical thinking. The infusion process incorporates particular objectives to apply critical thinking in an existing course. The immersion process invites students to reflect and make value judgments on any disciplinary courses without an explicit declaration, and, finally, the mixed method mixes the general principles of the infusion and immersion process.

According to Olivares and López (2016), critical thinking in health professionals is observed by the acquisition of information from different sources, integration and synthesis of information considering different treatment plans, communication with the patient, evidence based-decision making, and performance by identifying their own prejudices. The designed program included three sessions, which introduced participants to the evolution and trends of pedagogical methods, explained general requirements to teach in a clinical environment and provided practical methods to develop critical thinking in students.

Foster Learning in the Clinical Setting

Clinical learning occurs in diverse settings: during rounds, bedside, in the hallway, and alone in the library. It cannot be restricted as its development requires the adaptation to different cases that present or evolve in the clinic (Wilkerson, 1985). Martínez-González et al. (2008) and Aguirre Huacuja et al. (2012) consider the importance of mentoring students on diverse clinical settings. The program includes teaching approaches considering diverse contexts such as hospitals and healthcare centers.

Regarding medical education in a hospital setting, the bedside teaching approach during attending rounds has been used for generations as a common ritual for medical education. However, even if this routine is a powerful strategy for students to observe clinical skills, communication patterns, roles of the medical team and hospital management styles; it also generates tension among participants since it mixes education and work (Balmer, Master, Richards, Serwint & Giardino, 2010).

Harris et al. (2007) consider that faculty members in a health care center should balance the needs of individual/family with those of the students while providing patient-centered care. The teacher should also demonstrate how to function effectively in a managed care environment while preserving the educational mission.

The clinical context itself should be considered as a continuous learning experience where the student, faculty, nurses, technicians and the whole medical team has an implied learning role. Wilkerson (1985) advocates for it to be considered not as a teaching environment in which the faculty must prepare a lesson plan, but as an active environment were participants must be goal-oriented and be able to regulate their own learning strategies.

The module included techniques for faculty members to capitalize on every teachable moment in a clinical setting to promote clinical judgment and leadership in learners, considering the psychological characteristics of the millennial students. It considers more than supervising student performance, but it requires to be accessible (time and will) to help, and providing effective feedback to reinforce correct performance and attitudes.

Assess and Debrief Performance

Martínez-González et al. (2008), Aguirre Huacuja et al. (2012) and Harris et al. (2007) agree on the importance of evaluation. In order to measure the performance standards in students, a faculty member should consider expectations from both the higher education institution and the clinical setting. The educational program should describe the competencies and the desired graduate profile of students. The health care center usually has quality indicators that may help faculty members to establish metrics to deliver. Besides the grade, the students should receive proper feedback and debriefing from teachers in order to invite them to reflect on their achievements to improve their performance each time.

Larsen, Butler, Lawson, & Roediger III (2013) recommend Test Enhancing learning as an educational method to increase long-term retention. The purpose of this cognitive tool is to repeat the application of past exams to retrieve previous knowledge. Recent studies have inquired into the transferability of conceptual knowledge to clinical settings through testing clinical skills of students with standardized patients. Their results suggest that both written tests and repeated practice with simulated patients have direct implications on the retaining and application of knowledge on the clinical setting. For Cox and Irby (2007) written exams have the disadvantage of being time consuming and that they require training to develop items. Disadvantages for clinical simulation assessments are logistics and cost.

For Norcini (2003) written exams and simulation patients are useful for basic competences regarding knowledge and methods. However, it is not enough to prove performance and action, so he recommends the work based assessment to evaluate performance in actual clinical contexts. There are several ways to assess students in a clinical setting. Eardley, Bussey, Woodthorpe, Munsch and Beard (2013) recommend Case-Based Discussion, clinical evaluation exercises, direct observation of procedural skills, peer assessment tools, procedure based assessments and other workplace based assessments for surgical programs. Regarding the method, Norcini (2003) suggests involving several actors in the evaluation to improve reliability on the scores.

Some evaluations are related to the volume of work. Portfolios in healthcare are used for a range of purposes including the assessment of the amount of procedures applied on a range of time. According to Tochel et al. (2009) portfolios are a key connection between learning at organizational and individual levels. Today they may be in electronic formats where learners select the best available material to be scored.

Despite the type of assessment, there are some principles that should be considered by faculty members: a) Establish the goals of assessment, b) Determine what to assess, c) Decide how to assess, d) Pay attention of the unintended effects and e) Give performance feedback.

The module regarding assessment included how to design items for written exams, how to track performance and how to give feedback to students using the several applications of work based assessment such as: portfolios, direct observation, patient feedback, and 360 degree feedback.

Manage Healthcare Educational Technology

Harris et al. (2007) consider medical informatics as one of the important competences for medical educators. The authors recommend that clinicians should teach principles of medical reasoning, decision making, probability and evaluation of decision-making systems. They also should promote discussion on clinical informatics topics, including quality, accuracy and interpretation of medical data variables. And finally, they should understand management systems such as computerized medical records for clinical activity analysis and databases mining for research purposes.

In order to promote such analysis, it was included in the topic of Evidence-Based Medicine in the program. According to Barends and Briner (2014), evidence-based medicine teaches medical students how to learn on their own, specifically: how to formulate an answerable question (ask); how to search for evidence (acquire); how to critically appraise the evidence (appraise); how to apply the evidence on the clinical practice (apply) and how to monitor outcomes (assess). The course explains to clinical educators how to search in academic databases available at the School of Medicine and how to promote informational literacy competencies in students.

Information literacy embraces the incorporation of technology to obtain valuable information and knowledge, it assumes that the learner is able to critically assess the quality of the information (Sayed & Jager, 2014). For students to display this competency they should be able to locate resources of information, within a library. This action requires to utilize a computer and Internet to research on different databases.

In an academic environment, the use of educational platforms is also desired. The module introduced faculty members in the use of a Blackboard platform and encouraged them to prove other open access platforms as Schoology or Edmodo. Another technological advancement, simulation training is defined as the replacement of real patient encounters with either standardized patients or technologies that replicate clinical scenarios (Okuda, Bryson, DeMaria, Jacobson, Shen & Levine, 2009). The advantage of simulations is the creation on an ideal environment for learning activities, which may be predictable, consistent, standardized, safe and reproducible. Faculty members of the program received a general introduction on the types of simulation, from low fidelity models for basic manual skills, to high fidelity models to develop teamwork and problem solving abilities in a critical care environment.

Education Related to Bioethics and Citizenship

The importance of bioethical behavior and professionalism in medical educators is a consensus (Martínez-González et al., 2008; Aguirre et al., 2012; Nogueira Sotolongo et al., 2005). Cohen and Sherif (2014) consider that medical schools should include faculty professional development activities in order to encourage faculty members to develop reflection with students on topics of dignity, respect, and confidentiality amongst others.

Medicine is the integration of both biomedical and social sciences to provide a solution or treatment plan in the best benefit of the patient. According to Doukas, McCullough and Wear (2012), since the Flexner report an argument has been made in medicine for humanities education and the acquisition of humanistic skills. As students learn more about ethics and professionalism, they find knowledge and skills of reasoning and judgement that are essential to the professionalism and citizenship performance in medicine.

A multi-perspective frame of reference is needed when assessing a patient, providing a balance between the physician, patient or family of the patient perspectives. This skills or competence are patient-centered and enable the medical students to transit the path to become medical professionals.

According to Issenberg, Soo and Devine (2011) the care displayed by physicians must be compassionate, appropriate, and effective for the treatment of the actual health problems and the promotion of healthy lifestyles, as well. Clinician educators in this module were trained in the Konstanz Method of Dilemma Discussion (KMDD) proposed by Lind (2005). The KMDD educative dilemmas are tasks that do not affect anyone participating in a discussion, but are likely to cause real conflicts in the moral ideals of a person and at the same time may cause controversies among the participants. In the session, faculty members reflected on possibilities to apply dilemmas in their courses.

Promote Quality and Safety Patient Management

According to Kohn, Corrigan, & Donaldson (2000) every year between 44,000 to 98,000 people die in hospitals due to preventable medical errors. Some studies have shown the relevance on educating residents on quality and safety topics. After a 2-day patient safety course, Jansma, Wagner & Bijnen (2010) reported increased interest in residency students on improving patient safety through policies and communication. Similarly, Kelly et al. (2010) incorporated the concepts of quality and safety into a curriculum of Emergency Medicine residents.

Issenberg, Soo and Devine (2011) advocate for the commitment of the health and medical staff to carry with their professional responsibilities in adherence to ethical principles and a sensitivity to a diverse patient population. Patient safety becomes even more than the handling of a medical treatment, but the reporting of medical errors, and the system based practice approach.

Several authors (Ironside, Jeffries & Martin, 2009; Sullivan, Hirst, Cronenwett, 2009) define medical simulation as a comprehensive tool to foster quality and safety competence in undergraduate and residency programs.

Lee, An, Song, Jang and Park (2014) define seven key competencies of patient safety: recognize, respond to, and disclose adverse events; manage safety risks; communication; teamwork and understanding patient safety culture; understanding patient safety concept; informatics; and evidence-based practice. The authors define that these competencies must be acquired in 3 areas: knowledge, skills, and attitude.

This module introduced clinician educators on the importance of encouraging students in practicing quality and patient safety standards. Some topics included were: quality management basic concepts, continuous improvement quality tools and implementation of quality projects for improving patient care and safety. Some adverse cases were included where participants applied root cause analysis to provide corrective and preventive actions.

Assessment of the Implementation of the Program

The second phase of the mixed method consisted in running the pilot implementation, which included 18 face to face two hour sessions and online assignments. The assignments were used as proof of learning and improvement of the declared competencies. Sessions included dynamic activities and discussion among participants and facilitators. Each one was videotaped and shared through an online platform, promoting reflection and self-direction learning.

A total of 19 professors participated in the pilot, of which 11 were chair departments invited strategically to expand the program afterwards. At the end of the pilot participants shared experiences in a focus group session as part of the second moment of assessment of Pérez Juste (2000). This qualitative method is recommended as a feedback tool from customers and as a research instrument by Hernández, Fernández y Baptista (2003). Pilot participants expressed their level of satisfaction on collaborators, instructors, and content. Their feedback included suggestions to shorten the length of the program, to improve the interaction among participants and to invite more physicians as instructors.

Assessment from Faculty Experiences

The third phase of the mixed method was quantitative (Creswell & Plano, 2010). A questionnaire was selected and adapted to assess the overall satisfaction and the perceived effects of the program. Hernández et al. (2003) recommend this type of instrument when there's a need to collect information from a numbered population. To date, the six competence model has been offered to faculty members biannually, with a total of 96 graduates. The selected survey was designed by Herskovic et al. (2012). The authors study was prepared to assess whether clinical tutors perceived themselves as having made changes in their pedagogical practices after completing a program on teaching skills in clinical settings. The original survey included 13 questions related to four of the six competencies of the Development Program for Clinical Educators. This questionnaire was adapted for this study, including some questions to assess teaching and learning strategies not previously considered. Items related to principles of bioethics and citizenship and quality and safety patient management were also included. The perceived impact reported by professors by competency is presented in Table 3.

The competency that recorded highest influence was related to basic instructional skills from professors (74% reported major changes). The specific items were related to instruction of competency based education and critical thinking approaches. The least impact in the faculty practices were related to healthcare educational technology management (24% reported minor changes), specifically on items related with simulation training and library multimedia resources.

The instructional skills implemented by the professors included the development of critical thinking skills were they foster the interpretation and analysis of objective data for decision making processes. This is vital for clinical judgment where the health professionals must take life and death decision for

Table 3. Reported impact perceived by faculty experiences from practice

Competencies	Major	Similar	Minor	No Response
Apply basic instructional skills	74%	20%	1%	5%
Foster learning on the clinical setting	55%	30%	2%	13%
Assess and debrief performance	61%	24%	7%	8%
Manage healthcare educational technology	46%	27%	24%	3%
Educate bioethics and citizenship	55%	36%	0%	9%
Manage quality and patient safety	61%	30%	4%	5%
General				
Impact on faculty practices	70%	29%	2%	0%
Overall satisfaction	73%	15%	7%	5%

the best benefit of the patient. The changes related to healthcare educational technology management where the adoption of Learning Management Systems such as Schoology and Google Classroom to administrate learning resources, grades, and student interaction. In addition, apps, such as Nearpod and Kahoot, were incorporated to administer tests and short quizzes.

Institutionalization of the Program

The program has been programmed every semester. The presented results inspired an improvement of the program to assign participants to design and document an innovative project regarding medical education as part as their certification process. Starting in 2014, their ideas where sent for consideration to be shared on the *Conference of Innovation and Research in Education on the Academic Innovation in Health Track*. The first year 30 projects were developed, in 2015 about 38 works were published the congress presentation publications, and for 2016 the accepted presentations increased to 70, either for oral, poster or networking sessions.

SOLUTIONS AND RECOMMENDATIONS

The six competencies model has been assessed in the four moments proposed by Pérez Juste (2000). Quality management and medical education theories were combined to inquire about effectiveness of a pedagogical training program. This project can be transferred and replicated by other training programs for medical teachers if the contents are tailored specifically to their needs. It is recommendable to consider instructors rank, experience and influence on participants. The DPCE has been widely supported by leaders from both the School of Medicine and teaching hospitals. Recently, these authorities had been involved as instructors, which enhance the importance of educational and quality culture among physicians. Similarly to Conigliaro & Stratton (2010), the presented instruments and methods might be useful for identifying teachers who would most benefit from further development, either because they are new to the task or because they are operating well below the level of their peers.

FUTURE RESEARCH DIRECTIONS

Although participants reported increased knowledge in teaching techniques and educational principles, further research is needed to explore the long-time effects of the program in the teaching competencies from the medical faculty. There are also other issues to consider. According to Rashid and Siriwardena (2005) professionalization of medical educators has obvious benefits but there may also be considerable barriers. Similarly to the findings of their study, only a small proportion of the clinical professors have formal qualifications as educators. To manage such qualifications as a mandatory requisite for appointment, could have negative consequences on morale and retention for current teachers or recruitment of new faculty members.

The next step is to integrate competences on the training program in order to combine concepts and practices on two or more competences. Adamson et al. (2015) also recognized the importance to continue identifying skill sets necessary for a career as a clinician-educator and innovative approaches to develop a faculty program to formally train a subset of fellows in these skills.

Since technology management has a minor effect on participants, it has been incorporated as a transverse activity on several sessions. Future research will indicate if this upgrading has had an effect on actual teaching practices. Other important topic for future research is about millennial learning needs. Even when the DPCE already includes this information as an introduction, faculty members sense a rapid changing on effectiveness from traditional teaching methods, which should be taken into consideration for future editions of the program.

CONCLUSION

The need for faculty development programs to improve pedagogical practices in medical education is felt by every higher education institution. The challenge is to upgrade and update competencies on educators as rapid as emerging learning trends. Nevertheless the program has been mainly focused on the assurance and standardization of quality in medical education: in teaching, learning and educational process itself. However as this quality increases, the development of these clinical educator must keep up. The next step in this program should address themes regarding not only the challenges the student's must face tomorrow, but the challenges of society itself by integrating the whole educational organization: leaders, faculty, students, community, and in the health educational systems, the patient.

Millennial students will start university programs with different preparation from earlier generations and will require innovative environments and stimulus for learning. The situation is more critical to private universities which value added is highly demanded in return of investment from student sponsors.

The present program has evolved from a generic version to a customized design for clinical educators. This concept has increased enthusiasm and overall satisfaction from physicians to participate on a teaching role. However, medical programs design should develop an integral approach from several disciplines, perspectives and competences to graduate doctors for an uncertain future.

The awareness they gain of the impact their teaching and the responsibility they carry to challenge students, motivates grounded solutions that designed specifically to their context. They identify attributes such as a passion for teaching that allow them to view an educational setting from a multiple-perspective point of view. New students demand not only time for lectures or for feedback in the teacher' agenda, they also expect commitment. The educational program must prepare faculty, leaders and administrators to innovate and propose programs that are both perceived and assessed as relevant.

These results should promote such a reaction or impact in participants, which would guarantee the application of those methods in the future. Most importantly the changes should influence and provide evidence in results explicitly in the organizational system. An important ally in the assessment of educational methods and the effects on the student's learning is the teacher. As they become prepared to develop strategies, experiments and their respective instruments, they become part of the change itself.

The next step would professionalize the journey that faculty has started by designing a continuous program that could prepare them to develop structured educational experiments, the plan to implement an specific solution, and the support team to advise them with insight and future vision. The observed results have displayed a generation of enthusiastic and passionate teachers that are taking their first steps in the right direction: participating in seminars and educational congresses. We should provide them with means to share their vision and proposal in an academic showcase in prestigious journals that could detonate opportunities for them to work with colleges all-around the globe.

REFERENCES

Adamson, R., Richard, G., Kritek, P., Luks, A., Tonelli, M., & Benditt, J. (2015). Training the teachers: The clinician-Educator Track of the University of Washington Pulmonary and Critical Care Medicine Fellowhip Program. *Annals of the American Thoracic Society*, *12*(4), 480–485. doi:10.1513/AnnalsATS.201501-032OT PMID:25763811

Aguirre Huacuja, E., Castellanos Barrales, F., Galicia Negrete, H., González Torres, A., Fabián Jarquín, O., Ojeda Blanco, C.,... Vázquez Esquivel, J. (2012). Perfil por competencias docentes del profesor de medicina. Mexico: AMFEM Ed.

Atkinson, K., Ajjawi, R., & Cooling, N. (2011). Promoting clinical reasoning in general practice trainees: Role of the clinical teacher. *The Clinical Teacher*, *8*(1), 176–180. doi:10.1111/j.1743-498X.2011.00447.x PMID:21851565

Atkison, K., Ajjawi, R., & Cooling, N. (2011). Promoting clinical reasoning in general practice trainees: Role of the clinical teacher. *The Clinical Teacher*, *8*(1), 176–180. doi:10.1111/j.1743-498X.2011.00447.x PMID:21851565

Balmer, D. F., Master, C. L., Richards, B. F., Serwint, J. R., & Giardino, A. P. (2010). An ethnographic study of attending rounds in general paediatrics: Understanding the ritual. *Medical Education*, *44*(11), 1105–1116. doi:10.1111/j.1365-2923.2010.03767.x PMID:20946480

Barends, E., & Briner, R. (2014). Teaching Evidence-Based Practice: Lessons from the pioneers: An interview with Amanda Burls and Gordon Guyatt. *Academy of Management Learning & Education*, *13*(3), 476–483. doi:10.5465/amle.2014.0136

Boerebach, B., Lombarts, K., Keijzer, C., Heineman, M., & Arah, O. (2012). The teacher, the physician and the person: *How facultys teaching performance influences their role modelling. PLoS ONE*, *7*(3), 1–7. doi:10.1371/journal.pone.0032089 PMID:22427818

CAHSPR. (2016). *History of the Ted Freedman Award for Innovation in Education*. Retrieved May 10, 2016, from http://www.longwoods.com/pages/ted-freedman-award-history

Cantú-Delgado, H. (2006). *Desarrollo de una Cultura de Calidad* (3rd ed.). Mexico: Mc Graw-Hill.

Cohen, G. L., & Sherif, Y. A. (2014). Twelve tips on teaching and learning humanism in medical education. *Medical Teacher*, *36*(8), 680–684. doi:10.3109/0142159X.2014.916779 PMID:24965585

Conigliaro, R., & Stratton, T. (2010). The quality of clinical teaching. *The Clinical Teacher*, *7*(1), 143–146. PMID:20444073

Cox, M., Irby, D., & Epstein, R. M. (2007). Assessment in Medical Education. *The New England Journal of Medicine*, *356*(4), 387–396. doi:10.1056/NEJMra054784 PMID:17251535

Creswell, J. W., & Plano, C. (2010). *Designing and Conducting Mixed Methods Research*. Lincoln, NE: SAGE.

Doukas, D. J., McCullough, L. B., & Wear, S. (2012). Medical Education in Medical Ethics and Humanities as the Foundation for Developing Medical Professionalism. *Academic Medicine*, *87*(3), 334–341. doi:10.1097/ACM.0b013e318244728c PMID:22373629

Duvivier, R., Van Dalen, J., Vleuten, V., & Scherpbier, A. (2009). Teacher perceptions of desired qualities, competencies and strategies for clinical skill teachers. *Teaching Skills for Clinical Skills Teacher, 31*(1), 634-641.

Eardley, I., Bussey, M., Woodthorpe, A., Munsch, C., & Beard, J. (2013). Workplace-based assessment in surgical training: Experiences from the intercollegiate surgical curriculum programme. *The Australian and New Zealand Journal of Surgery*, *83*(6), 448–453. doi:10.1111/ans.12187 PMID:23656354

Ennis, R. H. (1992). John McPeck's Teaching Critical Thinking. *Educational Studies*, *23*(4), 462–472.

Evans, J., & Lindsay, W. L. (2014). *Administración y Control de la Calidad* (7th ed.). Mexico: Cengage Learning.

Facione, P. (1990). *The APA Delphi Report, Critical Thinking: A Statement of Expert Consensus for Purposes of Educational Assessment and Instruction 1*. The California Academic Press.

Finn, K., Chiappa, V., Puig, A., & Hunt, D. (2011). How to become a better clinical teacher: A collaborative peer observation process. *Medical Teacher*, *33*(1), 151–155. doi:10.3109/0142159X.2010.541534 PMID:21275544

Flexner, A. (1910). *Medical Education in United States and Canada*. The Carnegie Foundation for the Advancement of Teaching. Retrieved from http://archive.carnegiefoundation.org/pdfs/elibrary/Carnegie_Flexner_Report.pdf

Harris, D. L., Krause, K., Parish, D., & Smith, M. (2007). Academic Competencies for Medical Faculty. *Family Medicine*, *39*(5), 343–350. PMID:17476608

Hernández, R., Fernández, C., & Baptista, P. (2003). *Metodología de la Investigación* (3rd ed.). México: McGraw-Hill.

Herskovik, P., Miranda, T., Cortés, E., Delusshi, A., Gómez, P. A., Jiusán, A., & Puzant, M. etal. (2012). Creen haber cambiado los docentes un año después de un curso de docencia clínica. *Educación Médica*, *15*(3), 179–185.

Ibrahim, H., Stadler, D., Archuleta, S., Shah, N., Bertram, A., Nair, S., & Cofrancesco, J. (2015). Clinician-educators in emerging graduate medical education systems: Description, roles and perceptions. *Postgraduate Medical Journal*, *92*(1), 14–20. PMID:26512124

Ironside, P. M., Jeffries, P. R., & Martin, A. (2009). Fostering patient safety competencies using multiple-patient simulation experiences. *Nursing Outlook*, *57*(6), 332–337. doi:10.1016/j.outlook.2009.07.010 PMID:19942034

Issenberg, S. B., Soo, H., & Devine, L. A. (2011). Patient Safety Training Simulations Based on Competency Criteria of the Accreditation Council for Graduate Medical Education. *The Mount Sinai Journal of Medicine, New York*, *78*(1), 842–853. doi:10.1002/msj.20301 PMID:22069208

Jansma, J. D., Wagner, C., & Bijnen, A. B. (2010). Resident's intentions and actions after patient safety education. *BMC Health Services Research*, *10*(350), 1–9. PMID:20044945

Kelly, J. J., Thallner, E., Broida, R. I., Cheung, D., Meisl, H., Hamedani, A. G., & Beach, C. etal. (2010). Emergency Medicine Quality Improvement and Patient Safety Curriculum. *Academic Emergency Medicine*, *17*(2), 110–129. doi:10.1111/j.1553-2712.2010.00897.x PMID:21199092

Khan, C. B., & Chishti, S. (2012). Effects of Staff Training and Development on Professional Abilities of University Teachers in Distance Learning Systems. *Quarterly Review of Distance Education*, *13*(2), 87–94.

Kiani, Q., Umar, S., & Iqbal, M. (2014). What do medical students expect in a teacher? *The Clinical Teacher*, *11*(1), 203–208. doi:10.1111/tct.12109 PMID:24802922

Kohn, L. T., Corrigan, J., & Donaldson, M. S. (2000). *To err is human: Building a safer health system*. Washington, DC: National Academy Press.

Konerman, M., Alpert, C., & Shashank, S. (2016). Learning to be a clinician-educator. *Journal of the American College of Cardiology*, *67*(3), 338–342. doi:10.1016/j.jacc.2015.11.032 PMID:26796400

Larsen, D., Butler, A., Lawson, A., & Roediger, I. H. (2013). The importance of seeing the patient: Test-enhanced learning with standardized patients and written tests improves clinical application of knowledge. *Advances in Health Sciences Education: Theory and Practice*, *18*(3), 409–425. doi:10.1007/s10459-012-9379-7 PMID:22618856

Lee, N. J., An, J. Y., Song, T. M., Jang, H., & Park, S. Y. (2014). Psychometric evaluation of a patient safety competency self-evaluation tool for nursing students. *The Journal of Nursing Education*, *53*(10), 550–562. doi:10.3928/01484834-20140922-01 PMID:25275988

Lind, G. (2005). Moral Dilemma Discussion Revisited - The Konstanz Method. *Europes Journal of Psychology*, *1*(1), 1–5. doi:10.5964/ejop.v1i1.345

MacLeod, S. (2012). Walking the talk: The need for investment in educator development. *Education for Primary Care*, *23*(1), 242245. PMID:22925955

Malcolm Baldrige National Quality Awards. (2016). *Advocate Good Samaritan Hospital*. Available at: https://www.nist.gov/baldrige/advocate-good-samaritan-hospital

Martínez-González, A., López-Bárcena, J., Herrera Saint-Leu, P., Ocampo-Martínez, J., Petra, I., & Uribe-Martínez, G., … Morales-López, S. (2008). Modelo de competencias del profesor de medicina. *Educación Médica*, *11*(3), 157–10.

Marton, G., McCullough, B., & Ramnanan, C. (2014). A review of teaching skills development programmes for medical students. *Medical Education*, *49*(1), 149–160. PMID:25626746

Nilson, M., Pennbrant, S., Pilhammar, E., & Wenestarm, C.-G. (2010). Pedagogical strategies used in clinical medical education: Observational study. *BMC Medical Education*, *10*(9), 1–10. PMID:20074350

Nogueira Sotolongo, M., Rivera Michelena, C. N., & Blanco, F. (2005). Competencias docentes del médico de familia en el desempeño de la tutoría en la carrera de medicina. *Educación Médica Superior*, *19*(1), 1–1.

Norcini, J. J. (2003). Setting standards on educational tests. *Medical Education*, *37*(5), 464–474. doi:10.1046/j.1365-2923.2003.01495.x PMID:12709190

Okuda, Y., Bryson, E. O., DeMaria, S. Jr, Jacobson, L., Shen, B., & Levine, A. I. (2009). The Utility of Simulation in Medical Education: What Is the Evidence? *The Mount Sinai Journal of Medicine, New York*, *76*(4), 330–343. doi:10.1002/msj.20127 PMID:19642147

Olivares, S. (2016). Aprendizaje Centrado en las Perspectivas del Paciente. In S. Olivares, & J. Valdez-García (Eds.), *Aprendizaje Centrado en el Paciente: Cuatro perspectivas para un abordaje integral* (pp. 4-44). Ciudad de México: Editorial Médica Panamericana.

Olivares, S. L., & López, M. V. (2016). Evaluación de autopercepción del pensamiento crítico en estudiantes de medicina. *Revista Electrónica de Investigación Educativa*, *18*(3), 1–22.

Omid, A., & Haghani Fariba, A. P. (2016). Clinical teaching with emotional intelligence: A teaching toolbox. *Journal of Research in Medical Sciences*, *21*(1), 19–27.

Pérez Juste, R. (2000). La evaluación de programas educativos: Conceptos básicos, planteamientos generales y problemática. *Revista de Investigación Educativa*, *18*(2), 261–287.

Rashid, A., & Siriwardena, N. (2005). *The professionalisation of education an educators in postgraduate medicine. Education for Primary Care, 16*(1), 235-245.

Ross, M. (2014). Art in clinical teaching. *The Clinical Teacher*, *11*(1), 325–326. doi:10.1111/tct.12286 PMID:25041661

Sayed, Y., & Jager, K. (2014). Towards an investigation of information literacy in South African students. *South African Journal of Library and Information Science*, *65*(1), 5–12. doi:10.7553/65-1-1495

Singh, S., Pai, D. R., Sinha, N. K., Kaur, A., Kyaw Soe, A., & Barua, A. 5. (2013). Qualities of an effective teacher: What do medical teachers think? *BMC Medical Education*, *13*(128), 2–7. PMID:24044727

Sullivan, D. T., Hirst, D., & Cronenwett, L. (2009). Assessing quality and safety competencies of graduating prelicensure nursing students. *Nursing Outlook*, *57*(6), 323–331. doi:10.1016/j.outlook.2009.08.004 PMID:19942033

Taylor, S. J., & Bogdan, R. (1987). *Introducción a los métodos cualitativos de investigación*. Barcelona: Paidós.

Tochel, C., Haig, A., Hesketh, A., Cadzow, A., Beggs, K., Colthart, I., & Peacock, H. (2009). The effectiveness of portfolios for post-graduate assessment and education: BEME Guide No 12. *Medical Teacher*, *31*(4), 299–318. doi:10.1080/01421590902883056 PMID:19404890

Vogt, W. P. (2007). *Quantitative Research methods for Professionals*. Boston: Pearson.

Wilkerson, L., & Irby, D. (1998). Strategies for improving teaching practices: A comprehensive approach to faculty development. *Academic Medicine*, *73*(4), 387–396. doi:10.1097/00001888-199804000-00011 PMID:9580715

Wilkerson, L. A. (1985). Learning in a Clinical Setting. *To Improve the Academy, 4*, 120-133.

Yeates, P., Stewart, J., & Barton, R. (2008). What can we expect of clinical teachers? Establishing consensus on applicable skills, attitudes and practices. *Medical Education*, *42*(1), 134–142. doi:10.1111/j.1365-2923.2007.02986.x PMID:18230087

Zabar, S., Hanley, K., David, S. L., Kalet, A., Schwartz, M. D., Pearlman, E., & Lipkin, M. etal. (2004). Measuring the competence of residents as teachers. *Journal of General Internal Medicine*, *19*(2), 530–534. doi:10.1111/j.1525-1497.2004.30219.x PMID:15109318

KEY TERMS AND DEFINITIONS

Assessment: Refers to the tools and activities used to measure the performance of a person or an organization. This measure provides evidence to evaluate the improvement of the performance.

Clinical Educator: Refers to the high-skilled health personnel that besides their role in a healthcare environment work also as faculty in a university or hospital context, with the objective to provide training to the students.

Competence: Refers to the abilities, skills, or knowledge that empower an individual to provide an excellence performance in a determined activity or situation. It considers the joint application of knowledge and personality traits to perform.

Debriefing: Refers to the structured feedback performed after an educational activity. It is widely implemented in the clinical simulation environment to inquire on the students' performance deeper than the observed actions that were performed in the activity. This technique investigates the student's reasoning to understand the knowledge, experience, or reasoning that lead them to act a certain way.

Evaluation: Refers to the judgment or appraisal performed to measure the level of a person, program, or an organization.

Faculty Development Program: Refers to an educational program designed to provide faculty members with the knowledge and skills that they need to instruct, guide and mentor.

Medical Education: Refers to the educational activities that foster the transformative change in the student that enters the medical school into a physician. It is considered in both undergraduate (medical school) and graduate level (medical residency programs and fellowship).

Pedagogical Skills: Refers to the faculty skills needed to perform in the educational context. These involve the classroom management skills and disciplinary knowledge.

Quality Management: Refers to the approach that provides an organization with the opportunity to constantly assess the planning, control, and improvement of its performance. It incorporates the use of quality control tools to assure and accomplish a goal of reliable and constant quality level.

Simulation: Refers to the educational activity that is based on an artificial and controlled representation of reality were the student can perform through different clinical scenarios.

Compilation of References

Abrahamson, S., Denson, J. S., & Wolf, R. M. (1969). Effectiveness of a simulator in training anesthesiology residents. *Journal of Medical Education*, *44*, 515–519. PMID:5789592

Abu-Rish, E. B., Pfeifle, A., Jones, M., Hall, L. W., & Zierler, B. K. (2016). Findings from a mixed-methods study of an interprofessional faculty development program. *Journal of Interprofessional Care*, *30*(1), 83–89. doi:10.3109/13561820.2015.1051615 PMID:26576839

Accreditation Council for Graduate Medical Education. (2002). *ACGME Core Competencies*. Retrieved May 1, 2016, from http://www.ecfmg.org/echo/acgme-core-competencies.html

Accreditation Council for Graduate Medical Education. (2016). *ACGME common program requirements*. Retrieved from http://www.acgme.org/What-We-Do/Accreditation/Common-Program-Requirements

Accreditation Council for Graduate Medical Education. (2016). *What we do*. Retrieved May 21, 2016, from http://www.acgme.org/What-We-Do/Overview

Adamson, R., Richard, G., Kritek, P., Luks, A., Tonelli, M., & Benditt, J. (2015). Training the teachers: The clinician-Educator Track of the University of Washington Pulmonary and Critical Care Medicine Fellowhip Program. *Annals of the American Thoracic Society*, *12*(4), 480–485. doi:10.1513/AnnalsATS.201501-032OT PMID:25763811

Adnet, F., Borron, S. W., Dumas, J. L., Lapostolle, F., Cupa, M., & Lapandry, C. (2001). Study of the "sniffing position" by magnetic resonance imaging. *The Journal of the American Society of Anesthesiologists*, *94*(1), 83–86. PMID:11135726

Aebersold, M., & Tschannen, D. (2013). Simulation in nursing practice: The impact on patient care. *Online Journal of Issues in Nursing*, *18*(2). doi:10.3912/OJIN.Vol18No02Man06 PMID:23758424

Aggarwal, R., Soper, N., Ziv, A., Reznick, R., Mytton, O. T., Derbrew, M., . . . Morimoto, T. (2010). Training and simulation for patient safety. *Quality & Safety in Health Care, 19*(4), i34-i43. doi:10.1136/qshc.2009.038562

Aguirre Huacuja, E., Castellanos Barrales, F., Galicia Negrete, H., González Torres, A., Fabián Jarquín, O., Ojeda Blanco, C., . . . Vázquez Esquivel, J. (2012). Perfil por competencias docentes del profesor de medicina. Mexico: AMFEM Ed.

Ahmed, M., Sevdalis, N., Paige, J., Paragi-Gururaja, R., Nestel, D., & Arora, S. (2012). Identifying best practice guidelines for debrie ng in surgery: A tri-continental study. *American Journal of Surgery*, *203*(4), 523–529. doi:10.1016/j.amjsurg.2011.09.024 PMID:22450027

Ainsworth, H. L., & Eaton, S. E. (2010). *Formal, non-formal and informal learning in the sciences.* Retrieved May 1, 2016, from http://files.eric.ed.gov/fulltext/ED511414.pdf

Akaike, M., Fukutomi, M., Nagamune, M., Fujimoto, A., Tsuji, A., Ishida, K., & Iwata, T. (2012). Simulation-based medical education in clinical skills laboratory. *The Journal of Medical Investigation*, *59*(1-2), 28–35. doi:10.2152/jmi.59.28 PMID:22449990

Akhtar-Danesh, N., Baxter, P., Valaitis, R. K., Stanyon, W., & Sproul, S. (2009). Nurse faculty perceptions of simulation use in nursing education. *Western Journal of Nursing Research*, *31*(3), 312–329. doi:10.1177/0193945908328264 PMID:19176404

Albanese, M. A., Mejicano, G., Mullan, P., Kokotailo, P., & Gruppen, L. (2008). Defining characteristics of educational competencies. *Medical Education*, *42*(3), 248–255. doi:10.1111/j.1365-2923.2007.02996.x PMID:18275412

Al-Dahir, S., Bryant, K., Kennedy, K. B., & Robinson, D. S. (2014). Online virtual-patient cases versus traditional problem-based learning in advanced pharmacy practice experiences. *American Journal of Pharmaceutical Education*, *78*(4), 1–8. doi:10.5688/ajpe78476 PMID:24850938

Alessi, S. M., & Trollip, S. R. (2001). *Multimedia for learning: Methods and development* (3rd ed.). Boston, MA: Allyn & Bacon.

Alinier, G. (2010). Developing high-fidelity health care simulation scenarios: A guide for educators and professionals. *Simulation & Gaming*, *42*(1), 9–26. doi:10.1177/1046878109355683

Allen, I. E., & Seaman, J. (2016). *Online Report Card: Tracking Online Education in the United States*. Babson Park, MA: Babson Survey Research Group and Quahog Research Group. Retrieved July 20, 2016 from http://onlinelearningsurvey.com/reports/onlinereportcard.pdf

Almomen, R. K., Kaufman, D., Alotaibi, H., Al-Rowais, N. A., Albeik, M., & Albattal, S. M. (2016). Applying the ADDIE—Analysis, Design, Development, Implementation and Evaluation—Instructional Design Model to Continuing Professional Development for Primary Care Physicians in Saudi Arabia. *International Journal of Clinical Medicine*, *7*(08), 538–546. doi:10.4236/ijcm.2016.78059

American Association of College Nursing. (2014). *2014 annual report of the American Association of College Nursing*. Retrieved August 5, 2016 from http://www.aacn.nche.edu/aacn-publications/annual-reports/AnnualReport14.pdf

American Association of Colleges of Nursing. (2012). *White paper: Expectations for practice experiences in the RN-baccalaureate curriculum.* Retrieved October 26, 2016, from http://www.aacn.nche.edu/aacn-publications/white-papers/RN-BSN-White-Paper.pdf

American Association of Colleges of Nursing. (2015). *Degree Completion Programs for Registered Nurses: RN to Master's Degree and RN to Baccalaureate Programs*. Retrieved March 30, 2015 from http://www.aacn.nche.edu/media-relations/fact-sheets/degree-completion-programs

American Board of Anesthesiology. (2016). Retrieved from http://www.theaba.org/MOCA/About-MOCA-2-0

American Medical Association. (1995-2016). *Education center.* Retrieved October 26, 2016, from https://www.ama-assn.org/ama/pub/education-careers/education-center.page?

American Medical Association. (2015). *Accelerating change in medical education with visionary partners and bold innovations.* Retrieved April 22, 2016, from http://www.ama-assn.org/ama/pub/about-ama/strategic-focus/accelerating-change-in-medical-education/innovations.page-envisioning-expand

American Occupational Therapy Association, Inc. (2016). *Distance education entry-level occupational therapy (OT) educational programs.* Retrieved October 26, 2016, from http://www.aota.org/~/media/Corporate/Files/EducationCareers/Schools/DistanceEd/Distance_Education_Top_Percentage_OT_2014-2015.pdf

American Physical Therapy Association. (2015). *APTA Learning Center.* Retrieved October 26, 2016, from http://learningcenter.apta.org/default.aspx

Anderson, E., Smith, R., & Hammick, M. (2015). Evaluating an interprofessional education curriculum: A theory-informed approach. *Medical Teacher, 38*, 385–394. PMID:26079669

Anderson, L. W., Krathwohl, D. R., & Bloom, B. S. (2001). *A taxonomy for learning, teaching, and assessing: A revision of Bloom's taxonomy of educational objectives.* Allyn & Bacon.

Arnold, J. J., Johnson, L. M., Tucker, S. J., Chesak, S. S., & Dierkhising, R. A. (2011). Comparison of three simulation-based teaching methodologies for emergency response. *Clinical Simulation in Nursing, 9*(3), e85–e93. doi:10.1016/j.ecns.2011.09.004

Arnold, L., & Feighny, K. M. (1995). Students general learning approaches and performances in medical school: A longitudinal study. *Academic Medicine, 70*(8), 715–722. doi:10.1097/00001888-199508000-00016 PMID:7646748

Arnold, N., Ducate, L., & Kost, C. (2012). Collaboration or cooperation? Analyzing group dynamics and revision processes in wikis. *CALICO Journal, 29*(3), 431–448. doi:10.11139/cj.29.3.431-448

Ash, S. L., & Clayton, P. H. (2009). Generating, deepening, and documenting learning: The power of critical reflection in applied learning. *Journal of Applied Learning in Higher Education, 1*, 25-48. doi: 10.1097/NNE.0000000000000159

Ashton, K. S. (2012). Nurse Educators and the future of nursing. *Journal of Continuing Education in Nursing, 43*(3), 113–116. PMID:22263552

Association of American Medical Colleges. (2004). *Educating doctors to provide high quality medical care: A vision for medical education in the United States.* Washington, DC: Association of American Medical Colleges. Retrieved from https://members.aamc.org/eweb/upload/Educating%20Doctors%20to%20Provide%20July%202004.pdf

Association of American Medical Colleges. (2014). *Core entrustable professional activities for entering residency.* Washington, DC: Association of American Medical Colleges. Retrieved from http://www.aamc.org/cepaer

Association of American Medical Colleges. (2016). *Notable trends and five future forces.* AAMC.

Atkinson, K., Ajjawi, R., & Cooling, N. (2011). Promoting clinical reasoning in general practice trainees: Role of the clinical teacher. *The Clinical Teacher, 8*(1), 176–180. doi:10.1111/j.1743-498X.2011.00447.x PMID:21851565

Atkinson, R. C., & Shiffrin, R. M. (1968). Human memory: A proposed system and its control processes. In K. W. Spence & J. T. Spence (Eds.), *The psychology of learning and motivation: Advances in research and theory* (Vol. 2, pp. 89–195). New York: AcademicPress.

Australian Medical Council Limited. (2010). *Competence-based medical education AMC consultation paper.* Retrieved from http://www.amc.org.au/publications/policy

Authur. (1993). *Implicit learning and tacit knowledge: An essay on the cognitive unconscious.* Norwood, NJ: Oxford University Press.

Balmer, D. F., Master, C. L., Richards, B. F., Serwint, J. R., & Giardino, A. P. (2010). An ethnographic study of attending rounds in general paediatrics: Understanding the ritual. *Medical Education, 44*(11), 1105–1116. doi:10.1111/j.1365-2923.2010.03767.x PMID:20946480

Bandaranayake, R. C. (2011). *The integrated medical curriculum.* Radcliffe Publishing.

Bandiera, G., Boucher, A., Neville, A., Kuper, A., & Hodges, B. (2013). Integration and timing of basic and clinical sciences education. *Medical Teacher, 35*(5), 381–387. doi:10.3109/0142159X.2013.769674 PMID:23444888

Bandura, A. (1991). Social cognitive theory of self-regulation. *Organizational Behavior and Human Decision Processes, 50*(2), 248–287. doi:10.1016/0749-5978(91)90022-L

Barab, S., Warren, S. J., Del-Valle, R., & Fang, F. (2006). Coming to terms with communities of practice: A definition and operational criteria. In J. A. Pershing (Ed.), *Handbook of human performance technology: Principles, practices, and potential* (3rd ed.; pp. 640–664). San Francisco, CA: Pfeiffer.

Barends, E., & Briner, R. (2014). Teaching Evidence-Based Practice: Lessons from the pioneers: An interview with Amanda Burls and Gordon Guyatt. *Academy of Management Learning & Education, 13*(3), 476–483. doi:10.5465/amle.2014.0136

Barker, K. K., Bosco, C., & Oandasan, I. F. (2005). Factors in implementing interprofessional education and collaborative practice initiatives: Findings from key informant interviews. *Journal of Interprofessional Care, 19*(sup1), 166-176.

Barnett, S. M., & Ceci, S. J. (2002). When and where do we apply what we learn?: A taxonomy for far transfer. *Psychological Bulletin, 128*(4), 612–637. doi:10.1037/0033-2909.128.4.612 PMID:12081085

Barrows, H. S. (1986). A taxonomy of problem-based learning methods. *Medical Education, 20*(6), 481–486. doi:10.1111/j.1365-2923.1986.tb01386.x PMID:3796328

Barrows, H. S. (1996). Problem-based learning in medicine and beyond: A brief overview. *New Directions for Teaching and Learning, 1996*(68), 3–12. doi:10.1002/tl.37219966804

Barrows, H. S. (2002). Is it truly possible to have such a thing as dPBL? *Distance Education, 23*(1), 119–122. doi:10.1080/01587910220124026

Barrows, H. S., & Tamblyn, R. M. (1980). *Problem-based learning: An approach to medical education.* New York, NY: Springer.

Barzansky, B. (2013). *Medical school preparation for LCME accreditation.* Wayne State University School of Medicine. Retrieved June 6, 2015, from http://www.lcme.med.wayne.edu/intro.pdf

Batalden, P., Leach, D., Swing, S., Dreyfus, H., & Dreyfus, S. (2002). General competencies and accreditation in graduate medical education. *Health Affairs (Project Hope), 21*(5), 103–111. doi:10.1377/hlthaff.21.5.103 PMID:12224871

Baxter, L., Mattick, K., & Kuyken, W. (2013). Assessing health care students intentions and motivations for learning: The Healthcare Learning and Studying Inventory (HLSI). *Advances in Health Sciences Education: Theory and Practice, 18*(3), 451–462. doi:10.1007/s10459-012-9383-y PMID:22717990

Bearman, M., Cesnik, B., & Liddell, M. (2001). Random comparison of Virtual patient models in the context of teaching clinical communication skills. *Medical Education, 35*(9), 824–832. doi:10.1046/j.1365-2923.2001.00999.x PMID:11555219

Beaubien, J. M., & Baker, D. P. (2004). The use of simulation for training teamwork skills in health care: How low can you go? *Quality & Safety in Health Care, 13*(Supplement 1), i51–i56. doi:10.1136/qshc.2004.009845 PMID:15465956

Belfield, J. (2010). Using Gagnes theory to teach chest X-ray interpretation. *The Clinical Teacher, 7*(1), 5–8. doi:10.1111/j.1743-498X.2009.00329.x PMID:21134135

Benedict, N., & Schonder, K. (2011). Patient simulation software to augment an advanced pharmaceutics course. *American Journal of Pharmaceutical Education, 75*(2), 1–9. doi:10.5688/ajpe75221 PMID:21519411

Benor, D. E. (1982). Interdisciplinary integration in medical education: Theory and method. *Medical Education, 16*(6), 355–361. doi:10.1111/j.1365-2923.1982.tb00950.x PMID:7176983

Benumof, J. L. (2006). Corniculate cartilages are wrongly labeled arytenoid cartilages. *The Journal of the American Society of Anesthesiologists*, *104*(2), 377–377. PMID:16436864

Berney, S., Betrancourt, M., Molinari, G., & Hoyek, N. (2015). How spatial abilities and dynamic visualizations interplay when learning functional anatomy with 3D anatomical models. *Anatomical Sciences Education*, *8*(5), 452–462. doi:10.1002/ase.1524 PMID:25689057

Berwick, D. M., Nolan, T. W., & Whittington, J. (2008). The triple aim: Care, health, and cost. *Health Affairs*, *27*(3), 759–769. doi:10.1377/hlthaff.27.3.759 PMID:18474969

Bhandari, M., Montori, V., Devereaux, P. J., Dosanjh, S., Sprague, S., & Guyatt, G. H. (2003). Challenges to the practice of evidence-based medicine during residents surgical training: A qualitative study using grounded theory. *Academic Medicine*, *78*(11), 1183–1190. doi:10.1097/00001888-200311000-00022 PMID:14604884

Biocca, F., Harms, C., & Burgoon, J. K. (2003). Toward a more robust theory and measure of social presence: Review and suggested criteria. *Presence (Cambridge, Mass.)*, *12*(5), 456–480.

Bloom, B. S. (1956). *Taxonomy of educational objectives*. New York, NY: Longman.

Bloom, B. S. (1956). *Taxonomy of educational objectives: The classification of educational goals. Cognitive domain*. New York: David McKay.

Bloom, B. S. (1956). Taxonomy of educational objectives: Vol. 1. *Cognitive domain*. New York, NY: McKay.

Bloom, B. S. (1976). *Human characteristics and school learning*. New York: McGraw-Hill.

Bloom, B. S. (2005). Effects of continuing medical education on improving physician clinical care and patient health: A review of systematic reviews. *International Journal of Technology Assessment in Health Care*, *21*(3), 380–385. doi:10.1017/S026646230505049X PMID:16110718

Blue, A. V., Mitcham, M., Smith, T., Raymond, J., & Greenberg, R. (2010). Changing the future of health professions: Embedding interprofessional education within an academic health center. *Academic Medicine*, *85*(8), 1290–1295. doi:10.1097/ACM.0b013e3181e53e07 PMID:20671454

Blum, C. A., & Parcells, D. A. (2012). Relationship between high-fidelity simulation and patient safety in prelicensure nursing education: A comprehensive review. *The Journal of Nursing Education*, *51*(8), 429–U122. doi:10.3928/01484834-20120523-01 PMID:22624562

Boelen, C. (2002). A new paradigm for medical schools a century after Flexner's report. *Bulletin of the World Health Organization, 80*(7), 592-593. doi:S0042-96862002000700013

Boerebach, B., Lombarts, K., Keijzer, C., Heineman, M., & Arah, O. (2012). The teacher, the physician and the person: *How facultys teaching performance influences their role modelling. PLoS ONE*, *7*(3), 1–7. doi:10.1371/journal.pone.0032089 PMID:22427818

Botezatu, M., Hult, H., Tessma, M. K., & Fors, U. G. (2010). Virtual patient simulation for learning and assessment: Superior results in comparison with regular course exams. *Medical Teacher*, *32*(10), 845–850. doi:10.3109/01421591003695287 PMID:20854161

Boud, D., & Garrick, J. (1999). *Understanding learning at work*. London: Routledge.

Bower, B. L. (2016). *Distance education: Facing the faculty challenge*. Retrieved from http://www.westga.edu/distance/ojdla/summer42/bower42.html

Bradley, P. (2006). The history of simulation in medical education and possible future directions. *Medical Education, 40*(3), 254–262. doi:10.1111/j.1365-2929.2006.02394.x PMID:16483328

Branch, R. M. (2009). *Instructional design: The ADDIE approach* (Vol. 722). Springer Science & Business Media. doi:10.1007/978-0-387-09506-6

Brauer, D. G., & Ferguson, K. J. (2015). The integrated curriculum in medical education: AMEE guide no. 96. *Medical Teacher, 37*(4), 312–322. doi:10.3109/0142159X.2014.970998 PMID:25319403

Breen, H., & Jones, M. (2015). Experiential learning: Using virtual simulation in an online RN-to-BSN program. *The Journal of Continuing Education in Nursing, 46*(1), 27-33. doi:http://dx.doi.org.liblink.uncw.edu/10.3928/00220124-20141120-02

Bremner, M., Aduddell, K., Bennett, D., & VanGeest, J. (2006). The use of human patient simulators: Best practices with novice nursing students. *Nurse Educator, 31*(4), 170–174. doi:10.1097/00006223-200607000-00011 PMID:16855487

Bridge, P. D., Jackson, M., & Robinson, L. (2009). The effectiveness of streaming video on medical student learning: A case study. *Medical Education Online, 14*(0), 11. doi:10.3402/meo.v14i.4506 PMID:20165525

Bridges, D. R., Davidson, R. A., Odegard, P. S., Maki, I. V., & Tomkowiak, J. (2011). Interprofessional collaboration: Three best practice models of interprofessional education. *Medical Education Online, 16*(0), 6035. doi:10.3402/meo.v16i0.6035 PMID:21519399

Brooks, W. S., Woodley, K. T., Jackson, J. R., & Hoesley, C. J. (2015). Integration of gross anatomy in an organ system-based medical curriculum: Strategies and challenges. *Anatomical Sciences Education, 8*(3), 266–274. doi:10.1002/ase.1483 PMID:25132664

Brown, A. H., & Green, T. D. (2016). *The essentials of instructional design: Connecting fundamental principles with process and practice.* New York: Routledge.

Brown, J. S., Collins, A., & Duguid, P. (1989). Situated cognition and the culture of learning. *Education Researcher, 18*(1), 32–42. doi:10.3102/0013189X018001032

Bruno, I., & Santos, L. (2010). Written comments as a form of feedback. *Studies in Educational Evaluation, 36*(3), 111–120.

Bureau of Labor Statistics. (2013). *Occupations with the largest projected number of job openings due to growth and replacement needs, 2012 and projected 2022.* Retrieved from http://www.bls.gov/news.release/ecopro.t08.htm

Buring, S. M., Bhushan, A., Brazeau, G., Conway, S., Hansen, L., & Westberg, S. (2009). Interprofessional Education Supplement Keys to Successful Implementation of Interprofessional Education : Learning Location, Faculty Development, and Curricular Themes. *American Journal of Pharmaceutical Education, 73*(4), 60. doi:10.5688/aj730460 PMID:19657493

Buring, S. M., Bhushan, A., Broeseker, A., Conway, S., Duncan-Hewitt, W., Hansen, L., & Westberg, S. (2009). Interprofessional education: Definitions, student competencies, and guidelines for implementation. *American Journal of Pharmaceutical Education, 73*(4), 59. doi:10.5688/aj730459 PMID:19657492

Burneo, J. G., Jenkins, M. E., & Bussiere, M. (2006). Evaluating a formal evidence-based clinical practice curriculum in a neurology residency program. *Journal of the Neurological Sciences, 250*(1-2), 10–19. doi:10.1016/j.jns.2006.06.013 PMID:16859711

Buykx, P., Cooper, S., Kinsman, L., Endacott, R., Scholes, J., McConnell-Henry, T., & Cant, R. (2012). Patient deterioration simulation experiences: Impact on teaching and learning. *Collegian (Royal College of Nursing, Australia), 19*(3), 125–129. doi:10.1016/j.colegn.2012.03.011 PMID:23101346

Cahn, P. S. (2014). In and out of the curriculum: An historical case study in implementing interprofessional education. *Journal of Interprofessional Care*, *28*(2), 128–133. doi:10.3109/13561820.2013.872607 PMID:24383409

CAHSPR. (2016). *History of the Ted Freedman Award for Innovation in Education*. Retrieved May 10, 2016, from http://www.longwoods.com/pages/ted-freedman-award-history

Cain, J., & Fox, B. I. (2009). Web 2.0 and pharmacy education. *American Journal of Pharmaceutical Education*, *73*(7), 120. doi:10.5688/aj7307120 PMID:19960079

Cameron, A., Rennie, S., DiProspero, L., Langlois, S., Wagner, S., Potvin, M., & Reeves, S. et al. (2009). An introduction to teamwork findings from an evaluation of an interprofessional education experience for 1,000 first-year health science students. *Journal of Allied Health*, *38*(4), 220–226. PMID:20011821

Cannon-Bowers, J. A. (2008). Recent advances in scenario-based training for medical education. *Current Opinion in Anaesthesiology*, *21*(6), 784–789. doi:10.1097/ACO.0b013e3283184435 PMID:18997530

Cannon-Bowers, J. A., Burns, J. J., Salas, E., & Pruitt, J. S. (1998). Advanced technology in decision-making training. In J. A. Cannon-Bowers & E. Salas (Eds.), *Making decisions under stress: Implications for individual and team training* (pp. 365–374). Washington, DC: APA Press. doi:10.1037/10278-014

Cantú-Delgado, H. (2006). *Desarrollo de una Cultura de Calidad* (3rd ed.). Mexico: Mc Graw-Hill.

Carlisle, C., Cooper, H., & Watkins, C. (2004). Do none of you talk to each other?: The challenges facing the implementation of interprofessional education. *Medical Teacher*, *26*(6), 545–552. doi:10.1080/61421590410001711616 PMID:15763834

Carpenter-Aeby, T., & Aeby, V. G. (2013). Application of andragogy to instruction in an MSW practice class. *Journal of Instructional Psychology*, *40*(1-4), 3–13.

Carraccio, C. L., & Englander, R. (2013). From Flexner to competencies: Reflections on a decade and the journey ahead. *Academic Medicine*, *88*(8), 1067–1073. doi:10.1097/ACM.0b013e318299396f PMID:23807096

Carraccio, C., Englander, R., Van Melle, E., Ten Cate, O., Lockyer, J., Chan, M. K., & Snell, L. S et al.. (2016). Advancing competency-based medical education: A charter for clinician-educators. *Academic Medicine*, *91*(5), 645–649. doi:10.1097/ACM.0000000000001048 PMID:26675189

Carraccio, C., Wolfsthal, S. D., Englander, R., Ferentz, K., & Martin, C. (2002). Shifting paradigms: From Flexner to competencies. *Academic Medicine*, *77*(5), 361–367. doi:10.1097/00001888-200205000-00003 PMID:12010689

Carroll, J. B. (1989). The Carroll Model: A 25-Year retrospective and prospective view. *Educational Researcher*, *18*(1), 26–31. doi:10.3102/0013189X018001026

Carroll, M. W. (2013). Creative Commons and the Openness of Open Access. *The New England Journal of Medicine*, *368*(9), 789–791. doi:10.1056/NEJMp1300040 PMID:23445090

Case History: Case B. (n.d.). Retrieved from: http://learn.chm.msu.edu/neuropath/content/neuropath_cases/neuropathology_cases/CaseB.html

Causer, J., Barach, P., & Williams, A. M. (2014). Expertise in medicine: Using the expert performance approach to improve simulation training. *Medical Education*, *48*(2), 115–123. doi:10.1111/medu.12306 PMID:24528394

Cendan, J., & Lok, B. (2012). The use of virtual patients in medical school curricula. *Advances in Physiology Education*, *36*(1), 48–53. doi:10.1152/advan.00054.2011 PMID:22383412

Center for Workforce Development. (1998). *The teaching firm: Where productive work and learning converge. Report on research findings and implications*. Newton, MA: Education Development Center, Inc.

Chen, F., Delnat, C. C., & Gardner, D. (2015). The current state of academic centers for Interprofessional Education. *Journal of Interprofessional Care*, *29*(5), 497–498. doi:10.3109/13561820.2014.1002908 PMID:25586071

Chen, H. C., McNamara, M., Teherani, A., Cate, O. T., & OSullivan, P. (2016). Developing entrustable professional activities for entry into clerkship. *Academic Medicine*, *91*(2), 247–255. doi:10.1097/ACM.0000000000000988 PMID:26556295

Chen, H. C., van den Broek, W. E., & ten Cate, O. (2015). The case for use of entrustable professional activities in undergraduate medical education. *Academic Medicine*, *90*(4), 431–436. doi:10.1097/ACM.0000000000000586 PMID:25470310

Cherry, E., & Fenton, F. (2007). *The virtual heart.* Retrieved from http://thevirtualheart.org

Cherry, R. A., Williams, J., George, J., & Ali, J. (2007). The effectiveness of a human patient simulator in the ATLS shock skills station. *The Journal of Surgical Research*, *139*(2), 229–235. doi:10.1016/j.jss.2006.08.010 PMID:17161432

Cheston, C. C., Flickinger, T. E., & Chisolm, M. S. (2013). Social media use in medical education: A systematic review. *Academic Medicine*, *88*(6), 893–901. doi:10.1097/ACM.0b013e31828ffc23 PMID:23619071

Chiong, R., & Jovanovic, J. (2012). Collaborative Learning in Online Study Groups: An Evolutionary Game Theory Perspective. *Journal of Information Technology Education: Research*, *11*, 81–101.

Clapper, T. C. (2011). Interference in learning: What curriculum developers need to know. *Clinical Simulation in Nursing*, *7*(3), e77–e80. doi:10.1016/j.ecns.2010.08.001

Clark, R. C. (2008). *Building expertise: Cognitive methods for training and performance improvement.* San Francisco, CA: John Wiley & Sons.

Clark, R. C., & Mayer, R. E. (2011). *E-learning and the science of instruction: Proven guidelines for consumers and designers of multimedia learning.* San Francisco, CA: John Wiley & Sons. doi:10.1002/9781118255971

Cohen, G. L., & Sherif, Y. A. (2014). Twelve tips on teaching and learning humanism in medical education. *Medical Teacher*, *36*(8), 680–684. doi:10.3109/0142159X.2014.916779 PMID:24965585

Collins, A., Brown, J. S., & Holum, A. (1991). Cognitive apprenticeship: Making thinking visible. *American Educator*, *15*(3), 6–17.

Colwill, J. M., Cultice, J. M., & Kruse, R. L. (2008). Will generalist physician supply meet demands of an increasing and aging population?. *Health Affairs (Project Hope)*, *27*(3), w232–w241. doi:10.1377/hlthaff.27.3.w232 PMID:18445642

Colyer, H. (2008). Embedding interprofessional learning in pre-registration education in health and social care: Evidence of cultural lag. *Learning in Health and Social Care*, *7*(3), 126–133. doi:10.1111/j.1473-6861.2008.00185.x

Committee on the Roles of Academic Health Centers in the 21st Century, & Kohn, L. (2003). *Academic health centers: Leading change in the 21st century.* Washington, DC: The National Academies Press.

Conejo, P. E. (2010). *Faculty and student perceptions of preparation for and implementation of high fidelity simulation experiences in associate degree nursing programs* (Ph.D. Dissertation). Available from ProQuest Dissertations & Theses Full Text. (305210649). Retrieved from http://search.proquest.com.lp.hscl.ufl.edu/docview/305210649?accountid=10920

Conigliaro, R., & Stratton, T. (2010). The quality of clinical teaching. *The Clinical Teacher*, *7*(1), 143–146. PMID:20444073

Consorti, F., Mancuso, R., Nocioni, M., & Piccolo, A. (2012). Efficacy of virtual patients in medical education: A meta-analysis of randomized studies. *Computers & Education*, *59*(3), 1001–1008. doi:10.1016/j.compedu.2012.04.017

Cook, D. A. (2012). Revisiting cognitive and learning styles in computer-assisted instruction: Not so useful after all. *Academic Medicine*, *87*(6), 778–784. doi:10.1097/ACM.0b013e3182541286 PMID:22534603

Cook, D. A., Brydges, R., Hamstra, S. J., Zendejas, B., Szostek, J. H., Wang, A. T., & Hatala, R. et al. (2012). Comparative effectiveness of technology-enhanced simulation versus other instructional methods. *Simulation in Healthcare*, *7*(5), 308–320. doi:10.1097/SIH.0b013e3182614f95 PMID:23032751

Cook, D. A., Erwin, P. J., & Triola, M. M. (2010). Computerized virtual patients in health professions education: A systematic review and meta-analysis. *Academic Medicine*, *85*(10), 1589–1602. doi:10.1097/ACM.0b013e3181edfe13 PMID:20703150

Cook, D. A., Levinson, A. J., Garside, S., Dupras, D. M., Erwin, P. J., & Montori, V. M. (2008). Internet-based learning in the health professions: A meta-analysis. *Journal of the American Medical Association*, *300*(10), 1181–1196. doi:10.1001/jama.300.10.1181 PMID:18780847

Cook, D. A., & Triola, M. M. (2009). Virtual patients: A critical literature review and proposed next steps. *Medical Education*, *43*(4), 303–311. doi:10.1111/j.1365-2923.2008.03286.x PMID:19335571

Cooke, M., Irby, D. M., Sullivan, W., & Ludmerer, K. M. (2006). American medical education 100 years after the Flexner report. *The New England Journal of Medicine, 355*(13), 1339-1344. doi:355/13/1339

Cooper, J. B., & Taqueti, V. R. (2004). A brief history of the development of mannequin simulators for clinical education and training. *Quality & Safety in Health Care, 13*(Suppl 1), i11-i18. doi:13/suppl_1/i11

Cormack, R. S., & Lehane, J. (1984). Difficult tracheal intubation in obstetrics. *Anaesthesia*, *39*(11), 1105–1111. doi:10.1111/j.1365-2044.1984.tb08932.x PMID:6507827

Council on Social Work Education. (2016). *Accreditation: Online and distance education.* Retrieved October 26, 2016, from http://www.cswe.org/Accreditation/Information/OnlineandDistanceEducation.aspx

Covey, S. R. (1989). *The seven habits of highly effective people: Restoring the character ethic.* New York, NY: Fireside Books – Simon & Schuster.

Cox, M., Irby, D., & Epstein, R. M. (2007). Assessment in Medical Education. *The New England Journal of Medicine*, *356*(4), 387–396. doi:10.1056/NEJMra054784 PMID:17251535

Creswell, J. W., & Plano, C. (2010). *Designing and Conducting Mixed Methods Research.* Lincoln, NE: SAGE.

Cumin, D., & Merry, A. F. (2007). Simulators for use in anaesthesia. *Anaesthesia*, *62*(2), 151–162. doi:10.1111/j.1365-2044.2006.04902.x PMID:17223808

Cutrer, W. B., Castro, D., Roy, K. M., & Turner, T. L. (2011). Use of an expert concept map as an advance organizer to improve understanding of respiratory failure. *Medical Teacher*, *33*(12), 1018–1026. doi:10.3109/0142159X.2010.531159 PMID:22225439

Dabbagh, N., & Bannan-Ritland, B. (2005). *Online Learning: Concepts, Strategies, and Application.* Upper Saddle River, NJ: Pearson Education, Inc.

Dahle, L. O., Brynhildsen, J., Behrbohm Fallsberg, M., Rundquist, I., & Hammar, M. (2002). Pros and cons of vertical integration between clinical medicine and basic science within a problem-based undergraduate medical curriculum: Examples and experiences from Linkoping, Sweden. *Medical Teacher*, *24*(3), 280–285. doi:10.1080/01421590220134097 PMID:12098414

Daly, C. J., Bullock, J. M., Ma, M., & Aidulis, D. (2016). A comparison of animated versus static images in an instructional multimedia presentation. *Advances in Physiology Education*, *40*(2), 201–205. doi:10.1152/advan.00053.2015 PMID:27105738

Dankbaar, M. E. W., Alsma, J., Jansen, E. E. H., van Merrienboer, J. J. G., van Saase, J. L. C. M., & Schuit, S. C. E. (2015). An experimental study on the effects of a simulation game on students' clinical cognitive skills and motivation. *Advances in Health Sciences Education: Theory and Practice*, 1–17. doi:10.1007/s10459-015-9641-x PMID:26433730

Datta, C. (2012). The rise of E-learning and opportunities for Indian family physicians. *Journal of Family Medicine and Primary Care*, *1*(1), 7–9. doi:10.4103/2249-4863.94441 PMID:24478993

Davidson-Shivers, G. V. (2015). Universal design. In J. M. Spector (Ed.), *The SAGE encyclopedia of educational technology* (pp. 799–802). Thousand Oaks, CA: Sage Publication.

Davidson-Shivers, G. V., & Rasmussen, K. L. (2006). *Web-based learning: Design, implementation, and evaluation*. Upper Saddle River, NJ: Prentice Hall.

Davis, B. P., Clevenger, C. K., Posnock, S., Robertson, B. D., & Ander, D. S. (2015). Teaching the teachers: Faculty development in inter-professional education. *Applied Nursing Research*, *28*(1), 31–35. doi:10.1016/j.apnr.2014.03.003 PMID:24852452

Davis, D. A., Thomson, M. A., Oxman, A. D., & Haynes, R. B. (1995). Changing physician performance. A systematic review of the effect of continuing medical education strategies. *Journal of the American Medical Association*, *274*(9), 700–705. doi:10.1001/jama.1995.03530090032018 PMID:7650822

Davis, D., O'Brien, M. A., Freemantle, N., Wolf, F. M., Mazmanian, P., & Taylor-Vaisey, A. (1999). Impact of formal continuing medical education: Do conferences, workshops, rounds, and other traditional continuing education activities change physician behavior or health care outcomes? *Journal of the American Medical Association*, *282*(9), 867–874. doi:10.1001/jama.282.9.867 PMID:10478694

Davis, R., & Surajballi, V. (2014). Successful implementation and use of a learning management system. *Journal of Continuing Education in Nursing*, *45*(9), 379–381. doi:10.3928/00220124-20140825-12 PMID:25198116

de Divitiis, E., Cappabianca, P., & de Divitiis, O. (2004). The schola medica salernitana: The forerunner of the modern university medical schools. *Neurosurgery*, *55*(4), 722–745. doi:10.1227/01.NEU.0000139458.36781.31 PMID:15458581

de Gregorio, C., Arias, A., Navarrete, N., Cisneros, R., & Cohenca, N. (2015). Differences in disinfection protocols for root canal treatments between general dentists and endodontists: A Web-based survey. *The Journal of the American Dental Association*, *146*(7), 536–543. doi:10.1016/j.adaj.2015.01.027 PMID:26113101

de Hrussoczy-Wirth, D. (2010). *Simulation in undergraduate nursing education curriculum: An integrated review of the literature (Unpublished Master of Nursing)*. University of Victoria.

De La Harpe, B., & Radloff, A. (2000). Informed teachers and learners: The importance of assessing the characteristics needed for lifelong learning. *Studies in Continuing Education*, *22*(2), 169–182. doi:10.1080/713695729

deCharms, R. (1977). Students need not be pawns. *Theory into Practice*, *16*(4), 296–301. doi:10.1080/00405847709542716

Deladisma, A. M., Cohen, M., Stevens, A., Wagner, P., Lok, B., Bernard, T., & Dickerson, R. et al. (2007). Do medical students respond empathetically to a virtual patient? *American Journal of Surgery*, *193*(6), 756–760.

Dembo, M. H., & Howard, K. (2007). Advice about the use of learning styles: A major myth in education. *Journal of College Reading and Learning*, *37*(2), 101–109. doi:10.1080/10790195.2007.10850200

Dent, J., & Harden, R. M. (2013). *A practical guide for medical teachers*. London: Elsevier Health Sciences.

Denton, J. J., Armstrong, D. G., & Savage, T. V. (1980). Matching events of instruction to objectives. *Theory into Practice*, *19*(1), 10–14. doi:10.1080/00405848009542866

Dick, W., Carey, L., & Carey, J. (2009) The Systemic Design of Instruction (8th ed.). Boston, MA: Pearson e-text.

Dick, W., Carey, L., & Carey, J. O. (2015). *The systematic design of instruction* (8th ed.). Boston, MA: Pearson.

Dick, W., Carey, L., & Carey, J. O. (2015). *The Systematic Design of Instruction*. Upper Saddle River, NJ: Pearson.

Doherty-Restrepo, J. L., & Tivener, K. (2014). Current literature summary: Review of high-fidelity simulation in professional education. *Athletic Training Education Journal*, *9*(4), 190–192. doi:10.4085/0904190

Dolmans, D. H., Snellen-Balendong, H., & van der Vleuten, C. P. (1997). Seven principles of effective case design for a problem-based curriculum. *Medical Teacher*, *19*(3), 185–189. doi:10.3109/01421599709019379

Doukas, D. J., McCullough, L. B., & Wear, S. (2012). Medical Education in Medical Ethics and Humanities as the Foundation for Developing Medical Professionalism. *Academic Medicine*, *87*(3), 334–341. doi:10.1097/ACM.0b013e318244728c PMID:22373629

Downing, J., & Herrington, J. (2013, December). *Applied learning in online spaces: Traditional pedagogies informing educational design for today's learners.* Paper presented at the 30th Ascilite Conference, Sydney, Australia.

Drake, S. M. (2007). *Creating standards-based integrated curriculum: Aligning curriculum, content, assessment, and instruction*. Thousand Oaks, CA: Corwin Press, a SAGE Publications Company.

Dressel, P. L. (1958). The meaning and significance of integration. In N. B. Henry (Ed.), *The Integration of Educational Experiences* (pp. 3–25). Chicago, IL: University of Chicago Press.

Dreyfus, S. E. (2004). The five-stage model of adult skill acquisition. *Bulletin of Science, Technology & Society*, *24*(3), 177–181. doi:10.1177/0270467604264992

Driscoll, M. P. (2005). *Psychology of learning for instruction* (3rd ed.). Boston, MA: Allyn & Bacon.

Duffy, T. M., & Cunningham, D. J. (1996). Constructivism: Implications for the design and delivery of instruction. In D. J. Jonassen (Ed.), *Handbook of research for educational communication and technology* (pp. 170–198). New York, NY: McMillan.

Duque, G., Demontiero, O., Whereat, S., Gunawardene, P., Leung, O., Webster, P., & Sharma, A. (2013). Evaluation of a blended learning model in geriatric medicine: A successful learning experience for medical students. *Australasian Journal on Ageing*, *32*(2), 103–109. doi:10.1111/j.1741-6612.2012.00620.x PMID:23773249

Durham, C. F., & Alden, K. R. (2008). Enhancing patient safety in nursing education through patient simulation. In R. G. Hughes (Ed.), *Patient safety and quality: An evidence-based handbook for nurses* (pp. 221–260). Rockville, MD: Agency for Healthcare Research and Quality.

Dutile, C., Wright, N., & Beauchesne, M. (2011). Virtual clinical education: Going the full distance in nursing education. *Newborn and Infant Nursing Reviews; NAINR*, *11*(1), 43–48. doi:10.1053/j.nainr.2010.12.008

Duvivier, R., Van Dalen, J., Vleuten, V., & Scherpbier, A. (2009). Teacher perceptions of desired qualities, competencies and strategies for clinical skill teachers. *Teaching Skills for Clinical Skills Teacher, 31*(1), 634-641.

Dyer, J.-O., Hudon, A., Montpetit-Tourangeau, K., Charlin, B., Mamede, S., & van Gog, T. (2015). Example-based learning: Comparing the effects of additionally providing three different integrative learning activities on physiotherapy intervention knowledge. *BMC Medical Education*, *15*(1), 1–16. doi:10.1186/s12909-015-0308-3 PMID:25889066

Dyrbye, L. N., Starr, S. R., Thompson, G. B., & Lindor, K. D. (2011). A model for integration of formal knowledge and clinical experience: The advanced doctoring course at Mayo Medical School. *Academic Medicine*, *86*(9), 1130–1136. doi:10.1097/ACM.0b013e31822519d4 PMID:21785316

Eardley, I., Bussey, M., Woodthorpe, A., Munsch, C., & Beard, J. (2013). Workplace-based assessment in surgical training: Experiences from the intercollegiate surgical curriculum programme. *The Australian and New Zealand Journal of Surgery*, *83*(6), 448–453. doi:10.1111/ans.12187 PMID:23656354

Edwards, J. C., Kissling, G. E., Brannan, J. R., Plauche, W. C., & Marier, R. L. (1988). Study of teaching residents how to teach. *Academic Medicine*, *63*(8), 603–610. doi:10.1097/00001888-198808000-00003 PMID:3398015

Egerton, E. O., McConnell, E. S., Corazzini, K., Kitzmiller, R. R., & Crook, J. O. (2010). Birds of a Feather: Introducing a Virtual Learning Community for Geriatric Nurse Educators. *Journal of Continuing Education in Nursing*, *41*(5), 203–209. PMID:20481420

Ende, J. (1983). Feedback in clinical medical education. *Journal of the American Medical Association*, *250*(6), 777–781. doi:10.1001/jama.1983.03340060055026 PMID:6876333

Englander, R., Cameron, T., Ballard, A. J., Dodge, J., Bull, J., & Aschenbrener, C. A. (2013). Toward a common taxonomy of competency domains for the health professions and competencies for physicians. *Academic Medicine*, *88*(8), 1088–1094. doi:10.1097/ACM.0b013e31829a3b2b PMID:23807109

Englander, R., & Carraccio, C. (2014). From theory to practice: Making entrustable professional activities come to life in the context of milestones. *Academic Medicine*, *89*(10), 1321–1323. doi:10.1097/ACM.0000000000000324 PMID:24892405

Englander, R., Flynn, T., Call, S., Carraccio, C., Cleary, L., Fulton, T. B., & Aschenbrener, C. A. et al. (2016). Toward defining the foundation of the MD degree: Core entrustable professional activities for entering residency. *Academic Medicine*, *91*(10), 1352–1358; Advance online publication. doi:10.1097/ACM.0000000000001204 PMID:27097053

Ennis, R. H. (1992). John McPeck's Teaching Critical Thinking. *Educational Studies*, *23*(4), 462–472.

Eraut, M. (2000). Non-formal learning and tacit knowledge in professional work. *The British Journal of Educational Psychology*, *70*(Pt 1), 113–136. doi:10.1348/000709900158001 PMID:10765570

Eraut, M. (2004). Informal learning in the workplace. *Studies in Continuing Education*, *26*(2), 247–273. doi:10.1080/158037042000225245

Ertmer, P. A., & Newby, T. J. (1993). Behaviorism, cognitivism, constructivism: Comparing critical features from an instructional design perspective. *Performance Improvement Quarterly*, *6*(4), 50–72. doi:10.1111/j.1937-8327.1993.tb00605.x

Evans, J., & Lindsay, W. L. (2014). *Administración y Control de la Calidad* (7th ed.). Mexico: Cengage Learning.

Facione, P. (1990). *The APA Delphi Report, Critical Thinking: A Statement of Expert Consensus for Purposes of Educational Assessment and Instruction 1*. The California Academic Press.

Fanning, R. M., & Gaba, D. M. (2007). The role of debriefing in simulation-based learning. *Simulation in Healthcare*, *2*(2), 115–125. doi:10.1097/SIH.0b013e3180315539 PMID:19088616

Farnsworth, T. J., Peterson, T., Neill, K., Neill, M., & Lawson, J. (2015). Understanding the Structural, Human Resourcc, Political, and Symbolic Dimensions of Implementing and Sustaining Interprofessional Education. *Journal of Allied Health*, *44*(3), 152–157. PMID:26342612

Feingold, C. E., Calaluce, M., & Kallen, M. A. (2004). Computerized patient model and simulated clinical experience: Evaluation with baccalaureate nursing students. *The Journal of Nursing Education*, *43*(4), 156–163. PMID:15098909

Feltovich, P. J., Spiro, R. J., Coulson, R. L., & Feltovich, J. (1996). Collaboration within and among minds: Mastering complexity, individually, and in groups. In T. Koschmann (Ed.), *CSCL: Theory and practice of an emerging paradigm* (pp. 25–44). Mahwah, NJ: Erlbaum.

Ferguson, C., Inglis, S. C., Newton, P. J., Middleton, S., Macdonald, P. S., & Davidson, P. M. (2016). Education and practice gaps on atrial fibrillation and anticoagulation: A survey of cardiovascular nurses. *BMC Medical Education*, *16*(1), 1–10. doi:10.1186/s12909-015-0504-1 PMID:26758627

Fieschi, M., Soula, G., Giorgi, R., Gouvernet, J., Fieschi, D., Botti, G., & Berland, Y. (2002). Experimenting with new paradigms for medical education and the emergence of a distance learning degree using the internet: Teaching evidence-based medicine. *Medical Informatics and the Internet in Medicine*, *27*(1), 1–11. doi:10.1080/14639230110105301 PMID:12509118

Filichia, L., Halan, S., Blackwelder, E., Rossen, B., Lok, B., Korndorffer, J., & Cendan, J. (2011). Description of web-enhanced virtual character simulation system to standardize patient hand-offs. *The Journal of Surgical Research*, *166*(2), 176–181. doi:10.1016/j.jss.2010.04.052 PMID:20828726

Finn, K., Chiappa, V., Puig, A., & Hunt, D. (2011). How to become a better clinical teacher: A collaborative peer observation process. *Medical Teacher*, *33*(1), 151–155. doi:10.3109/0142159X.2010.541534 PMID:21275544

Flexner, A. (1910). *Medical education in the United States and Canada*. Retrieved from http://archive.carnegiefoundation.org/publications/medical-education-united-states-and-canada-bulletin-number-four-flexner-report-0

Flexner, A. (1910). *Medical Education in United States and Canada*. The Carnegie Foundation for the Advancement of Teaching. Retrieved from http://archive.carnegiefoundation.org/pdfs/elibrary/Carnegie_Flexner_Report.pdf

Fook, J., dAvray, L., Norrie, C., Psoinos, M., Lamb, B., & Ross, F. (2013). Taking the long view: Exploring the development of interprofessional education. *Journal of Interprofessional Care*, *27*(4), 286–291. doi:10.3109/13561820.2012.759911 PMID:23659644

Forsberg, E., Georg, C., Ziegert, K., & Fors, U. (2011). Virtual patients for assessment of clinical reasoning in nursing: A pilot study. *Nurse Education Today*, *31*(8), 757–762. doi:10.1016/j.nedt.2010.11.015 PMID:21159412

Foster, A., Chaudhary, N., Murphy, J., Lok, B., Waller, J., & Buckley, P. F. (2014). The use of simulation to teach suicide risk assessment to health profession Trainees—Rationale, methodology, and a proof of concept demonstration with a virtual patient. *Academic Psychiatry*, 1–10. PMID:25026950

Fox, R. D., & Bennett, N. L. (1998). Continuing medical education: Learning and change: Implications for continuing medical education. *British Medical JournalJ*, *316*(7129), 466–468. doi:10.1136/bmj.316.7129.466 PMID:9492684

Frank, J. R., & Danoff, D. (2007). The CanMEDS initiative: Implementing an outcomes-based framework of physician competencies. *Medical Teacher*, *29*(7), 642–647. doi:10.1080/01421590701746983 PMID:18236250

Frank, J. R., Mungroo, R., Ahmad, Y., Wang, M., De Rossi, S., & Horsley, T. (2010a). Toward a definition of competency-based education in medicine: A systematic review of published definitions. *Medical Teacher*, *32*(8), 631–637. doi:10.3109/0142159X.2010.500898 PMID:20662573

Frank, J. R., Snell, L. S., Cate, O. T., Holmboe, E. S., Carraccio, C., Swing, S. R., & Harris, K. A. et al. (2010b). Competency-based medical education: Theory to practice. *Medical Teacher*, *32*(8), 638–645. doi:10.3109/0142159X.2010.501190 PMID:20662574

Freeth, D., Hammick, M., Reeves, S., Koppel, I., & Barr, H. (2008). *Effective interprofessional education: development, delivery, and evaluation*. Oxford, UK: Wiley-Blackwell.

Friedlander, M. J., Andrews, L., Armstrong, E. G., Aschenbrenner, C., Kass, J. S., Ogden, P., & Viggiano, T. R. et al. (2011). What can medical education learn from the neurobiology of learning? *Academic Medicine*, *86*(4), 415–420. doi:10.1097/ACM.0b013e31820dc197 PMID:21346504

Furney, S. L., Orsini, A. N., Orsetti, K. E., Stern, D. T., Gruppen, L. D., & Irby, D. M. (2001). Teaching the one-minute preceptor. *Journal of General Internal Medicine*, *16*(9), 620–624. doi:10.1046/j.1525-1497.2001.016009620.x PMID:11556943

Gaba, D. M. (2004). The future vision of simulation in health care. *Quality & Safety in Health Care*, *13*(suppl_1), i2–i10. doi:10.1136/qshc.2004.009878 PMID:15465951

Gagne, R. M. (1985). *The conditions of learning and theory of instruction*. New York, NY: Holt, Rinehart and Winston.

Gagné, R. M., Wager, W. W., Golas, K., & Keller, J. M. (2005). *Principles of Instructional Design* (5th ed.). Boston, MA: Cengage Learning.

Gardner, H. (1999). *Intelligence reframed: Multiple intelligences for the 21st century*. New York: Basic Books.

Gardner, S. F., Chamberlin, G. D., Heestand, D. E., & Stowe, C. D. (2002). Interdisciplinary didactic instruction at Academic Health Centers in the United States: Attitudes and barriers. *Advances in Health Sciences Education: Theory and Practice*, *7*(3), 179–190. doi:10.1023/A:1021144215376 PMID:12510140

Ge, X., Huang, D., Zhang, H., & Bowers, B. (2013). Three-dimension design for mobile learning: Pedagogical, design, and technological considerations and implications. In Z. L. Berge & L. Y. Muilenburg (Eds.), *Handbook of mobile learning* (pp. 329–345). New York, NY: Routledge.

Gigante, J., Dell, M., & Sharkey, A. (2010). Beyond good job: How to give effective feedback. *Pediatrics*, *127*(2), 205–207. doi:10.1542/peds.2010-3351 PMID:21242222

Gilbert, J. H. (2005). Interprofessional learning and higher education structural barriers. *Journal of Interprofessional Care, 19*(sup1), 87-106.

Gilbert, J. H. V. (2005). Interprofessional learning and higher education structural barriers. *Journal of Interprofessional Care*, *19*(sup1), 87–106. doi:10.1080/13561820500067132 PMID:16096148

Gilbert, J. H., Yan, J., & Hoffman, S. J. (2010). A WHO report: Framework for action on interprofessional education and collaborative practice. *Journal of Allied Health*, *39*(Supplement 1), 196–197. PMID:21174039

Gilbert, S. D. (2001). *How to be a successful online student*. New York, NY: McGraw-Hill.

Gilligan, C., Outram, S., & Levett-Jones, T. (2014). Recommendations from recent graduates in medicine, nursing, and pharmacy on improving interprofessional education in university programs: A qualitative study. *BMC Medical Education*, *14*(1), 52–62. doi:10.1186/1472-6920-14-52 PMID:24636554

Goldman, E., & Schroth, W. S. (2012). Perspective: Deconstructing integration: A framework for the rational application of integration as a guiding curricular strategy. *Academic Medicine*, *87*(6), 729–734. doi:10.1097/ACM.0b013e318253cad4 PMID:22534596

Good, M. L. (2003). Patient simulation for training basic and advanced clinical skills. *Medical Education*, *37*(s1), 14–21. doi:10.1046/j.1365-2923.37.s1.6.x PMID:14641634

Gordon, J. A., Wilkerson, W. M., Shaffer, D. W., & Armstrong, E. G. (2001). Practicing medicine without risk: Students and educators response to high-fidelity patient simulation. *Academic Medicine*, *76*(5), 469–472. doi:10.1097/00001888-200105000-00019 PMID:11346525

Grabowski, B. L. (2004). Generative learning contributions to the design of instruction and learning. In D. H. Jonassen (Ed.), *Handbook of Research on Educational Communications and Technology* (2nd ed.; pp. 719–743). Lawrence Earlbaum.

Green, E. H. (2006). *SOAPS to SAFER: A model for teaching and evaluating oral case presentations.* Retrieved April 24, 2016, from https://www.med.unc.edu/aging/fellowship/current/presentations/giving-feedback-on-oral-presentations/making-soaps-safer

Green, M. L. (2000). Evidence-based medicine training in internal medicine residency programs: A national survey. *Journal of General Internal Medicine*, *15*(2), 129–133. doi:10.1046/j.1525-1497.2000.03119.x PMID:10672117

Greiner, A., & Knebel, E. (2003). *Committee on the Health Professions Education Summit. Health Professions Education: A Bridge to Quality*. The National Academic Press.

Griffin-Sobel, J. P. (2009). The ENTREE model for integrating technologically rich learning strategies in a school of nursing. *Clinical Simulation in Nursing*, *5*(2), e73–e78. doi:10.1016/j.ecns.2009.01.008

Griffin-Sobel, J. P., Acee, A., Sharoff, L., Cobus-Kuo, L., Woodstock-Wallace, A., & Dornbaum, M. (2010). A transdisciplinary approach to faculty development in nursing education technology. *Nursing Education Perspectives*, *31*(1), 41–43. doi:10.1043/1536-5026-31.1.41 PMID:20397480

Gruppen, L. D., & Stansfield, R. B. (in press). *Personal and institutional components of the medical school education environment*. Academic Press.

Gruppen, L., Rytting, M., & Marti, K. (in press). *The educational environment.* Academic Press.

Grymonpre, R., van Ineveld, C., Nelson, M., Jensen, F., De Jaeger, A., Sullivan, T., & Booth, A. et al. (2010). See it – do it – learn it: Learning interprofessional collaboration in the clinical context. *Journal of Research in Interprofessional Practice and Education*, *1*(2), 127–144.

Guerrasio, J., Brooks, E., Rumack, C. M., Christensen, A., & Aagaard, E. M. (2016). Association of characteristics, deficits, and outcomes of residents placed on probation at one institution, 20022012. *Academic Medicine*, *91*(3), 382–387. doi:10.1097/ACM.0000000000000879 PMID:26352762

Guimond, M. E., Sole, M. L., & Salas, E. (2011). Getting ready for simulation-based training: A checklist for nurse educators. *Nursing Education Perspectives*, *32*(3), 179–185. doi:10.5480/1536-5026-32.3.179 PMID:21834380

Guise, V., Chambers, M., Conradi, E., Kavia, S., & Välimäki, M. (2012). Development, implementation and initial evaluation of narrative virtual patients for use in vocational mental health nurse training. *Nurse Education Today*, *32*(6), 683–689. doi:10.1016/j.nedt.2011.09.004 PMID:22056146

Hafferty, F. W. (1998). Beyond curriculum reform: Confronting medicine's hidden curriculum. *Academic Medicine*, *73*(4), 403–407. doi:10.1097/00001888-199804000-00013 PMID:9580717

Halic, O., Lee, D., Paulus, T., & Spence, M. (2010). To blog or not to blog: Student perceptions of blog effectiveness for learning in a college-level course. *The Internet and Higher Education*, *13*(4), 206–213. doi:10.1016/j.iheduc.2010.04.001

Hall, L. W., & Zierler, B. K. (2015). Interprofessional Education and Practice Guide No. 1; Developing faculty to effectively facilitate interprofessional education. *Journal of Interprofessional Care*, *29*(1), 3–7. doi:10.3109/13561820.2014.937483 PMID:25019466

Hall, W. A. (2006). Developing clinical placements in times of scarcity. *Nurse Education in Practice*, *6*(6), 319–325. doi:10.1016/j.nepr.2006.07.005 PMID:19040897

Hammick, M., Freeth, D., Koppel, I., Reeves, S., & Barr, H. (2007). A best evidence systematic review of interprofessional education: BEME Guide no. 9. *Medical Teacher*, *29*(8), 735–751. doi:10.1080/01421590701682576 PMID:18236271

Hannafin, M. J., Hannafin, K. M., Land, S. M., & Oliver, K. (1997). Grounded practice and the design of constructivist learning environments. *Educational Technology Research and Development*, *45*(3), 101–117.

Hannafin, M. J., Land, S., & Oliver, K. (1999). Open learning environments: Foundations and models. In C. Reigeluth (Ed.), *Instructional design theories and models: A new paradigm of instructional theory* (pp. 115–140). Mahwah, NJ: Erlbaum.

Harden, R. M. (2000). The integration ladder: A tool for curriculum planning and evaluation. *Medical Education, 34*(7), 551-557. doi:med697

Harden, R. M. (1999). AMEE guide no. 14: Outcome-based education: Part 1-an introduction to outcome-based education. *Medical Teacher*, *21*(1), 7–14. doi:10.1080/01421599979969

Harden, R. M., Davis, M. H., & Crosby, J. R. (1997). The new Dundee medical curriculum: A whole that is greater than the sum of the parts. *Medical Education*, *31*(4), 264–271. doi:10.1111/j.1365-2923.1997.tb02923.x PMID:9488841

Harden, R. M., & Gleeson, F. A. (1979). Assessment of clinical competence using an objective structured clinical examination (OSCE). *Medical Education*, *13*(1), 39–54. doi:10.1111/j.1365-2923.1979.tb00918.x PMID:763183

Harder, B. N. (2009). Evolution of simulation use in health care education. *Clinical Simulation in Nursing*, *5*(5), e169–e172. doi:10.1016/j.ecns.2009.04.092

Harris, D. L., Krause, K., Parish, D., & Smith, M. (2007). Academic Competencies for Medical Faculty. *Family Medicine*, *39*(5), 343–350. PMID:17476608

Harris, J. M., Kutob, R. M., Surprenant, Z. J., Maiuro, R. D., & Delate, T. A. (2002). Can internet-based education improve physician confidence in dealing with domestic violence? *Family Medicine*, *34*(4), 287–292. PMID:12017143

Hattie, J., & Timperley, H. (2007). The power of feedback. *Review of Educational Research*, *77*(1), 81–112. doi:10.3102/003465430298487

Hauer, K. E., Ten Cate, O., Boscardin, C., Irby, D. M., Iobst, W., & O'Sullivan, P. S. (2014). Understanding trust as an essential element of trainee supervision and learning in the workplace. *Advances in Health Sciences Education: Theory and Practice*, *19*(3), 435–456. doi:10.1007/s10459-013-9474-4 PMID:23892689

Hayden, J. K., Smily, R. A., Raij, A., Kardong-Edgren, S., & Jeffries, P. R. (2014). The NCSBN national simulation study: A longitudinal, randomized, controlled Study Replacing clinical hours with simulation in Prelicensure nursing education. *Journal of Nursing Regulation*, *5*(2Supplement.).

Hayes, R., & Singer, M. J. (1989). *Simulation fidelity in training system design: Bridging the gap between reality and training*. New York, NY: Springer-Verlag. doi:10.1007/978-1-4612-3564-4

Health Resources and Services Administration. (2013). *The U.S. nursing workforce: Trends in supply and education.* Rockville, MD: National Center for Health Workforce Analysis.

Hean, S., Clark, J. M., Adams, K., & Humphris, D. (2006). Will opposites attract? Similarities and differences in students perceptions of the stereotype profiles of other health and social care professional groups. *Journal of Interprofessional Care*, *20*(2), 162–181. doi:10.1080/13561820600646546 PMID:16608718

Hernández, R., Fernández, C., & Baptista, P. (2003). *Metodología de la Investigación* (3rd ed.). México: McGraw-Hill.

Herskovik, P., Miranda, T., Cortés, E., Delusshi, A., Gómez, P. A., Jiusán, A., & Puzant, M. et al. (2012). Creen haber cambiado los docentes un año después de un curso de docencia clínica. *Educación Médica*, *15*(3), 179–185.

Hii, P.-C., & Chung, W.-Y. (2011). A comprehensive ubiquitous healthcare solution on an Android™ mobile device. *Sensors (Basel, Switzerland)*, *11*(7), 6799–6815. doi:10.3390/s110706799 PMID:22163986

Hill, A. G., Yu, T. C., Barrow, M., & Hattie, J. (2009). A systematic review of resident-as-teacher programmes. *Medical Education*, *43*(12), 1129–1140. doi:10.1111/j.1365-2923.2009.03523.x PMID:19930503

Hinderer, K. A., Klima, D., Truong, H.-A., Rangel, A. G., Brown, V., Talley, W., & Joyner, R. L. Jr et al.. (2016). Faculty Perceptions, Knowledge, and Attitudes Toward Interprofessional Education and Practice. *Journal of Allied Health*, *45*(1), 1E–4E. PMID:26937886

Hind, M., Norman, I., Cooper, S., Gill, E., Hilton, R., Judd, P., & Jones, S. C. (2003). Interprofessional perceptions of health care students. *Journal of Interprofessional Care*, *17*(1), 21–34. doi:10.1080/1356182021000044120 PMID:12772467

Hmelo-Silver, C. E. (2004). Problem-based learning: What and how do students learn? *Educational Psychology Review*, *16*(3), 235–266. doi:10.1023/B:EDPR.0000034022.16470.f3

Hodgins, M. W., & Lovell, K. L. (1988). CNS Neoplasms - Interactive videodisc instructional unit. *Bulletin of Pathology Education*, *13*, 89–90.

Hojat, M., Veloski, J. J., & Gonnella, J. S. (2009). Measurement and correlates of physicians' lifelong learning. *Academic Medicine*, *84*(8), 1066–1074. doi:10.1097/ACM.0b013e3181acf25f PMID:19638773

Ho, K., Jarvis-Selinger, S., Borduas, F., Frank, B., Hall, P., Handfield-Jones, R., & Rouleau, M. et al. (2008). Making interprofessional education work: The strategic roles of the academy. *Academic Medicine*, *83*(10), 934–940. doi:10.1097/ACM.0b013e3181850a75 PMID:18820523

Holford, J., & van der Veen, R. (2003). *Lifelong learning, governance and active citizenship in Europe*. Guildford: ETGACE.

Holmboe, E. S. (2015). Realizing the promise of competency-based medical education. *Academic Medicine*, *90*(4), 411–413. doi:10.1097/ACM.0000000000000515 PMID:25295967

Holmboe, E., Ginsburg, S., & Bernabeo, E. (2011). The rotational approach to medical education: Time to confront our assumptions? *Medical Education*, *45*(1), 69–80. doi:10.1111/j.1365-2923.2010.03847.x PMID:21155870

Holtslander, L. F., Racine, L., Furniss, S., Burles, M., & Turner, H. (2012). Developing and piloting an online graduate nursing course focused on experiential learning of qualitative research methods. *The Journal of Nursing Education*, *51*(6), 345–348. doi:10.3928/01484834-20120427-03 PMID:22533499

Hommes, J., Rienties, B., de Grave, W., Bos, G., Schuwirth, L., & Scherpbier, A. (2012). Visualising the invisible: A network approach to reveal the informal social side of student learning. *Advances in Health Sciences Education: Theory and Practice*, *17*(5), 743–757. doi:10.1007/s10459-012-9349-0 PMID:22294429

Horak, B. J., OLeary, K. C., & Carlson, L. (1998). Preparing health care professionals for quality improvement: The George Washington University/George Mason University experience. *Quality Management in Health Care*, *6*(2), 21–30. doi:10.1097/00019514-199806020-00003 PMID:10178156

Horsburgh, M., Lamdin, R., & Williamson, E. (2001). Multiprofessional learning : The attitudes of medical, nursing and pharmacy students to sharnces, Health Education, Keywordsed learning. *Medical Education*, *35*(9), 876–883. doi:10.1046/j.1365-2923.2001.00959.x PMID:11555226

Howard Hughes Medical Institute. (2016). *Neurophysiology virtual lab*. Retrieved from http://www.hhmi.org/biointeractive/neurophysiology-virtual-lab

Howard, V. M., Englert, N., Kameg, K., & Perozzi, K. (2011). Integration of simulation across the undergraduate curriculum: Student and faculty perspectives. *Clinical Simulation in Nursing*, *7*(1), e1–e10. doi:10.1016/j.ecns.2009.10.004

Hoyek, N., Collet, C., Di Rienzo, F., De Almeida, M., & Guillot, A. (2014). Effectiveness of three-dimensional digital animation in teaching human anatomy in an authentic classroom context. *Anatomical Sciences Education*, *7*(6), 430–437. doi:10.1002/ase.1446 PMID:24678034

Huang, K., Ge, X., & Bowers, B. (2006). *The Virtual Clinic: Simulated ethical decision making in nursing education*. Paper presented at the annual convention of Association of Educational Communications and Technology, Dallas, TX.

Huang, G., Reynolds, R., & Candler, C. (2007). Virtual patient simulation at U.S. and canadian medical schools. *Academic Medicine*, *82*(5), 446–451. doi:10.1097/ACM.0b013e31803e8a0a PMID:17457063

Hung, W. (2006). The 3C3R model: A conceptual framework for designing problems in PBL. *The Interdisciplinary Journal of Problem-Based Learning*, *1*(1), 55–77. doi:10.7771/1541-5015.1006

Hung, W. (2009). The 9-step problem design process for problem-based learning: Application of the 3C3R model. *Educational Research Review*, *4*(2), 118–141. doi:10.1016/j.edurev.2008.12.001

Hung, W. (2013). Problem-based learning: A learning environment for enhancing learning transfer. *New Directions for Adult and Continuing Education*, *2013*(137), 27–38. doi:10.1002/ace.20042

Ibrahim, H., Stadler, D., Archuleta, S., Shah, N., Bertram, A., Nair, S., & Cofrancesco, J. (2015). Clinician-educators in emerging graduate medical education systems: Description, roles and perceptions. *Postgraduate Medical Journal*, *92*(1), 14–20. PMID:26512124

Institute of Medicine (IOM). (2015). *Measuring the impact of interprofessional education on collaborative practice and patient outcomes*. Washington, DC: The National Academies Press.

Institute of Medicine Committee on Quality of Health Care in America. (2001). *Crossing the Quality Chasm: A New Health System for the 21st Century*. Retrieved May 30, 2016, from http://www.ncbi.nlm.nih.gov/pubmed/25057539

Institute of Medicine. (2015). *Measuring the impact of Interprofessional Education (IPE) on collaborative practice and patient outcomes*. Retrieved from http://nationalacademies.org/hmd/reports/2015/impact-of-ipe.aspx#sthash.nrPQl0Ah.dpuf

Interprofessional Education Collaborative Expert Panel. (2011). *Core competencies for interprofessional collaborative practice: Report of an expert panel*. Washington, DC: Interprofessional Education Collaborative.

Interprofessional Education Collaborative Expert Panel. (2016). *Core competencies for interprofessional collaborative practice: 2016 update*. Washington, DC: Interprofessional Education Collaborative.

Irby, D. M., Aagaard, E., & Teherani, A. (2004). Teaching points identified by preceptors observing one-minute preceptor and traditional preceptor encounters. *Academic Medicine*, *79*(1), 50–55. doi:10.1097/00001888-200401000-00012 PMID:14690997

Irby, D. M., & Wilkerson, L. (2008). Teaching rounds: Teaching when time is limited. *BMJ: British Medical Journal*, *336*(7640), 384–387. doi:10.1136/bmj.39456.727199.AD PMID:18276715

Ironside, P. M., Jeffries, P. R., & Martin, A. (2009). Fostering patient safety competencies using multiple-patient simulation experiences. *Nursing Outlook*, *57*(6), 332–337. doi:10.1016/j.outlook.2009.07.010 PMID:19942034

Issenberg, S. B., & McGaghie, W. C. (2013). Looking to the future. In W. C. McGaghie (Ed.), *International best practices for evaluation in the health professions* (pp. 341–359). London: Radcliffe Publishing.

Issenberg, S. B., McGaghie, W. C., Petrusa, E. R., Gordon, D. L., & Scalese, R. J. (2005). Features and uses of high-fidelity medical simulations that lead to effective learning: A BEME systematic review. *Medical Teacher*, *27*(1), 10–28. doi:10.1080/01421590500046924 PMID:16147767

Issenberg, S. B., Soo, H., & Devine, L. A. (2011). Patient Safety Training Simulations Based on Competency Criteria of the Accreditation Council for Graduate Medical Education. *The Mount Sinai Journal of Medicine, New York*, *78*(1), 842–853. doi:10.1002/msj.20301 PMID:22069208

Janda, M. S., Mattheos, N., Nattestad, A., Wagner, A., Nebel, D., Färbom, C., & Attström, R. et al. (2004). Simulation of patient encounters using a virtual patient in periodontology instruction of dental students: Design, usability, and learning effect in History-Taking skills. *European Journal of Dental Education*, *8*(3), 111–119. doi:10.1111/j.1600-0579.2004.00339.x PMID:15233775

Jansen, D. A., Berry, C., Brenner, G. H., Johnson, N., & Larson, G. (2010). A collaborative project to influence nursing faculty interest in simulation. *Clinical Simulation in Nursing*, *6*(6), e223-e229. http://dx.doi.org.lp.hscl.ufl.edu/10.1016/j.ecns.2009.08.006

Jansma, J. D., Wagner, C., & Bijnen, A. B. (2010). Resident's intentions and actions after patient safety education. *BMC Health Services Research*, *10*(350), 1–9. PMID:20044945

Jeffries, P. R. (2005). A framework for designing, implementing, and evaluating simulations used as teaching strategies in nursing. *Nursing Education Perspectives*, *26*(2), 96. PMID:15921126

Jeffries, P. R. (2005). A framework for designing, implementing, and evaluating: Simulations used as teaching strategies in nursing. *Nursing Education Perspectives*, *26*(2), 96–103. PMID:15921126

Jewett, L. S., Greenberg, L. W., & Goldberg, R. M. (1982). Teaching residents how to teach: A one-year study. *Academic Medicine*, *57*(5), 361–366. doi:10.1097/00001888-198205000-00002 PMID:7069756

Johnsen, K., Raij, A., Stevens, A., Lind, D. S., & Lok, B. (2007). The validity of a virtual human experience for interpersonal skills education. In *Proceedings of the SIGCHI Conference on Human Factors in Computing Systems*, (pp. 1049-1058). doi:10.1145/1240624.1240784

Johnson, A. (2008). A Nursing Faculty's Transition to Teaching Online. *Nursing Education Perspectives*, *29*(1), 17–22. PMID:18330417

Jonassen, D. (1999). Constructivism and computer-mediated communication in distance education. *American Journal of Distance Education*, *9*(2), 7–26.

Jonassen, D. H. (1999). Designing constructivist learning environments. In C. M. Reigeluth (Ed.), *Instructional design theories and models: A new paradigm of instructional technology* (Vol. 2, pp. 215–239). Mahwah, NJ: Lawrence Erlbaum Associates.

Jonassen, D. H. (1999). Designing constructivist learning environments. In C. M. Reigeluth (Ed.), *Instructional design theories and models: A new paradigm of instructional theory* (Vol. 2, pp. 215–239). Mahwah, NJ: Lawrence Erlbaum Associates.

Jonassen, D. H. (2011). *Learning to solve problems: A handbook for designing problem-solving learning environments*. New York, NY: Routledge.

Jordan, J., Jalali, A., Clarke, S., Dyne, P., Spector, T., & Coates, W. (2013). Asynchronous vs didactic education: Its too early to throw in the towel on tradition. *BMC Medical Education*, *13*(1), 105–105. doi:10.1186/1472-6920-13-105 PMID:23927420

Kahaleh, A. A., Danielson, J., Franson, K. L., Nuffer, W. A., & Umland, E. M. (2015). An interprofessional education panel on development, implementation, and assessment strategies. *American Journal of Pharmaceutical Education*, *79*(6), 78. doi:10.5688/ajpe79678 PMID:26430265

Kardong-Edgren, S. E., Starkweather, A. R., & Ward, L. D. (2008). The integration of simulation into a clinical foundations of nursing course: Student and faculty perspectives. *International Journal of Nursing Education Scholarship*, *5*(1), 1–16. doi:10.2202/1548-923X.1603 PMID:18673294

Karpicke, J. D., & Blunt, J. R. (2011). Retrieval practice produces more learning than elaborative studying with concept mapping. *Science*, *331*(6018), 772–775. doi:10.1126/science.1199327 PMID:21252317

Karpicke, J. D., & Roediger, H. L. (2008). The critical importance of retrieval for learning. *Science*, *319*(5865), 966–968. doi:10.1126/science.1152408 PMID:18276894

Kassam, R., Kwong, M., & Collins, J. (2013). Role-emergent model: An effective strategy to address clinical placement shortages. *The Internet Journal of Allied Health Sciences and Practice*, *11*(4).

Kavamoto, C. A., Wen, C. L., Battistella, L. R., & Bohm, G. M. (2005). A Brazilian model of distance education in physical medicine and rehabilitation based on videoconferencing and internet learning. *Journal of Telemedicine and Telecare*, *11*(Supplementary 1), 80-82.

Keedy, A. W., Durack, J. C., Sandhu, P., Chen, E. M., OSullivan, P. S., & Breiman, R. S. (2011). Comparison of traditional methods with 3D computer models in the instruction of hepatobiliary anatomy. *Anatomical Sciences Education*, *4*(2), 84–91. doi:10.1002/ase.212 PMID:21412990

Keller, J. M. (1979). Motivation and instructional design: A theoretical perspective. *Journal of Instructional Development*, *2*(4), 26–34. doi:10.1007/BF02904345

Keller, J. M. (2008). First principles of motivation to learn and e3-learning. *Distance Education*, *29*(2), 175–185. doi:10.1080/01587910802154970

Keller, J. M. (2010). *Motivational Design for Learning and Performance: The ARCS Model Approach*. NY: Springer. doi:10.1007/978-1-4419-1250-3

Kelley, A., & Aston, L. (2011). An evaluation of using champions to enhance inter-professional learning in the practice setting. *Nurse Education in Practice*, *11*(1), 36–40. doi:10.1016/j.nepr.2010.06.003 PMID:20630804

Kelley, C. G. (2015). Using a virtual patient in an advanced assessment course.[doi]. *The Journal of Nursing Education*, *54*(4), 228–231. doi:10.3928/01484834-20150218-13 PMID:25692279

Kelly, J. J., Thallner, E., Broida, R. I., Cheung, D., Meisl, H., Hamedani, A. G., & Beach, C. et al. (2010). Emergency Medicine Quality Improvement and Patient Safety Curriculum. *Academic Emergency Medicine*, *17*(2), 110–129. doi:10.1111/j.1553-2712.2010.00897.x PMID:21199092

Kelsey, N. C., & Claus, S. (2016). Embedded, in situ simulation improves ability to rescue. *Clinical Simulation in Nursing*, *12*(11), 522–527. doi:10.1016/j.ecns.2016.07.009

Kena, G., Musu-Gillette, L., Robinson, J., Wang, X., Rathbun, A., Zhang, J., . . . Dunlop Velez, E. (2015). The condition of education 2015 (NCES 2015-144). Washington, DC: U.S. Department of Education, National Center for Education Statistics. Retrieved from http://nces.ed.gov/pubsearch

Kenny, P. G., Parsons, T. D., Gratch, J., & Rizzo, A. A. (2008). Evaluation of justina: A virtual patient with PTSD. In *Intelligent Virtual Agents*, (pp. 394-408). doi:10.1007/978-3-540-85483-8_40

Kenny, P. G., Parsons, T. D., Gratch, J., Leuski, A., & Rizzo, A. A. (2007). *Virtual patients for clinical therapist skills training*. Berlin: Springer Berlin Heidelberg; doi:10.1007/978-3-540-74997-4_19

Kenny, P. G., Parsons, T. D., & Rizzo, A. A. (2009). *Human computer interaction in virtual standardized patient systems. In Human-computer interaction. interacting in various application domains* (pp. 514–523). Springer. doi:10.1007/978-3-642-02583-9_56

Kern, D. E., Thomas, P. A., & Hughes, M. T. (Eds.). (2010). *Curriculum development for medical education: a six-step approach*. Baltimore, MD: JHU Press.

Khadjooi, K., Rostami, K., & Ishaq, S. (2011). How to use Gagne's model of instructional design in teaching psychomotor skills. *Gastroenterology and Hepatology from Bed to Bench*, *4*(3), 116. PMID:24834168

Khalil, M. K., & Elkhider, I. A. (2016). Applying learning theories and instructional design models for effective instruction. *Advances in Physiology Education*, *40*(2), 147–156. doi:10.1152/advan.00138.2015 PMID:27068989

Khan, C. B., & Chishti, S. (2012). Effects of Staff Training and Development on Professional Abilities of University Teachers in Distance Learning Systems. *Quarterly Review of Distance Education*, *13*(2), 87–94.

Kiani, Q., Umar, S., & Iqbal, M. (2014). What do medical students expect in a teacher? *The Clinical Teacher*, *11*(1), 203–208. doi:10.1111/tct.12109 PMID:24802922

Kiegaldie, D., & White, G. (2006). The virtual patient: Development, implementation and evaluation of an innovative computer simulation for postgraduate nursing students. *Journal of Educational Multimedia and Hypermedia*, *15*(1), 31–47.

Kleinert, H. L., Sanders, C., Mink, J., Nash, D., Johnson, J., Boyd, S., & Challman, S. (2007). Improving student dentist competencies and perception of difficulty in delivering care to children with developmental disabilities using a virtual patient module. *Journal of Dental Education*, *71*(2), 279-286. doi:71/2/279

Kleinheksel, A. J. (2014). Transformative learning through virtual patient simulations: Predicting critical student reflections. *Clinical Simulation in Nursing*, *10*(6), e301–e308. doi:10.1016/j.ecns.2014.02.001

Kleinheksel, A. J. (2015). *Measuring the adoption and integration of virtual patient simulations in nursing education: An exploratory factor analysis (Unpublished PhD Dissertation)*. University of Florida.

Knill, R. L. (1993). Difficult laryngoscopy made easy with a BURP. *Canadian Journal of Anaesthesia*, *40*(3), 279–282. doi:10.1007/BF03037041 PMID:8467551

Knowles, M. S. (1970). *The modern practice of adult education: Andragogy versus pedagogy*. New York: Association Press.

Knowles, M. S., Holton, E. F. III, & Swanson, R. A. (2014). *The adult learner: The definitive classic in adult education and human resource development*. New York, NY: Routledge.

Kohn, L. T., Corrigan, J. M., & Donaldson, M. S. (2002). *To err is human: building a safer health system*. Washington, DC: National Academy Press.

Kohn, L. T., Corrigan, J., & Donaldson, M. S. (2000). *To err is human: Building a safer health system*. Washington, DC: National Academy Press.

Kolb, D. A., Boyatzis, R. E., & Mainemelis, C. (2001). Experiential learning theory: Previous research and new directions. *Perspectives on Thinking, Learning, and Cognitive Styles*, *1*, 227-247.

Kolb, A. Y., & Kolb, D. A. (2012). Experiential learning theory. In *Encyclopedia of the Sciences of Learning*. New York, NY: Springer.

Kolb, D. (1984). *Experiential learning: experience as the source of learning and development*. Englewood Cliffs, NJ: Prentice Hall.

Konerman, M., Alpert, C., & Shashank, S. (2016). Learning to be a clinician-educator. *Journal of the American College of Cardiology*, *67*(3), 338–342. doi:10.1016/j.jacc.2015.11.032 PMID:26796400

Kreijns, K. M., Kirschner, P. A., Jochems, W., & van Buuren, H. (2004). Determining sociability, social space, and social presence in (a)synchronous collaborative groups. *Cyberpsychology & Behavior*, *7*(2), 155–172. PMID:15140359

Kreitzer, M. J., Kligler, B., & Meeker, W. C. (2009). Health professions education and integrative healthcare. *Explore (New York, N.Y.)*, *5*(4), 212–227. doi:10.1016/j.explore.2009.05.012 PMID:19608111

Kroboth, P., Crismon, L. M., Daniels, C., Hogue, M., Reed, L., Johnson, L., & Maine, L. L. et al. (2007). Getting to solutions in interprofessional education: Report of the 2006-2007 professional affairs committee. *American Journal of Pharmaceutical Education*, *71*(19), 1–8. PMID:17429501

Krouse, A. (2015). Instructional design: More important than ever! *The Journal of Nursing Education*, *54*(6), 304–305. PMID:26057423

Kulasegaram, K. M., Martimianakis, M. A., Mylopoulos, M., Whitehead, C. R., & Woods, N. N. (2013). Cognition before curriculum: Rethinking the integration of basic science and clinical learning. *Academic Medicine*, *88*(10), 1578–1585. doi:10.1097/ACM.0b013e3182a45def PMID:23969375

Kulasegaram, K., Min, C., Howey, E., Neville, A., Woods, N., Dore, K., & Norman, G. (2015). The mediating effect of context variation in mixed practice for transfer of basic science. *Advances in Health Sciences Education: Theory and Practice*, *20*(4), 953–968. doi:10.1007/s10459-014-9574-9 PMID:25524224

Lajoie, S. (2005). Extending the scaffolding metaphor. *Instructional Science*, *33*(5), 541–557. doi:10.1007/s11251-005-1279-2

Langton, H. (2009). Interprofessional education in higher education institutions: models, pedagogies, and realities. In P. Bluteau & A. Jackson (Eds.), *Interprofessional Education: Making it Happen* (pp. 37–58). Basingstoke, UK: Palgrave Macmillan.

Larsen, D. P., Butler, A. C., & Roediger, H. L. III. (2008). Test-enhanced learning in medical education. *Medical Education*, *42*(10), 959–966. doi:10.1111/j.1365-2923.2008.03124.x PMID:18823514

Larsen, D., Butler, A., Lawson, A., & Roediger, I. H. (2013). The importance of seeing the patient: Test-enhanced learning with standardized patients and written tests improves clinical application of knowledge. *Advances in Health Sciences Education: Theory and Practice*, *18*(3), 409–425. doi:10.1007/s10459-012-9379-7 PMID:22618856

Lau, K. H. V. (2014). Computer-based teaching module design: Principles derived from learning theories. *Medical Education*, *48*(3), 247–254. doi:10.1111/medu.12357 PMID:24528459

Lave, J., & Wenger, E. (1991). *Situated Learning: Legitimate Peripheral Participation*. Cambridge, UK: Cambridge University Press. doi:10.1017/CBO9780511815355

Lawlis, T. R., Anson, J., & Greenfield, D. (2014). Barriers and enablers that influence sustainable interprofessional education: A literature review. *Journal of Interprofessional Care*, *28*(4), 305–310. doi:10.3109/13561820.2014.895977 PMID:24625198

Leaviss, J. (2000). Exploring the perceived effects of an undergraduate multiprofessional education intervention. *Medical Education*, *34*(6), 483–486. doi:10.1046/j.1365-2923.2000.00678.x PMID:10792692

Lee, N. J., An, J. Y., Song, T. M., Jang, H., & Park, S. Y. (2014). Psychometric evaluation of a patient safety competency self-evaluation tool for nursing students. *The Journal of Nursing Education, 53*(10), 550–562. doi:10.3928/01484834-20140922-01 PMID:25275988

Leppink, J., & van den Heuvel, A. (2015). The evolution of cognitive load theory and its application to medical education. *Perspectives on Medical Education, 4*(3), 119-127.

Levinson, A. J. (2010). Where is evidence-based instructional design in medical education curriculum development? *Medical Education, 44*(6), 536–537. doi:10.1111/j.1365-2923.2010.03715.x PMID:20604847

Lewis, R. A. (2009). *The effect of virtual clinical gaming simulations on student learning outcomes in medical-surgical nursing education courses* (Ed.D. Dissertation). Available from ProQuest Dissertations & Theses Full Text. (305123049). Retrieved from http://search.proquest.com.lp.hscl.ufl.edu/docview/305123049?accountid=10920

Lewis, E. J., Baernholdt, M., & Hamric, A. B. (2013). Nurses experience of medical errors: An integrative literature review. *Journal of Nursing Care Quality, 28*(2), 153–161. doi:10.1097/NCQ.0b013e31827e05d1 PMID:23222195

Liaison Committee on Medical Education. (2016). *Functions and structure of a medical school.* Retrieved May 14, 2016, from http://lcme.org/publications/

Liaison Committee on Medical Education. (2016). *Functions and structure of a medical school: Standards for accreditation of medical education programs leading to the MD degree.* Retrieved from http://lcme.org/publications/

Liaison Committee on Medical Education. (2016). *Functions and Structure of a Medical School: Standards for Accreditation of Medical Education Programs Leading to the MD Degree.* Retrieved March 15, 2016, from http://lcme.org/publications/

Liew, S.-C., Sidhu, J., & Barua, A. (2015). The relationship between learning preferences (styles and approaches) and learning outcomes among pre-clinical undergraduate medical students. *BMC Medical Education, 15*(1), 44. doi:10.1186/s12909-015-0327-0 PMID:25889887

Lind, G. (2005). Moral Dilemma Discussion Revisited - The Konstanz Method. *Europes Journal of Psychology, 1*(1), 1–5. doi:10.5964/ejop.v1i1.345

Lin, K. Y., & Shen, Y. F. (2013). The nursing students attitude toward using blogs in a nursing clinical practicum in Taiwan: A 3-R framework. *Nurse Education Today, 33*(9), 1079–1082. doi:10.1016/j.nedt.2012.03.019 PMID:22520239

Linzer, M. (1987). The journal club and medical education: Over one hundred years of unrecorded history. *Postgraduate Medical Journal, 63*(740), 475–478. doi:10.1136/pgmj.63.740.475 PMID:3324090

Liu, J. C., & Stewart, M. G. (2007). Teaching evidence-based medicine in otolaryngology. *Otolaryngologic Clinics of North America, 40*(6), 1261–1274. doi:10.1016/j.otc.2007.07.006 PMID:18021839

Livingstone, D. (1999). Exploring the iceberg of adult learning: Findings of the first Canadian survey of informal learning practices. *Canadian Journal for the Study of Adult Education, 13*(2), 49–72.

Lovell, K. L., & Hodgins, M. W. (2001). Implementation and evaluation of neuroscience technology resources for second-year medical students. In *Proceedings of Slice of Life/Computers in Health Care Annual Meeting.* Salt Lake City, UT: University of Utah.

Lovell, K. L., Haf, J., & Hodgins, M. (1991). Development of neuropathology interactive videodisc instructional units. *Teaching and Learning in Medicine, 3*(3), 156–158. doi:10.1080/10401339109539501

Lovell, K. L., Parkhurst, P. E., Sprafka, S. A., Hodgins, M. W., & Bean, P. L. (1993). Quantitative and qualitative evaluation of interactive videodisc instructional modules in preclinical neuropathology education. *Teaching and Learning in Medicine*, *5*(1), 3–9. doi:10.1080/10401339309539579

Luke, R., Solomon, P., Baptiste, S., Hall, P., Orchard, C., Rukholm, E., & Carter, L. (2009). Online interprofessional health sciences education: From theory to practice. *The Journal of Continuing Education in the Health Professions*, *29*(3), 161–167. doi:10.1002/chp.20030 PMID:19728380

Lutfiyya, M. N., Brandt, B. F., & Cerra, F. (2016). Reflections From the Intersection of Health Professions Education and Clinical Practice. *Academic Medicine*, *91*(6), 766–771. doi:10.1097/ACM.0000000000001139 PMID:26959223

Lytle, R. (2011, November 11). Study: Online education continues growth. *US News and World Report.* Retrieved from http://www.usnews.com/education/online-education/articles/2011/11/11/study-online-education-continues-growth

Macdonald, R., & Savin-Baden, M. (2004). *A briefing on assessment in problem-based learning*. LTSN Generic Centre Assessment Series No 7. York, England: LTSN Generic Centre. Retrieved from http://www.ltsn.ac.uk/application.asp?app=resources.asp&process=full_ record&section=generic&id=349

MacLeod, S. (2012). Walking the talk: The need for investment in educator development. *Education for Primary Care*, *23*(1), 242245. PMID:22925955

Magill, I. W. (1931). Technique in Endotracheal Anesthesia. *Anesthesia and Analgesia*, *10*(4), 164–168.

Malcolm Baldrige National Quality Awards. (2016). *Advocate Good Samaritan Hospital*. Available at: https://www.nist.gov/baldrige/advocate-good-samaritan-hospital

Malik, A. S., & Malik, R. H. (2011). Twelve tips for developing an integrated curriculum. *Medical Teacher*, *33*(2), 99–104. doi:10.3109/0142159X.2010.507711 PMID:20874013

Mallampati, S. R., Gatt, S. P., Gugino, L. D., Desai, S. P., Waraksa, B., Freiberger, D., & Liu, P. L. (1985). A clinical sign to predict difficult tracheal intubation; a prospective study. *Canadian Anaesthetists Society Journal*, *32*(4), 429–434. doi:10.1007/BF03011357 PMID:4027773

Malone, T. W. (1981). Toward a theory of intrinsically motivating instruction. *Cognitive Science*, *5*(4), 333–369. doi:10.1207/s15516709cog0504_2

Mancuso-Murphy, J. (2007). Distance education in nursing: An integrated review of online nursing students' experiences with technology-delivered instruction. *The Journal of Nursing Education*, *46*(6), 252–260. PMID:17580737

Mangels, J. A., Butterfield, B., Lamb, J., Good, C., & Dweck, C. S. (2006). Why do beliefs about intelligence influence learning success? A social cognitive neuroscience model. *Social Cognitive and Affective Neuroscience*, *1*(2), 75–86. doi:10.1093/scan/nsl013 PMID:17392928

Mann, K. V. (1999). Motivation in medical education: How theory can inform our practice. *Academic Medicine*, *74*(3), 237–239. doi:10.1097/00001888-199903000-00011 PMID:10099642

Marsick, V. J., Watkins, K., Callahan, M., & Volpe, M. (2009). Informal and incidental learning in the workplace. In M. C. Smith & DeFrates-Densch (Eds.), Handbook of research on adult learning and development (pp. 570-599). New York, NY: Routledge.

Marsick, V. J. (2009). Toward a unifying framework to support informal learning theory, research and practice. *Journal of Workplace Learning*, *21*(4), 265–275. doi:10.1108/13665620910954184

Marsick, V. J., & Volpe, M. (1999). The nature and need for informal learning. *Advances in Developing Human Resources*, *1*(3), 1–9. doi:10.1177/152342239900100302

Marsick, V. J., & Watkins, K. E. (2001). Informal and incidental learning. *New Directions for Adult and Continuing Education*, *89*(89), 25–34. doi:10.1002/ace.5

Martínez-González, A., López-Bárcena, J., Herrera Saint-Leu, P., Ocampo-Martínez, J., Petra, I., & Uribe-Martínez, G., … Morales-López, S. (2008). Modelo de competencias del profesor de medicina. *Educación Médica*, *11*(3), 157–10.

Martinez, M. E. (2010). *Learning and Cognition: The design of the mind*. Upper Saddle River, NJ: Pearson Education, Inc.

Marton, G., McCullough, B., & Ramnanan, C. (2014). A review of teaching skills development programmes for medical students. *Medical Education*, *49*(1), 149–160. PMID:25626746

Mast, L. J., Rahman, A., Schatzman, B. I., Bridges, D., & Horsley, N. (2015). Innovations in continuing professional education: A model to impact interprofessional collaboration. *International Public Health Journal*, *7*(1), 65–77.

Mavis, B. E., Lovell, K. L., & Ogle, K. S. (1998). Why Johnnie cant apply neuroscience: Testing alternative hypotheses using performance-based assessment. *Advances in Health Science Education*, *3*(3), 165–175. doi:10.1023/A:1009794026466 PMID:12386438

Mayer, R. E. (2008). Applying the science of learning: Evidence-based principles for the design of multimedia instruction. *The American Psychologist*, *63*(8), 760–769. doi:10.1037/0003-066X.63.8.760 PMID:19014238

Mayer, R. E. (2010). Applying the science of learning to medical education. *Medical Education*, *44*(6), 543–549. doi:10.1111/j.1365-2923.2010.03624.x PMID:20604850

Mayer, R. E. (2011). *Applying the science of learning*. Upper Saddle River, NJ: Pearson.

Mayer, R. E., & Moreno, R. (2010). Nine ways to reduce cognitive load in multimedia learning. *Educational Psychologist*, *38*(1), 43–52. doi:10.1207/S15326985EP3801_6

McFadyen, A. K., Maclaren, W. M., & Webster, V. S. (2007). The Interdisciplinary Education Perception Scale (IEPS): an alternative remodelled sub-scale structure and its reliability. *Journal of Interprofessional Care*, *21*(4), 433–443.

McFadyen, A. K., Webster, V., Strachan, K., Figgins, E., Brown, H., & McKechnie, J. (2005). The Readiness for Interprofessional Learning Scale: A possible more stable sub-scale model for the original version of RIPLS. *Journal of Interprofessional Care*, *19*(6), 595–603. doi:10.1080/13561820500430157 PMID:16373215

McGaghie, W. C., Issenberg, S. B., Cohen, E. R., Barsuk, J. H., & Wayne, D. B. (2011). Does simulation-based medical education with deliberate practice yield better results than traditional clinical education? A meta-analytic comparative review of evidence. *Academic Medicine*, *86*(6), 706–711. doi:10.1097/ACM.0b013e318217e119 PMID:21512370

McGaghie, W. C., Issenberg, S. B., Petrusa, E. R., & Scalese, R. J. (2010). A critical review of simulation-based medical education research: 20032009. *Medical Education*, *44*(1), 50–63. doi:10.1111/j.1365-2923.2009.03547.x PMID:20078756

McKeon, L. M., Norris, T., Cardell, B., & Britt, T. (2009). Developing patient-centered care competencies among prelicensure nursing students using simulation. *The Journal of Nursing Education*, *48*(12), 711–715. doi:10.3928/01484834-20091113-06 PMID:20000255

McNair, R. P. (2005). The case for educating health care students in professionalism as the core content of interprofessional education. *Medical Education*, *39*(5), 456–464. doi:10.1111/j.1365-2929.2005.02116.x PMID:15842679

Means, T. B., Jonassen, D. H., & Dwyer, F. M. (1997). Enhancing relevance: Embedded ARCS strategies vs. purpose. *Educational Technology Research and Development*, *45*(1), 5–17. doi:10.1007/BF02299610

Medel-Anonuevo, C., Ohsako, T., & Mauch, W. (2001). *Revisiting lifelong learning for the 21st century*. UNESCO Institute for Education. Retrieved March 1, 2016, from http://www.unesco.org/education/uie/pdf/revisitingLLL.pdf

Medina, L., Racadio, J., & Schwid, H. (2000). Computers in radiology. *Pediatric Radiology*, *30*(5), 299–305. doi:10.1007/s002470050744 PMID:10836590

Megroth, E., & Washburne, V. (1949). Integration in education. *The Journal of Educational Research*, *43*(2), 81–92. doi:10.1080/00220671.1949.10881753

Merrill, M. D. (2002). First principles of instruction. *Educational Technology Research and Development*, *50*(3), 43–59. doi:10.1007/BF02505024

Merrill, M. D., Drake, L., Lacy, M. J., & Pratt, J. (1996). Reclaiming instructional design (PDF). *Educational Technology*, *36*(5), 5–7.

Meticulous Research. (2014). *Global virtual patient simulation market to reach $508.7 million by 2019* [Press Release]. Meticulous Research.

Miller, J. (1978). *Living Systems*. New York, NY: McGraw-Hill.

Miller, M., & Jensen, R. (2014). Avatars in nursing: An integrative review. *Nurse Educator*, *39*(1), 38–41. doi:10.1097/01.NNE.0000437367.03842.63 PMID:24300258

Misch, D. A. (2002). Andragogy and medical education: Are medical students internally motivated to learn? *Advances in Health Sciences Education: Theory and Practice*, *7*(2), 153–160. doi:10.1023/A:1015790318032 PMID:12075147

Morrison, J. L. (2000). *Challenges in implementing distance learning programs*. Retrieved from htttp://horizon.unc.edu/projects/resources/44items.html

Morrison, E. H., Friedland, J. A., Boker, J., Rucker, L., Hollingshead, J., & Murata, P. (2001). Residents-as-teachers: Training in US residency programs and offices of graduate medical education. *Academic Medicine*, *76*(10Supplement), S1–S4. doi:10.1097/00001888-200110001-00002 PMID:11597856

Morrison, G. R., Ross, S. M., Kalman, H. K., & Kemp, J. E. (2013). *Designing Effective Instruction* (7th ed.). Hoboken, NJ: John Wiley & Sons, Inc.

Morrison, G., Ross, S., & Kemp, J. (2007). *Designing effective instruction*. Hoboken, NJ: Jonh Wiley & Sons.

Motola, I., Devine, L. A., Chung, H. S., Sullivan, J. E., & Issenberg, S. B. (2013). Simulation in healthcare education: A best evidence practical guide. *Medical Teacher*, *35*(10), 1511–1530. doi:10.3109/0142159X.2013.818632 PMID:23941678

Muller, J. H., Jain, S., Loeser, H., & Irby, D. M. (2008). Lessons learned about integrating a medical school curriculum: Perceptions of students, faculty and curriculum leaders. *Medical Education*, *42*(8), 778–785. doi:10.1111/j.1365-2923.2008.03110.x PMID:18627445

Muller, S. (1984). Physicians for the twenty-first century: Report of the project panel on the general professional education of the physician and college preparation for medicine. *Journal of Medical Education*, *59*, 1–208. PMID:6492116

Murray, T. A. (2013). Innovations in nursing education: The state of the art. *Journal of Nursing Regulation*, *3*(4), 25–31. doi:10.1016/S2155-8256(15)30183-6

Nasca, T. J., Philibert, I., Brigham, T., & Flynn, T. C. (2012). The next GME accreditation systemrationale and benefits. *The New England Journal of Medicine*, *366*(11), 1051–1056. doi:10.1056/NEJMsr1200117 PMID:22356262

National League for Nursing. (2005). *Core competencies of nurse educators*. Available at http://www.nln.org/professional-development-programs/competencies-for-nursing-education/nurse-educator-core-competency

National Society for Experiential Education. (2009). *Eight principles of good practice for all experiential learning activities.* Retrieved August 17, 2016 from http://www.nsee.org/8-principles

National Society for Experiential Education. (2013). *Guiding principles of ethical practice.* Retrieved August 17, 2016 from http://www.nsee.org/guiding-principles

Nehring, W. M., & Lashley, F. R. (2009). Nursing simulation: A review of the past 40 years. *Simulation & Gaming, 40*(4), 528–552. doi:10.1177/1046878109332282

Nendaz, M. R., & Tekian, A. (1999). Assessment in problem-based learning medical schools: A literature review. *Teaching and Learning in Medicine, 11*(4), 232–243. doi:10.1207/S15328015TLM110408

Neville, A. J. (2009). Problem-based learning and medical education forty years on. *Medical Principles and Practice, 18*(1), 1–9. doi:10.1159/000163038 PMID:19060483

Nguyen, D. N., Zierler, B., & Nguyen, H. Q. (2011). A survey of nursing faculty needs for training in use of new technologies for education and practice. *The Journal of Nursing Education, 50*(4), 181–189. doi:10.3928/01484834-20101130-06 PMID:21117532

Nilson, M., Pennbrant, S., Pilhammar, E., & Wenestarm, C.-G. (2010). Pedagogical strategies used in clinical medical education: Observational study. *BMC Medical Education, 10*(9), 1–10. PMID:20074350

Nisbet, G., Lincoln, M., & Dunn, S. (2013). Informal interprofessional learning: An untapped opportunity for learning and change within the workplace. *Journal of Interprofessional Care, 27*(6), 469–475. doi:10.3109/13561820.2013.805735 PMID:23789898

Nogueira Sotolongo, M., Rivera Michelena, C. N., & Blanco, F. (2005). Competencias docentes del médico de familia en el desempeño de la tutoría en la carrera de medicina. *Educación Médica Superior, 19*(1), 1–1.

Norcini, J. J. (2003). Setting standards on educational tests. *Medical Education, 37*(5), 464–474. doi:10.1046/j.1365-2923.2003.01495.x PMID.12709190

Norman, G. R., & Schmidt, H. G. (2000). Effectiveness of problem-based learning curricula: Theory, practice and paper darts. *Medical Education, 34*(9), 721–728. doi:10.1046/j.1365-2923.2000.00749.x PMID:10972750

Northouse, P. G. (2015). *Introduction to leadership concepts and practices* (3rd ed.). Thousand Oaks, CA: Sage.

Nothnagle, M., Anandarajah, G., Goldman, R. E., & Reis, S. (2011). Struggling to be self-directed: Residents paradoxical beliefs about learning. *Academic Medicine, 86*(12), 1539–1544. doi:10.1097/ACM.0b013e3182359476 PMID:22030764

Oandasan, I., & Reeves, S. (2005). Key elements for interprofessional education. Part 1: The learner, the educator and the learning context. *Journal of Interprofessional Care, 19*(sup1), 21-38.

Oandasan, I., & Reeves, S. (2005a). Key elements for interprofessional education. Part 1: The learner, the educator and the learning context. *Journal of Interprofessional Care, 19*(sup1s1), 21–38. doi:10.1080/13561820500083550 PMID:16096143

Oandasan, I., & Reeves, S. (2005b). Key elements of interprofessional education. Part 2: Factors, processes and outcomes. *Journal of Interprofessional Care, 19*(sup1s1), 39–48. doi:10.1080/13561820500081703 PMID:16096144

Okuda, Y., Bryson, E. O., DeMaria, S., Jacobson, L., Quinones, J., Shen, B., & Levine, A. I. (2009). The utility of simulation in medical education: what is the evidence?. *Mount Sinai Journal of Medicine: A Journal of Translational and Personalized Medicine, 76*(4), 330-343.

Okuda, Y., Bond, W., Bonfante, G., McLaughlin, S., Spillane, L., Wang, E., & Gorden, J. A. et al. (2008). National growth in simulation training within emergency medicine residency programs, 2003–2008. *Academic Emergency Medicine*, *15*(11), 1113–1116. doi:10.1111/j.1553-2712.2008.00195.x PMID:18717652

Okuda, Y., Bryson, E. O., DeMaria, S. Jr, Jacobson, L., Shen, B., & Levine, A. I. (2009). The Utility of Simulation in Medical Education: What Is the Evidence? *The Mount Sinai Journal of Medicine, New York*, *76*(4), 330–343. doi:10.1002/msj.20127 PMID:19642147

Olivares, S. (2016). Aprendizaje Centrado en las Perspectivas del Paciente. In S. Olivares, & J. Valdez-García (Eds.), *Aprendizaje Centrado en el Paciente: Cuatro perspectivas para un abordaje integral* (pp. 4-44). Ciudad de México: Editorial Médica Panamericana.

Olivares, S. L., & López, M. V. (2016). Evaluación de autopercepción del pensamiento crítico en estudiantes de medicina. *Revista Electrónica de Investigación Educativa*, *18*(3), 1–22.

Omid, A., & Haghani Fariba, A. P. (2016). Clinical teaching with emotional intelligence: A teaching toolbox. *Journal of Research in Medical Sciences*, *21*(1), 19–27.

Orsmond, P., & Zvauya, R. (2015). Community of learners: Charting learning in first year graduate entry medical students during problem-based learning (PBL) study. *Advances in Health Sciences Education: Theory and Practice*, *20*(2), 479–497. doi:10.1007/s10459-014-9542-4 PMID:25118861

Ottestad, E., Boulet, J., & Lighthall, G. (2007). Evaluating the management of septic shock using patient simulation. *Critical Care Medicine*, *35*(3), 769–775. doi:10.1097/01.CCM.0000256849.75799.20 PMID:17235260

Ozolins, I., Hall, H., & Peterson, R. (2008). The student voice: Recognising the hidden and informal curriculum in medicine. *Medical Teacher*, *30*(6), 606–611. doi:10.1080/01421590801949933 PMID:18608968

Paas, F., Renkl, A., & Sweller, J. (2010). Cognitive load theory and instructional design: Recent developments. *Educational Psychologist*, *38*(1), 1–4. doi:10.1207/S15326985EP3801_1

Palincsar, A. S. (1986). The role of dialogue in providing scaffolded instruction. *Educational Psychologist*, *21*(1-2), 73–98. doi:10.1080/00461520.1986.9653025

Parkhurst, P. E., Lovell, K. L., Sprafka, S. A., Hodgins, M. W., & Bean, P. L. (1991). Evaluation of interactive videodisc instructional modules in preclinical neuropathology education. *Journal of Medical Education Technology*, *2*, 17–21.

Parks, D. J. (2010). Lest we forget our past: A leader in curriculum development—Ralph Winfred Tyler. *The Educational Forum*, *75*(1), 80–86. doi:10.1080/00131725.2010.528549

Passiment, M., Sacks, H., & Huang, G. (2011). *Medical simulation in medical education: Results of an AAMC Survey*. Washington, DC: Association of American Medical Colleges.

Pate, A., Smaldino, S., Mayall, H. J., & Luetkehans, L. (2009). Questioning the Necessity of Nonacademic Social Discussion Forums within Online Courses. *Quarterly Review of Distance Education*, *10*(1), 1–8.

Paver-Erzen, V., & Cimerman, M. (2007) The value of clinical simulation-based training. In T. Jarm, P. Kramar, & A. Zupanic (Eds.), *11th Mediterranean Conference on Medical and Biomedical Engineering and Computing 2007* (pp. 327-328). Berlin, Germany: Springer. doi:10.1007/978-3-540-73044-6_82

Pecukonis, E., Doyle, O., & Bliss, D. L. (2008). Reducing barriers to interprofessional training: Promoting interprofessional cultural competence. *Journal of Interprofessional Care*, *22*(4), 417–428. doi:10.1080/13561820802190442 PMID:18800282

Peeters, J., Backer, F. D., Buffel, T., Kindekens, A., Struyven, K., Zhu, C., & Lombaerts, K. (2014). Adult learners' informal learning experiences in formal education setting. *Journal of Adult Development*, *21*(3), 181–192. doi:10.1007/s10804-014-9190-1

Pérez Juste, R. (2000). La evaluación de programas educativos: Conceptos básicos, planteamientos generales y problemática. *Revista de Investigación Educativa*, *18*(2), 261–287.

Pian-Smith, M. C., Simon, R., Minehart, R. D., Podraza, M., Rudolph, J., Walzer, T., & Raemer, D. (2009). Teaching residents the two-challenge rule: A simulation-based approach to improve education and patient safety. *Simulation in Healthcare*, *4*(2), 84–91. doi:10.1097/SIH.0b013e31818cffd3 PMID:19444045

Pina, A. A., & Mizell, A. P. (2014). *Real-life distance education: Case studies in practice*. Charlotte, NC: Information Age.

Prober, C. G., & Heath, C. (2012). Lecture halls without lectures—a proposal for medical education. *The New England Journal of Medicine*, *366*(18), 1657–1659. doi:10.1056/NEJMp1202451 PMID:22551125

Ramani, S. (2003). Twelve tips to improve bedside teaching. *Medical Teacher*, *25*(2), 112–115. doi:10.1080/0142159031000092463 PMID:12745516

Rashid, A., & Siriwardena, N. (2005). *The professionalisation of education an educators in postgraduate medicine. Education for Primary Care, 16*(1), 235-245.

Reber, A. (1993). *Implicit Learning and Tacit Knowledge*. Oxford, UK: Oxford University Press.

Reed, S. J., & Edmunds, D. (2015). Use of a blog in an undergraduate nursing leadership course. *Nurse Education in Practice*, *15*(6), 537–542. doi:10.1016/j.nepr.2015.07.010 PMID:26299700

Reeves, S., Boet, S., Zierler, B., & Kitto, S. (2015). Interprofessional Education and Practice Guide No. 3: Evaluating interprofessional education. *Journal of Interprofessional Care*, *29*(4), 305–312. doi:10.3109/13561820.2014.1003637 PMID:25671416

Reeves, S., Goldman, J., & Oandasan, I. (2007). Key factors in planning and implementing interprofessional education in health care settings. *Journal of Allied Health*, *36*(4), 231–235. PMID:18293805

Reeves, S., Perrier, L., Goldman, J., Freeth, D., & Zwarenstein, M. (2013). Interprofessional education: Effects on professional practice. *Cochrane Database of Systematic Reviews*, (3): 1–21. doi:10.1002/14651858.CD002213.pub3 PMID:23543515

Reeves, T. C., Herrington, J., & Oliver, R. (2005). Design research: A socially responsible approach to instructional technology research in higher education. *Journal of Computing in Higher Education*, *16*(2), 96–115.

Reigeluth, C. M. (1983). Meaningfulness and instruction: Relating what is being learned to what a student knows. *Instructional Science*, *12*(3), 197–218. doi:10.1007/BF00051745

Reigeluth, C. M. (1999). *The elaboration theory: Guidance for scope and sequence decisions. In Instructional design theories and models: A new paradigm of instructional theory* (Vol. 2, pp. 425–453). Mahwah, NJ: Lawrence Erlbaum Associates.

Reigeluth, C. M., & Moore, J. (1999). Cognitive education and the cognitive domain. In C. M. Reigeluth (Ed.), *Instructional design theories and models: A new paradigm of instructional theory* (Vol. 2, pp. 51–68). Mahwah, NJ: Lawrence Erlbaum Associates.

Reiser, R. A. (2001). A history of instructional design and technology: Part II: A history of instructional design. *Educational Technology Research and Development*, *49*(2), 57–67. doi:10.1007/BF02504928

Remington, T. L., Foulk, M. A., & Williams, B. C. (2006). Evaluation of evidence for interprofessional education. *American Journal of Pharmaceutical Education, 70*(3), 66. doi:10.5688/aj700366 PMID:17136186

Richey, R. C. (2000). *The legacy of Robert M. Gagne*. Syracuse, NY: ERIC Clearinghouse on Information & Technology.

Richey, R. C., Klein, J. D., & Tracey, M. W. (2010). *The instructional design knowledge base: Theory, research, and practice*. New York, NY: Routledge.

Rienties, B., Toetenel, L., & Bryan, A. (2015, March). Scaling up learning design: Impact of learning design activities on LMS behavior and performance. In *Proceedings of the Fifth International Conference on Learning Analytics And Knowledge* (pp. 315-319). ACM. doi:10.1145/2723576.2723600

Robb, A., White, C., Cordar, A., Wendling, A., Lampotang, S., & Lok, B. (2015). A comparison of speaking up behavior during conflict with real and virtual humans. *Computers in Human Behavior, 52*, 12–21. doi:10.1016/j.chb.2015.05.043

Roberts, N. K., Brenner, M. J., Williams, R. G., Kim, M. J., & Dunnington, G. L. (2012). Capturing the teachable moment: A grounded theory study of verbal teaching interactions in the operating room. *Surgery, 151*(5), 643–650. doi:10.1016/j.surg.2011.12.011 PMID:22244182

Rogers, P. C., Graham, C. R., & Mayes, C. T. (2007). Cultural competence and instructional design: Exploration research into the delivery of online instruction cross-culturally. *Educational Technology Research and Development, 55*(2), 197–217. doi:10.1007/s11423-007-9033-x

Rogers, P. L., Jacob, H., Thomas, E. A., Harwell, M., Willenkin, R. L., & Pinsky, M. R. (2000). Medical students can learn the basic application, analytic, evaluative, and psychomotor skills of critical care medicine. *Critical Care Medicine, 28*(2), 550–554. doi:10.1097/00003246-200002000-00043 PMID:10708198

Rohrer, D., & Pashler, H. (2010). Recent research on human learning challenges conventional instructional strategies. *Educational Researcher, 39*(5), 406–412. doi:10.3102/0013189X10374770

Rosen, K. R. (2008). The history of medical simulation. *Journal of Critical Care, 23*(2), 157–166. doi:10.1016/j.jcrc.2007.12.004 PMID:18538206

Rossett, A. (1995). Needs assessment. In G. Anglin (Ed.), *Instructional technology: Past, present and future* (2nd ed.; pp. 183–196). Englewood, CO: Libraries Unlimited, Inc.

Rossett, A. (1999). Knowledge management meets analysis. *Training & Development, 53*, 62–68.

Ross, M. (2014). Art in clinical teaching. *The Clinical Teacher, 11*(1), 325–326. doi:10.1111/tct.12286 PMID:25041661

Royal College of General Practitioners. (2016). *The RCGP curriculum: Core curriculum statement*. Retrieved from http://www.rcgp.org.uk/training-exams/gp-curriculum-overview/document-version.aspx

Ruiz, J. G., Cook, D. A., & Levinson, A. J. (2009). Computer animations in medical education: A critical literature review. *Medical Education, 43*(9), 838–846. doi:10.1111/j.1365-2923.2009.03429.x PMID:19709008

Ruiz, J. G., Mintzer, M. J., & Leipzig, R. M. (2006). The impact of e-learning in medical education. *Academic Medicine, 81*(3), 207–212. doi:10.1097/00001888-200603000-00002 PMID:16501260

Ruiz, M. G., Ezer, H., & Purden, M. (2013). Exploring the nature of facilitating interprofessional learning: Findings from an exploratory study. *Journal of Interprofessional Care, 27*(6), 489–495. doi:10.3109/13561820.2013.811640 PMID:23859380

Sackett, D. L., Rosenberg, W. M., Gray, J. A., Haynes, R. B., & Richardson, W. S. (1996). Evidence based medicine: What it is and what it isn't. *British Medical Journal, 312*(7023), 71–72. doi:10.1136/bmj.312.7023.71 PMID:8555924

Sackett, D. L., Straus, S. E., Richardson, W. S., & Rosenberg, W. (2000). *Evidence-based medicine: How to practice and teach EBM* (2nd ed.). New York, NY: Churchill Livingstone.

Saettler, P. (1990). *The evolution of American educational technology*. Englewood Cliffs, NJ: Libraries Unlimited.

Salas, E., Wilson, K. A., Burke, C. S., & Priest, H. A. (2005). Using simulation-based training to improve patient safety: What does it take? *Joint Commission Journal on Quality and Patient Safety*, *31*(7), 363–371. doi:10.1016/S1553-7250(05)31049-X PMID:16130979

Salsberg, E., & Grover, A. (2006). Physician workforce shortages: Implications and issues for academic health centers and policymakers. *Academic Medicine*, *81*(9), 782–787. doi:10.1097/00001888-200609000-00003 PMID:16936479

Sanders, C. L., Kleinert, H. L., Free, T., King, P., Slusher, I., & Boyd, S. (2008). Developmental disabilities: Improving competence in care using virtual patients. *The Journal of Nursing Education*, *47*(2), 66–73. doi:10.3928/01484834-20080201-05 PMID:18320957

Sargeant, J. (2009). Theories to aid understanding and implementation of interprofessional education. *The Journal of Continuing Education in the Health Professions*, *29*(3), 178–184. doi:10.1002/chp.20033 PMID:19728383

Sargeant, J., Hill, T., & Breau, L. (2010). Development and testing of a scale to assess interprofessional education (IPE) facilitation skills. *The Journal of Continuing Education in the Health Professions*, *30*(2), 126–131. doi:10.1002/chp.20069 PMID:20564701

Savery, J. (2005). Be VOCAL: Characteristics of successful online instructors. *Journal of Interactive Online Learning*, *4*(2), 141–152.

Sayed, Y., & Jager, K. (2014). Towards an investigation of information literacy in South African students. *South African Journal of Library and Information Science*, *65*(1), 5–12. doi:10.7553/65-1-1495

Schank, R. (2002). *Designing world-class e-learning*. New York, NY: McGraw-Hill.

Schank, R. C., Berman, T. R., & Macpherson, K. A. (1999). Learning by doing. In C. M. Reigeluth (Ed.), *Instructional design theories and models: A new paradigm of instructional technology* (Vol. 2, pp. 161–182). Mahwah, NJ: Lawrence Erlbaum Associates.

Schardt, C. (2001). Evidence-based medicine and the hospital librarian. *Journal of Hospital Librarianship*, *1*(2), 1–14. doi:10.1300/J186v01n02_01

Schmidmaier, R., Ebersbach, R., Schiller, M., Hege, I., Holzer, M., & Fischer, M. R. (2011). Using electronic flashcards to promote learning in medical students: Retesting versus restudying. *Medical Education*, *45*(11), 1101–1110. doi:10.1111/j.1365-2923.2011.04043.x PMID:21988625

Schmidt, E., Goldhaber-Fiebert, S. N., Ho, L. A., & McDonald, K. M. (2013). Simulation exercises as a patient safety strategy: A systematic review. *Annals of Internal Medicine*, *158*(5 Pt 2), 426–426. doi:10.7326/0003-4819-158-5-201303051-00010 PMID:23460100

Schmidt, H. G. (1983). Problem-based learning: Rationale and description. *Medical Education*, *17*(1), 11–16. doi:10.1111/j.1365-2923.1983.tb01086.x PMID:6823214

Schmidt, H. G., Machiels-Bongaerts, M., Hermans, H., ten Cate, T. J., Venekamp, R., & Boshuizen, H. P. (1996). The development of diagnostic competence: Comparison of a problem-based, an integrated, and a conventional medical curriculum. *Academic Medicine*, *71*(6), 658–664. doi:10.1097/00001888-199606000-00021 PMID:9125924

Schmitz, C. C., & Cullen, M. J. (2015, March 20). *Evaluating interprofessional education and collaborative practice: What should I consider when selecting a measurement tool?* Retrieved from https://nexusipe.org/informing/resource-center/evaluating-ipecp

Schon, D. A. (1983). *The reflective practitioner: How professionals think in action.* New York: Basic Books.

Schrock, J. W., & Cydulka, R. K. (2006). Lifelong learning. *Emergency Medicine Clinics of North America, 24*(3), 785–795. doi:10.1016/j.emc.2006.05.012 PMID:16877143

Schugurensky, D. (2000). *The forms of informal learning: Towards a conceptualization of the field.* Centre for the Study of Education and Work.

Schumacher, D. J., Englander, R., & Carraccio, C. (2013). Developing the master learner: Applying learning theory to the learner, the teacher, and the learning environment. *Academic Medicine, 88*(11), 1635–1645. doi:10.1097/ACM.0b013e3182a6e8f8 PMID:24072107

Schwartzman, R., & Henry, K. (2009). From celebration to critical investigation: Charting the course of scholarship in applied learning. *Journal of Applied Learning in Higher Education, 1*, 3–23.

Schwen, T. M. (1973). Learner analysis. *AV Communication Review, 21*(1), 44–72. doi:10.1007/bf02770828

Shear, T., Greenberg, S., & Tokarczyk, A. (2013). Does training with human patient simulation translate to improved patient safety and outcome? *Current Opinion in Anaesthesiology, 26*(2), 159–163. doi:10.1097/ACO.0b013e32835dc0af PMID:23339975

Sheridan, S., & Williams, P. (2011). Developing individual goals, shared goals, and the goals of others: Dimensions of constructive competition in learning contexts. *Scandinavian Journal of Educational Research, 55*(2), 145–164. doi:10.1080/00313831.2011.554694

Sherry, L. (1995). Issues in distance learning. *International Journal of Educational Telecommunications, 1*(4), 337–365.

Shin, H., Sok, S., Hyun, D. S., & Kim, M. J. (2015). Competency and an active learning program in undergraduate nursing education. *Journal of Advanced Nursing, 71*(3), 591–598. doi: 101111/jan.12564

Shrader, S., Mauldin, M., Hammad, S., Mitcham, M., & Blue, A. (2015). Developing a comprehensive faculty development program to promote interprofessional education, practice and research at a free-standing academic health science center. *Journal of Interprofessional Care, 29*(2), 165–167. doi:10.3109/13561820.2014.940417 PMID:25051084

Shute, V. J. (2008). Focus on formative feedback. *Review of Educational Research, 78*(1), 153–189. doi:10.3102/0034654307313795

Silver, I. L., & Leslie, K. (2009). Faculty development for continuing interprofessional education and collaborative practice. *The Journal of Continuing Education in the Health Professions, 29*(3), 172–177. doi:10.1002/chp.20032 PMID:19728382

Simpson, J. G., Furnace, J., Crosby, J., Cumming, A. D., Evans, P. A., Friedman Ben David, M., & MacPherson, S. G. et al. (2002). The Scottish doctorlearning outcomes for the medical undergraduate in Scotland: A foundation for competent and reflective practitioners. *Medical Teacher, 24*(2), 136–143. doi:10.1080/01421590220120713 PMID:12098432

Singh, S., Pai, D. R., Sinha, N. K., Kaur, A., Kyaw Soe, A., & Barua, A. 5. (2013). Qualities of an effective teacher: What do medical teachers think? *BMC Medical Education, 13*(128), 2–7. PMID:24044727

Skule, S. (2004). Learning conditions at work: A framework to understand and assess informal learning in the workplace. *International Journal of Training and Development, 8*(1), 8–20. doi:10.1111/j.1360-3736.2004.00192.x

Skule, S., Stuart, M., & Nyen, T. (2002). International briefing 12: Training and development in Norway. *International Journal of Training and Development*, *6*(4), 263–276. doi:10.1111/1468-2419.00164

Slagter van Tryon, P. J., & Bishop, M. J. (2006). Identifying e-mmediacy strategies for webbased instruction: A Delphi study. *Quarterly Review of Distance Education*, *7*(1), 49–62.

Slagter van Tryon, P. J., & Bishop, M. J. (2009). Theoretical foundations for enhancing social connectedness in online learning environments. *Distance Education*, *30*(3), 291–315.

Slagter van Tryon, P. J., & Bishop, M. J. (2012). Evaluating social connectedness online: The design and development of the Social Perceptions in Learning contexts Instrument. *Distance Education*, *33*(3), 347–364.

Smaldino, S. (1999). Instructional design for distance education. *TechTrends*, *43*(5), 9–13. doi:10.1007/BF02818158

Smaldino, S. E., Lowther, D. L., & Russell, J. D. (2008). *Instructional Technology and Media for Learning* (9th ed.). Upper Saddle River, NJ: Pearson.

Smith, P. L., & Ragan, T. J.(2005). *Instructional design* (3rd ed.). Hoboken, NJ: John Wiley & Sons, Inc.

Smith, S. F., Roberts, N. J., & Partridge, M. R. (2009). UK respiratory trainees' views about implementing e-learning into postgraduate training. *THORAX, 64*(Supplementary 4). doi:10.1136/thx.2009.127191z

Smith, A. R., Cavanaugh, C., & Moore, W. A. (2011). Instructional multimedia: An investigation of student and instructor attitudes and student study behavior. *BMC Medical Education*, *11*(1), 38–38. doi:10.1186/1472-6920-11-38 PMID:21693058

Smith, C. A., Ganschow, P. S., Reilly, B. M., Evans, A. T., McNutt, R. A., Osei, A., & Yadav, S. et al. (2000). Teaching residents evidence-based medicine skills. *Journal of General Internal Medicine*, *15*(10), 710–715. doi:10.1046/j.1525-1497.2000.91026.x PMID:11089714

Smith, C. S., Gerrish, W. G., Nash, M., Fisher, A., Brotman, A., Smith, D., & Dreffin, M. et al. (2015). Professional equipoise: Getting beyond dominant discourses in an interprofessional team. *Journal of Interprofessional Care*, *29*(6), 603–609. doi:10.3109/13561820.2015.1051216 PMID:26652633

Smith, G. G., Passmore, D., & Faught, T. (2009). The challenges of online nursing education. *The Internet and Higher Education*, *12*(2), 98–103. doi:10.1016/j.iheduc.2009.06.007

Smith, P. L., & Ragan, T. J. (1999). *Instructional design*. New York, NY: Wiley.

Smith, S. D., Dunham, L., Dekhtyar, M., Dinh, A., Lanken, P. N., Moynahan, K. F., & Skochelak, S. E. et al. (2016). Medical Student Perceptions of the Learning Environment: Learning Communities Are Associated With a More Positive Learning Environment in a Multi-Institutional Medical School Study. *Academic Medical Documentation*. doi:10.1097/ACM.0000000000001214

Song, H. S., Kalet, A. L., & Plass, J. L. (2011). Assessing medical students self-regulation as aptitude in computer-based learning. *Advances in Health Sciences Education: Theory and Practice*, *16*(1), 97–107. doi:10.1007/s10459-010-9248-1 PMID:20872071

Spaulding, W. B. (1991). *Revitalizing medical education, McMaster medical school: The early years, 1965–1974*. Hamilton, Canada: Decker.

Spiro, R. J., Coulson, R. L., Feltovich, P. J., & Anderson, D. K. (1988). *Cognitive flexibility theory: Advanced knowledge acquisition in ill- structured domains. In 10th Annual Conference of the Cognitive Science Society* (pp. 375–383). Hillsdale, NJ: Erlbaum.

Spiro, R., Feltovich, P., Jacobson, M., & Coulson, R. (1991). Knowledge representation, content specification, and the development of skill in situation-specific knowledge assembly: Some constructivist issues as they relate to cognitive flexibility theory and hypertext. *Educational Technology*, *31*(9), 22–25.

Squad, S. (2016). *Wisdom tooth extraction.* Retrieved form http://www.surgerysquad.com/surgeries/virtual-wisdom-tooth-extraction/

Stanley, D., & Latimer, K. (2011). *'The ward': A simulation game for nursing students.* Academic Press. doi:10.1016/j.nepr.2010.05.010

Steelman, V. M. (2016). The Iowa model. *AORN Journal*, *103*(1), 5. doi:10.1016/j.aorn.2015.11.020 PMID:26746021

Steinert, Y., Mann, K., Centeno, A., Dolmans, D., Spencer, J., Gelula, M., & Prideaux, D. (2006). A systematic review of faculty development initiatives designed to improve teaching effectiveness in medical education: BEME Guide No. 8. *Medical Teacher*, *28*(6), 497–526. doi:10.1080/01421590600902976 PMID:17074699

Sternberger, C. S. (2012). Interactive learning environment: Engaging students using clickers. *Nursing Education Perspectives*, *33*(2), 121–124. doi:10.5480/1536-5026-33.2.121 PMID:22616412

Stevens, A., Hernandez, J., Johnsen, K., Dickerson, R., Raij, A., & Harrison, C. (2006). *The use of virtual patients to teach medical students history taking and communication skills.* Academic Press.

Stewart, S., Hansen, T. S., Pope, D., Schmidt, B., Thyes, J. G., Jambunathan, J., & Berthold, T. (2010). Developing a second life campus for online accelerated BSN students. *Computers, Informatics, Nursing*, *28*(5), 253–258. doi:10.1097/01.NCN.0000388348.29174.9f PMID:20736721

Stroup, C. (2014). Simulation usage in nursing fundamentals: Integrative literature review. *Clinical Simulation in Nursing, 10*(3), e155-e164. http://dx.doi.org.lp.hscl.ufl.edu/10.1016/j.ecns.2013.10.004

Stull, C. L., & Blue, C. M. (2016). Examining the influence of professional identity formation on the attitudes of students towards interprofessional collaboration. *Journal of Interprofessional Care*, *30*(1), 90–96. doi:10.3109/13561820.2015.1066318 PMID:26833108

Sullivan, D. T., Hirst, D., & Cronenwett, L. (2009). Assessing quality and safety competencies of graduating prelicensure nursing students. *Nursing Outlook*, *57*(6), 323–331. doi:10.1016/j.outlook.2009.08.004 PMID:19942033

Swanwick, T. (2005). Informal learning in postgraduate medical education: From cognitivism to culturism. *Medical Education*, *39*(8), 859–865. doi:10.1111/j.1365-2929.2005.02224.x PMID:16048629

Sweigart, L., Burden, M., Carlton, K. H., & Fillwalk, J. (2014). Virtual simulations across curriculum prepare nursing students for patient interviews. *Clinical Simulation in Nursing, 10*(3), e139-e145. http://dx.doi.org.lp.hscl.ufl.edu/10.1016/j.ecns.2013.10.003

Sweller, J. (1994). Cognitive load theory, learning difficulty, and instructional design. *Learning and Instruction*, *4*(4), 295–312. doi:10.1016/0959-4752(94)90003-5

Sweller, J. (2008). Human cognitive architecture. In J. M. Spector, M. D. Merrill, J. van Merrienboer, & M. P. Driscoll (Eds.), *Handbook of Research on Educational Communications and Technology* (3rd ed.; pp. 369–381). New York: Lawrence Erlbaum Associates.

Sweller, J., van Merrienboer, J. J. G., & Paas, F. G. W. C. (1998). Cognitive architecture and instructional design. *Educational Psychology Review*, *10*(3), 251–296. doi:10.1023/A:1022193728205

Swing, S. R. (2007). The ACGME outcome project: Retrospective and prospective. *Medical Teacher*, *29*(7), 648–654. doi:10.1080/01421590701392903 PMID:18236251

Swing, S. R., Beeson, M. S., Carraccio, C., Coburn, M., Iobst, W., Selden, N. R., & Vydareny, K. et al. (2013). Educational milestone development in the first 7 specialties to enter the next accreditation system. *Journal of Graduate Medical Education*, *5*(1), 98–106. doi:10.4300/JGME-05-01-33 PMID:24404235

Takaya, K. (2008). Jerome Bruners theory of education: From early Bruner to later Bruner. *Interchange*, *39*(1), 1–19. doi:10.1007/s10780-008-9039-2

Tang, K. S. (2015). The PRO instructional strategy in the construction of scientific explanations. *Teaching Science: The Journal of the Australian Science Teachers Association*, *61*(4), 14–24.

Taylor, S. J., & Bogdan, R. (1987). *Introducción a los métodos cualitativos de investigación*. Barcelona: Paidós.

ten Cate, O. (2005). Entrustability of professional activities and competency-based training. *Medical Education*, *39*(12), 1176-1177. doi:MED2341

ten Cate, O., & Scheele, F. (2007). Competency-based postgraduate training: Can we bridge the gap between theory and clinical practice? *Academic Medicine*, *82*(6), 542–547. doi:10.1097/ACM.0b013e31805559c7 PMID:17525536

The Arnold P. Gold Foundation. (2013). *About us: Overview*. Retrieved May 1, 2016, from http://humanism-in-medicine.org/about-us/

The Blue Ridge Academic Health Group. (2003). *Reforming medical education: Urgent priority for the academic health center in the new century*. Retrieved from http://www.whsc.emory.edu/blueridge/publications/reports.html

The Commonwealth Fund Task Force on Academic Health Centers. (2002). *Training tomorrow's doctors: The medical education mission of academic health centers*. The Commonwealth Fund. Retrieved from http://www.commonwealthfund.org/publications/fund-reports/2002/apr/training-tomorrows-doctors--the-medical-education-mission-of-academic-health-centers

The Organisation for Economic Co-operation and Development. (2010). *Recognition of Non-formal and Informal Learning*. Retrieved April 29, 2016, from http://www.oecd.org/edu/skills-beyond school/recognitionofnon-formalandinformallearning-home.htm

Thistlethwaite, J. (2012). Interprofessional education: A review of context, learning and the research agenda. *Medical Education*, *46*(1), 58–70. doi:10.1111/j.1365-2923.2011.04143.x PMID:22150197

Thistlethwaite, J., Kumar, K., Moran, M., Saunders, R., & Carr, S. (2015). An exploratory review of pre-qualification interprofessional education evaluations. *Journal of Interprofessional Care*, *29*(4), 292–297. doi:10.3109/13561820.2014.985292 PMID:25431833

Thornock, S. B. (2013). *Satisfaction of outcome achievement with web-enhanced teaching strategies in nursing education* (Ed.D. Dissertation). Available from ProQuest Dissertations & Theses Full Text. (1400228888). Retrieved from http://search.proquest.com.lp.hscl.ufl.edu/docview/1400228888?accountid=10920

Tochel, C., Haig, A., Hesketh, A., Cadzow, A., Beggs, K., Colthart, I., & Peacock, H. (2009). The effectiveness of portfolios for post-graduate assessment and education: BEME Guide No 12. *Medical Teacher*, *31*(4), 299–318. doi:10.1080/01421590902883056 PMID:19404890

Toma, C., & Butera, F. (2015). Cooperation versus competition effects on information sharing and use in group decision-making. *Social and Personality Psychology Compass*, *9*(9), 455–467. doi:10.1111/spc3.12191

Tough, A. M. (2002). *The iceberg of informal adult learning*. NALL Working Paper, 49. Retrieved May 2, 2016, from http://nall.oise.utoronto.ca/res/49AllenTough.pdf

Tough, A. M. (1979). *The adult's learning projects: A fresh approach to theory and practice in adult learning* (2nd ed.). Austin, TX: Learning Concepts.

Trafton, P. R., & Midgett, C. (2001). Learning through problems: A powerful approach to teaching mathematics. *Teaching Children Mathematics*, *7*(9), 532–536.

Travaglia, J. F., Nugus, P., Greenfield, D., Westbrook, J., & Braithwaite, J. (2011). Contested innovation: The diffusion of interprofessionalism across a health system. *International Journal for Quality in Health Care*, *23*(6), 629–636. doi:10.1093/intqhc/mzr064 PMID:22003045

Triola, M. M. (2016). *Eduational innovation in a continuously learning health care system.* Keynote address delivered at the conference of the Central Group on Educational Affair, Ypsilanti, MI.

Triola, M., Feldman, H., Kalet, A. L., Zabar, S., Kachur, E. K., Gillespie, C., . . . Lipkin, M. (2006). *A randomized trial of teaching clinical skills using virtual and live standardized patients*. Academic Press. doi:10.1111/j.1525-1497.2006.00421.x

Triola, M. M., & Pusic, M. V. (2012). The education data warehouse: A transformative tool for health education research. *Journal of Gradudate Medical Education*, *4*(1), 113–115. doi:10.4300/JGME-D-11-00312.1 PMID:23451320

Tworek, J., Jamniczky, H., Jacob, C., Hallgrimsson, B., & Wright, B. (2013). The LINDSAY virtual human project: An immersive approach to anatomy and physiology. *Anatomical Sciences Education*, *6*(1), 19–28. doi:10.1002/ase.1301 PMID:22791664

University of Kentucky Office of Medical Education. (2016. April 22). *Medical Education Goals*. Retrieved from http://www.meded.med.uky.edu/medical-education-goals

van Merrienboer, J. J. G. (2007). Alternate models of instructional design: Holistic design approaches and complex learning. In R. A. Reiser & J. Dempsey (Eds.), *Trends and issues in instructional design and technology* (2nd ed., pp. 72–81). Upper Saddle River, NJ: Merrill/Prentice Hall.

van Merrienboer, J. J. G., & Kirschner, P. A. (2001). Three worlds of instructional design: State of the art and future directions. *Instructional Science*, *29*(4/5), 429–441. doi:10.1023/A:1011904127543

Van Merrienboer, J. J. G., & Sweller, J. (2010). Cognitive load'theory in health professional education: Design principles and strategies. *Medical Education*, *44*, 85–93. doi:10.1111/j.1365-2923.2009.03498.x PMID:20078759

van Mook, W. N., de Grave, W. S., Gorter, S. L., Muijtjens, A. M., Zwaveling, J. H., Schuwirth, L. W., & van der Vleuten, C. P. (2010). Fellows' in intensive care medicine views on professionalism and how they learn it. *Intensive Care Medicine*, *36*(2), 296–303. doi:10.1007/s00134-009-1644-8 PMID:19771410

Vogt, W. P. (2007). *Quantitative Research methods for Professionals*. Boston: Pearson.

Wagner, N. L., Wagner, P. J., & Jayachandran, P. (2005). Distance learning courses in occupational medicine: Methods and good practice. *Indian Journal of Occupational and Environmental Medicine*, *9*(2), 57. doi:10.4103/0019-5278.16742

Wald, D., Peet, A., Cripe, J., & Kinloch, M. (2016). *A simulated night on call experience for graduating medical students*. MedEdPORTAL Publications. Retrieved from https://doi.org/10.15766/mep_2374-8265.10483

Walsh, M. (2011). *Narrative pedagogy and simulation: Future directions for nursing education*. Academic Press.

Waltz, C. F., Jenkins, L. S., & Han, N. (2014). The use and effectiveness of active learning methods in nursing and health professions education: A literature review. *Nursing Education Perspectives*, *35*(6), 392–400. doi:10.5480/13-1168

Wamsley, M. A., Julian, K. A., & Wipf, J. E. (2004). A literature review of resident-as-teacher curricula. *Journal of General Internal Medicine*, *19*(5 Pt. 2), 574–581. doi:10.1111/j.1525-1497.2004.30116.x PMID:15109328

Warm, E. J., Mathis, B. R., Held, J. D., Pai, S., Tolentino, J., Ashbrook, L., & Mueller, C. et al. (2014). Entrustment and mapping of observable practice activities for resident assessment. *Journal of General Internal Medicine*, *29*(8), 1177–1182. doi:10.1007/s11606-014-2801-5 PMID:24557518

Weaver, S. J., Salas, E., & King, H. B. (2011). Twelve best practices for team training evaluation in health care. *Joint Commission Journal on Quality and Patient Safety*, *37*(8), 341–349. doi:10.1016/S1553-7250(11)37044-4 PMID:21874969

Webster, M. R. (2009). An innovative faculty toolkit: Simulation success. *Nurse Educator*, *34*(4), 148–149. doi:10.1097/NNE.0b013e3181aabdf9 PMID:19574848

Weiss, R. E. (2003). Designing problems to promote higher-order thinking. In D. S. Knowlton & D. C. Sharp (Eds.), *Problem-based learning in the information age* (pp. 25–31). San Francisco, CA: Jossey-Bass.

Wenger, E. (1998). *Communities of practice: Learning, meaning, and identify*. New York, NY: Cambridge University Press. doi:10.1017/CBO9780511803932

Werquin, P. (2010). *Recognizing non-formal and informal learning: Outcomes, Policies and Practices.* Retrieved April 25, 2016, from http://www.eucen.eu/sites/default/files/OECD_RNFIFL2010_Werquin.pdf

White, C. B., Bassali, R. W., & Heery, L. B. (1997). Teaching residents to teach: An instructional program for training pediatric residents to precept third-year medical students in the ambulatory clinic. *Archives of Pediatrics & Adolescent Medicine*, *151*(7), 730–735. doi:10.1001/archpedi.1997.02170440092016 PMID:9232050

Wiecha, J., & Barrie, N. (2002). Collaborative online learning: A new approach to distance CME. *Academic Medicine*, *77*(9), 928–929. doi:10.1097/00001888-200209000-00031 PMID:12228097

Wiggins, G. P., & McTighe, J. (2005). *Understanding by design*. Alexandria, VA: Assoc. for Supervision and Curriculum Development.

Wijnen-Meijer, M., Cate, O. T., Rademakers, J. J., Van Der Schaaf, M., & Borleffs, J. C. (2009). The influence of a vertically integrated curriculum on the transition to postgraduate training. *Medical Teacher*, *31*(11), e528–e532. doi:10.3109/01421590902842417 PMID:19909031

Wilkerson, L. A. (1985). Learning in a Clinical Setting. *To Improve the Academy, 4*, 120-133.

Wilkerson, L., & Irby, D. (1998). Strategies for improving teaching practices: A comprehensive approach to faculty development. *Academic Medicine*, *73*(4), 387–396. doi:10.1097/00001888-199804000-00011 PMID:9580715

Wilson, F. C. (2007). Teaching by residents. *Clinical Orthopaedics and Related Research*, *454*, 247–250. doi:10.1097/BLO.0b013e31802b4944 PMID:17091017

Wilt, K. E., & King, M. (2012). Time well spent: Integrating simulation into an accelerated 1-year BSN program. *Clinical Simulation in Nursing, 8*(3), e103-e107. http://dx.doi.org.lp.hscl.ufl.edu/10.1016/j.ecns.2010.10.002

Winn, W. (2004). Cognitive perspective in psychology. In D. H. Jonassen (Ed.), *Handbook of Research on Educational Communications and Technology* (2nd ed.; pp. 79–112). Lawrence Earlbaum.

Wolpaw, T. M., Wolpaw, D. R., & Papp, K. K. (2003). SNAPPS: A learner-centered model for outpatient education. *Academic Medicine*, *78*(9), 893–898. doi:10.1097/00001888-200309000-00010 PMID:14507619

Wolters, C. A., & Benzon, M. B. (2013). Assessing and predicting college students use of strategies for the self-regulation of motivation. *Journal of Experimental Education*, *81*(2), 199–221. doi:10.1080/00220973.2012.699901

Wong, G., Greenhalgh, T., & Pawson, R. (2010). Internet-based medical education: A realist review of what works, for whom and in what circumstances. *BMC Medical Education*, *10*(1), 12–12. doi:10.1186/1472-6920-10-12 PMID:20122253

Wood, D. J., Bruner, J. S., & Ross, G. (1976). The role of tutoring in problem solving. *Journal of Child Psychology and Psychiatry, and Allied Disciplines*, *17*(2), 89–100. doi:10.1111/j.1469-7610.1976.tb00381.x PMID:932126

Woods, N. N., Neville, A. J., Levinson, A. J., Howey, E. H., Oczkowski, W. J., & Norman, G. R. (2006). The value of basic science in clinical diagnosis. *Academic Medicine*, *81*(10 Suppl), S124-7. doi:00001888-200610001-00031

Wood, T. (2009). Assessment not only drives learning, it may also help learning. *Medical Education*, *43*(1), 5–6. doi:10.1111/j.1365-2923.2008.03237.x PMID:19140992

Wood, T. J., Cunnington, J. P. W., & Norman, G. R. (2000). Assessing the measurement properties of a clinical reasoning exercise. *Teaching and Learning in Medicine*, *12*(4), 196–200. doi:10.1207/S15328015TLM1204_6 PMID:11273369

World Health Organization. (2011). *Framework for action on interprofessional education and collaborative practice*. Geneva: World Health Organization.

Yeates, P., Stewart, J., & Barton, R. (2008). What can we expect of clinical teachers? Establishing consensus on applicable skills, attitudes and practices. *Medical Education*, *42*(1), 134–142. doi:10.1111/j.1365-2923.2007.02986.x PMID:18230087

Yerkes, R. M., & Dodson, J. D. (1908). The relation of strength of stimulus to rapidity of habit-formation. *The Journal of Comparative Neurology and Psychology*, *18*(5), 459–482. doi:10.1002/cne.920180503

Young, J. R. (2008). When professors create social networks for classes, some students see a 'Creepy Treehouse'. *The Chronical of Higher Education*. Retrieved April 1, from http://chronicle.com/blogs/wiredcampus/when-professors-create-social-networks-for-classes-some-students-see-a-creepy-treehouse/4176

Yukselturk, E., & Top, E. (2013). Exploring the link among entry characteristics, participation behaviors and course outcomes of online learners: An examination of learner profile using cluster analysis. *British Journal of Educational Technology*, *44*(5), 716–728. doi:10.1111/j.1467-8535.2012.01339.x

Zabar, S., Hanley, K., David, S. L., Kalet, A., Schwartz, M. D., Pearlman, E., & Lipkin, M. et al. (2004). Measuring the competence of residents as teachers. *Journal of General Internal Medicine*, *19*(2), 530–534. doi:10.1111/j.1525-1497.2004.30219.x PMID:15109318

Zimmerman, B. J. (2002). Becoming a self-regulated learner: An overview. *Theory into Practice*, *41*(2), 64–72. doi:10.1207/s15430421tip4102_2

Zorek, J., & Raehl, C. (2013). Interprofessional education accreditation standards in the USA: A comparative analysis. *Journal of Interprofessional Care*, *27*(2), 123–130. doi:10.3109/13561820.2012.718295 PMID:22950791

About the Contributors

Jill E. Stefaniak is an Assistant Professor of Instructional Design and Technology at Old Dominion University. Prior to joining Old Dominion University, Jill was the Director of Education Training at the Oakland University William Beaumont School of Medicine. An experienced educator, Jill has trained medical students to become physician educators in community and hospital environments. She received her Ph.D. from Wayne State University in Instructional Technology, and holds a designation as a Certified Professional in Learning & Performance. Previously, she earned a Masters of Training and Development with a double concentration in Instructional Design & Technology and Organizational Development & Leadership from Oakland University in 2008 and a Bachelors of Commerce from the University of Windsor in 2006. Her research interests include learner-centered instruction, cognitive apprenticeships, informal learning environments, and medical simulation.

* * *

Jason Bates is a Master's prepared Instructional Designer and Healthcare Simulation Manager with over 10 years of experience developing simulation based education in medicine. He currently serves as Training and Simulation Manager at The University of Maryland Medical Center leading the development of medical simulation programs within the Shock Trauma Center. He has an extensive background in the design, development and implementation of simulation based training over a wide array of delivery mechanisms and simulation modalities. He has applied Interactive Multi-Media Instruction principles to virtual world, serious game and e-learning development. He has led project development, instructional systems development and validation processes to ensure the complete life cycle of training development is carried out.

Gayle V. Davidson-Shivers is a professor of Instructional Design and Development at the University of South Alabama. Her MA and PhD are from the University of Minnesota-Twin Cities and her BS in education is from Western Oregon University. She teaches instructional design models, needs assessment, and human performance improvement among other topics and supervises doctoral and master's students. Being first in her program to teach online, she began focusing her research interests on online learning and instruction. She co-authored with Karen Rasmussen, Web-based learning: Design, implementation, and evaluation. Her publications include book chapters, journal articles and proceedings papers. She is a program coordinator and served on the USA Faculty Senate. Other service includes university committees, editorial board for the British Journal of Educational Technology, membership on the AACE Ed Media Executive Committee, AECT Definitions and Terms Committee, AECT D&D Division Board, and the Advisory Board for Penelope House.

Joy Doll, OTD, OTR/L, is an Associate Professor of Occupational Therapy at Creighton University. She is the Executive Director of the Creighton Center for Inteprofessional Practice, Education and Research. She is one of the leaders of interprofessional education at Creighton University.

Elizabeth A. Gazza is an associate professor of nursing at UNCW. She has served as chief nursing administrator and faculty for undergraduate through doctoral level nursing education programs. She has taught in fully online nursing education programs for 8 years and has completed research, presented, and published on topics related to the faculty role, including online teaching and facilitating writer development.

Xun Ge, Ph.D., is Professor of Instructional Psychology and Technology with the Department of Educational Psychology, the University of Oklahoma. She received her doctorate in Instructional Systems from the Pennsylvania State University. Dr. Ge's research focuses on ill-structured problem solving, self-regulation, and designing scaffolds for open learning environments to support students' problem solving. She is particularly interested in the impact of technology affordances (e.g., games, simulations, and mobile technology) on learners' ill-structured problem solving. Dr. Ge has published extensively, including numerous articles in top-tier journals, two edited books and multiple book chapters with highly regarded publishers. She has been serving on the editorial board for several leading journals in her field, including Educational Technology Research & Development, Interdisciplinary Journal of Problem-based Learning, and Technology, and Knowledge and Learning. Dr. Ge has been recognized for several awards in her field, including "Young Scholar" award and "Outstanding Journal Article" award.

Kun Huang, Ph.D., is an Assistant Professor in the Department of Instructional Systems and Workforce Development at the Mississippi State University. She received her Ph.D. in Instructional Psychology and Technology from the University of Oklahoma. She has extensive experience with research and practice in simulation-based learning, including its application to medical education. Prior to her faculty career, she had six years of experience working as an instructional designer at two academic health science centers, where she helped to design and facilitate learning with high-fidelity simulations. Dr. Huang's research interests focus on problem-based learning, simulation-based learning, and students' beliefs and motivation in technology-supported learning environments. Her research has been published in refereed journals such as Educational Technology Research and Development, Journal of Educational Computing Research, Teaching and Teacher Education, Interdisciplinary Journal of Problem-based Learning, and Journal of Educational Multimedia and Hypermedia.

Kathryn N. Huggett, PhD, Professor of Medicine at the University of Vermont. She is the inaugural Larner Endowed Professor in Medical Education and directs the Teaching Academy at the University of Vermont's Robert M. Larner, M.D. College of Medicine. Prior to her appointment at the University of Vermont, Katie served as co-chair of the IPE Steering Committee at Creighton University as part of her role at Creighton University in the School of Medicine.

Margaret Jergenson is the department chair and Associate Professor within the School of Dentistry at Creighton University. Maggie served on the Interprofessional Education Steering Committee at Creighton University.

Barbara Joyce, Ph.D., is an Associate Professor of Biomedical Science and Director of Curriculum Evaluation at Oakland University William Beaumont School of Medicine Dr. Joyce's experience has spanned the continuum of medical education although her current focus is at the undergraduate medical education level. Dr. Joyce joined Oakland University William Beaumont School of Medicine (OUWB) in 2010 as an Associate Professor of Biomedical Science and Director of Curriculum Evaluation. She is also the Course Director for the Behavioral Science course. Prior to OUWB, Dr. Joyce was Director of Instructional Design at Henry Ford Health System and a Clinical Associate Professor in the Department of Family Medicine at Wayne State University. At Henry Ford Health System she designed, implemented, and evaluated curricula, assessment tools, and program improvement processes for 45 ACGME accredited residency and fellowship training programs. Previously, she was Senior Project Manager at the ACGME, and worked on the Outcome Project providing faculty development on the ACGME competencies. She has a PH.D. from Wayne State University in Educational and Clinical Psychology.

A. J. Kleinheksel completed her undergraduate education at Michigan State University. After serving as an AmeriCorps VISTA, Dr. Kleinheksel earned a Master of Education in Educational Leadership and Policy, and a Ph.D. in Educational Technology from the University of Florida. She currently serves as the Director of Instructional Design at Shadow Health, a company that develops digital standardized patients for health professions education.

Thomas Lamey is a doctoral student in the Instructional Design and Development (IDD) department at the University of South Alabama (USA). In 2008, Thomas received his Bachelor of Science in Cardiorespiratory Care from USA. In 2012, Thomas completed his Master of Science in IDD from USA. He is a Registered Respiratory Therapist and Certified-Asthma Educator with 8 years of clinical and preceptor experience in a large 600 bed urban hospital.

Victor Law is an Assistant Professor at the University of New Mexico in the Program of Organization, Information, and Learning Sciences. He received his PhD in Educational Psychology from the University of Oklahoma. His research explores the social aspects of self-regulation in collaborative learning environments. In addition, he has been conducting studies examining the effects of different scaffolding approaches, including massively multiplayer online games, computer-based simulation, and dynamic modeling, on students' complex problem-solving learning outcomes. Dr. Law has published empirical studies in national and international refereed journals, such as Computers and Education, Computers in Human Behaviors, Journal of Educational Computing Research, Journal of Educational Technology & Society, Interdisciplinary Journal of Problem-based Learning, Technology, Knowledge and Learning, Technology, Instruction, Cognition, and Learning, and International Journal of Knowledge Management and E-Learning.

Anna Lerant, MD, CHSE, is a non-clinical professor of anesthesiology and the managing director of the Simulation and Interprofessional Education Center at the University of Mississippi Medical Center in Jackson, Mississippi. She received her MD degree from the Semmelweis University School of Medicine, Budapest Hungary in 1992. In 1999, she joined the faculty of the School of Medicine at the University of Mississippi Medical Center and received numerous awards for excellence in teaching. She had been involved in simulation-based education for medical and other healthcare professionals since 2005 as educator, curriculum developer and facilitator.

Mildred Vanessa López Cabrera is currently the Coordinator of Innovation and Academic Quality at the National School of Medicine Tecnológico de Monterrey, where she is responsible for the proposal and coordination of educational innovation projects and their respective broadcast in national and international forums and scientific journals, monitoring indicators academic quality, the organization of national and international conventions, conferences and meetings of medical education, and strengthening the research and educational innovation by advising teachers in the documentation of their experiences on educational innovation. She participates in different projects at institutional level for innovation in teaching learning, and the inclusion of technology in the classroom and in clinical settings. Which she combines with her teaching practice at a undergraduate and graduate level of engineering and medical specialty in Clinical Care Quality.

Kathryn Lovell is a Professor, Depts, Neurology and Radiology, Colleges of Human and Osteopathic Medicine, Michigan State University.

Anna Maio, MD, is a physician in general internal medicine and an educator for the Creighton University School of Medicine. She is one of the leaders of interprofessional education and collaborative practice at Creighton University.

Misa Mi is an associate professor and health information specialist in the Department of Biomedical Sciences at the Oakland University William Beaumont School of Medicine. She has been designing and providing training for learners across the spectrum of medical education over the past two decades. She earned her Ph.D. in Learning Design & Technology and a Masters of Library & Information Science from Wayne State University and was trained in the Program for Educators in Health Professions at the Harvard Macy Institute, Harvard University. She is a distinguished member of the Academy of Health Information Professionals of the Medical Library Association.

Rebecca Moote is an Associate Professor at the Regis University School of Pharmacy. Regis SOP was the first program to use an integrated Team-Based Learning (TBL) approach to teaching throughout the pharmacy doctorate curriculum. She has an interest in TBL facilitation skills and how expert facilitation enhances learning in the classroom. She has a strong interprofessional focus and has worked to evaluate the impact of collaboration across disciplines of learning.

W. Bosseau Murray, M.B., Ch.B., MD, is a clinical anesthesiologist at Pennsylvania State University College of Medicine, Hershey, PA. He has 40 years of clinical experience (including Level 1 Trauma Centers) in South Africa, Great Britain, Canada and the USA. He is an ACLS and an ATLS instructor. He has 16 years of experience teaching in the Clinical Simulation Center at Pennsylvania State University College of Medicine. He is a founding member of the Society for Simulation in Health Care (SSH) and a regular Faculty Member at the International Meeting for Simulation in Health Care (IMSH). He is the author of 80+ peer reviewed papers, many on simulation for health-care education. He is co-author (with Richard Kyle) of the book "Clinical Simulation: Operations, Management and Engineering."

Silvia Lizett Olivares Olivares, MsC, PhD., is the Academic Dean of the School of Medicine at Tecnológico de Monterrey. She is associate professor, researcher and academic leader on topics related with medical education and quality management. As Academic Dean, she leads curriculum design, programs accreditation, faculty development, medical education research, international programs, ethics and professionalism, students' assessment and clinical simulation for graduate and undergraduate medical programs. She participates as senior examiner for the Nuevo León Quality Award, as secretary of the Quality Board of the Mexican Association for Medical Schools (AMFEM by its initials in Spanish) and she is member of the Latin Association for Clinical Simulation (ALASIC by its initials in Spanish). She has been examiner for the National Quality Award in Mexico and the Latin American Quality Award. She has received international recognition by Reimagine Education QS Awards, national medical associations and institutional distintions.

Jeffrey D. Orledge, MD, FACEP, is an associate professor of Emergency Medicine and the medical director of the Simulation and Interprofessional Education Center at the University of Mississippi Medical Center, Jackson, MS. Dr. Orledge has been involved in simulation-based education for over 15 years. He contributed to development of high fidelity simulations that are used in the Advanced Disaster Life Support course, the emergency medicine residents' "boot camp", as well as several other student and provider courses.

Beth Oyarzun earned her PhD in Instructional Design and Technology from Old Dominion University. Beth has worked as an instructional designer in the Office of eLearning at the University of North Carolina Wilmington (UNCW) since 2010. She previously worked as the technology liaison at the Watson College of Education also at UNCW. She has worked in the higher education environment teaching and training online pedagogy for more than ten years. Beth was previously a high school mathematics teacher for nine years in various counties surrounding the Wilmington, NC area.

Katie Packard, PharmD, MS, is an Associate Professor of Pharmacy Practice at Creighton University. She served on the Interprofessional Education Steering Committee.

Karen Paschal, PT, DPT, MS, is a Professor of Physical Therapy at Creighton University. She served on the Interprofessional Education Steering Committee.

Meghan Potthoff, PhD, APRN, is an Assistant Professor in the Creighton University College of Nursing. She will be serving as the Chair of the IPE Curriculum Committee.

Robin Rockhold, following receipt of a baccalaureate degree from Kenyon College in 1973, was awarded the Ph.D. in pharmacology from the University of Tennessee Center for the Health Sciences in 1978. Initial post-doctoral training at the Pharmakologishes Institut, der Universitat Heidelberg was followed by a second post-doctoral period in the Department of Physiology & Biophysics, an initial appointment as Assistant Professor in that department, and subsequent appointments as Assistant, Associate and full Professor in the Department of Pharmacology & Toxicology at the University of Mississippi Medical Center (UMMC). He began administrative duties in 2005 and currently serves as Deputy Chief Academic Officer. With over 100 peer-reviewed publications and book chapters, Dr. Rockhold has served as Principal Investigator, Co-Investigator or Investigator on 42 awards since 1983, with over $18 million being awarded. He has been responsible for strategic oversight of UMMC simulation-based education since 2008.

Ann Ryan Haddad is a Professor Pharmacy Practice and Director of the Office of Interprofessional Scholarship, Service and Education at Creighton University. She is a leader in the development of the interprofessonal education curriculum at Creighton University.

Patricia J. Slagter van Tryon is an Associate Professor in the Department of Mathematics, Science, and Instructional Technology Education at East Carolina University where she teaches graduate courses in instructional technology in a 100% online Master of Arts in Education program. Her research interests include the design of instruction for online and blended learning environments and social cognition and schema revision strategies through instructional e-mmediacy in online learning environments.

Bill Solomonson, CPT, is Associate Professor in the Department of Organizational Leadership at Oakland University in Rochester, Michigan. His research interests include the client-consultant relationship, multi-media learning theory, online learning pedagogy, and organizational performance improvement. Bill's current research explores the factors affecting trust and relationship commitment in the client-consultant relationship.

Tina M. Souders, MSW, LCSW, JD, is a Clinical Associate Professor at the University of North Carolina at Chapel Hill, School of Social Work. She is the Director of the Winston-Salem Distance Education MSW Program. She teaches courses in Social Work Practice with Organizations and Communities, Social Work and the Law, and assists faculty in the development of online instruction.

Stephanie M. Swanberg, MSI, AHIP, is Assistant Professor, Information Literacy and eLearning Librarian in the Department of Biomedical Sciences at Oakland University William Beaumont School of Medicine (OUWB). She received her Master of Science in Information degree from The University of Michigan School of Information and worked at The University of Michigan Taubman Health Sciences Library prior to joining OUWB. Ms. Swanberg instructs medical students in information searching, evaluation, and management within the research and evidence-based medicine courses as well as designs faculty development seminars for basic science and clinical faculty members in information mastery. Her research interests include information literacy instruction, medical education, evidence-based medicine, and community health.

Dominique Thomas received her M.Ed. in Instructional Psychology and Technology from the University of Oklahoma in 2004. She is currently a Technical Trainer at CACI International where she designs and develops front-end user interfaces, rich multimedia content, and gamification techniques to enhance computer-based training for tactical systems. She is interested in research in serious games and simulations for mobile devices.

Martha Todd, PhD, APRN-NP, is an Associate Professor in the College of Nursing at Creighton University. She served on the IPE Steering Committee.

Jorge Eugenio Valdez García is a medical doctor graduated from the School of Medicine of Tecnológico de Monterrey, also specialist in Ophtalmology, with a fellowship in Cornea and Refractive Surgery from the Institute of Ophtalmology UNAM. Master in Arts in Medical Science from Boston University School of Medicine. Currently the Dean of the School of Medicine and Health Sciences of

Tecnológico de Monterrey. Fellow of the Academia Mexicana de Cirugía. National Researcher Level I, National System of Researchers (CONACYT). Fellow of the National Academy of Medical Education (President of the Northern Chapter). Member of the Executive Board of Mexican Association of Faculties and Schools of Medicine (AMFEM). He has authored: 3 books, 7 chapters, 68 scientific articles, and 50 abstracts published both nationally and internationally. Teaching and research Award from Tecnológico de Monterrey, 2008. National Award in Ophtalmology, 1993 and 2016 from the Mexican Society of Ophtalmology.

Qian Wang is a graduate student pursuing her Ph.D. degree in Instructional Psychology and Technology at the University of Oklahoma. Her research interests include scaffolding students' cognition and metacognition through enhancing their motivation, as well as developing cognitive tools to support their reasoning, ill-structured problem solving, and decision making.

Index

A

accreditation 53-54, 57, 164-166, 178, 183, 188, 194, 197, 209-212, 216-217, 220, 224-225, 278
Accreditation Council for Graduate Medical Education (ACGME) 165, 183
accreditation standards 188, 194, 209-210, 216, 220, 224
administration 44, 65, 68, 140, 194, 199, 201, 209, 212, 215, 245, 284
advance organizers 10, 27, 36
analysis 1-2, 4-5, 8-9, 12-13, 19, 21-23, 27-28, 35, 37, 39-40, 51-52, 55, 66, 83, 86, 101-102, 107-111, 114-115, 117, 120-122, 124-126, 128, 130, 136, 138-139, 155, 237, 253, 280, 285, 291-293
andragogy 4, 172, 183
applied learning 150-152, 154-156, 158-161, 163
assessment 1, 4-5, 11-13, 15, 18, 20, 22, 32, 35, 41-42, 44, 53-55, 57-59, 61, 65-67, 69-71, 76, 90-91, 99, 111, 115, 122, 133-136, 138-142, 145, 165, 178, 180, 186, 188, 193, 196-198, 200-201, 215-216, 219-220, 237-239, 247-249, 251, 253-254, 268, 277, 279, 282, 284, 286-287, 290, 292-293, 295, 300
asynchronous 11, 13-15, 27, 150-152, 155-156, 248-251, 253-254, 261
Asynchronous Learning 27
Atlanto-Occipital Extension 115, 132

B

Backward Design 53-54, 61, 67-69, 71, 76
Behaviorism 2, 174
Big Data 237, 243
blended learning 45, 51, 107, 109, 135, 145

C

champions 192, 212, 214-217, 221, 224
clinical competence 85, 168, 183
clinical educator 280, 286, 288, 295, 300
cognitive load 10, 27, 36, 262, 264, 270, 272-273, 276
cognitivism 3
collaboration 7, 17, 40, 58, 62, 65, 67, 140-142, 188-189, 191, 193, 209-212, 214, 216-217, 221, 232, 234-235, 237, 286
collaborative practice 186, 188, 193, 195, 200-201, 205, 209, 220, 224
Communities of Practice 151, 233-234, 243
competence 7, 55, 57, 66, 82, 85-86, 88, 90, 111-112, 160, 168, 173, 175, 183, 192, 231, 265, 273, 280, 288, 292-293, 300
competencies 53-59, 61, 63, 68, 70-71, 76, 78, 133-134, 136, 139, 143, 164, 173, 187-188, 224, 231, 236, 277-280, 284-286, 288, 290-295
competency-based education 55-57, 65, 69-70, 76
Computer Mediated Communication 145
computer-assisted instruction 249-250, 260
computer-based simulation 79, 86, 88, 90, 99
computer-based teaching module 276
concept maps 10, 27, 66
Contextualization 43, 51
Core Competencies for Interprofessional Collaborative Practice 188, 224
Creative Commons 263, 265-266, 276
curriculum 12-13, 22, 35, 37, 53-55, 57-58, 60-66, 69-71, 76, 82, 101-102, 129-130, 133-136, 155, 158, 166, 177-178, 180, 191, 197-198, 200, 209, 212-217, 219, 221, 225-226, 229-230, 234, 236-239, 251-254, 263, 270-271, 282, 284, 286, 292
Curriculum Integration 76

D

debriefing 78, 89-91, 99-100, 123, 130, 199, 228, 232, 253, 280, 287, 290, 300
Delivery strategies 31-32, 34, 43, 51
Design Research 142, 145

designing 1, 8, 14, 37, 54-55, 67, 70-71, 76-79, 81-83, 90, 99, 111, 133-135, 154-156, 160, 172, 177-178, 186-187, 210, 215, 232, 234, 253, 264, 295
development 2-3, 5, 10, 14, 21-23, 31-32, 34-37, 45, 55, 57-58, 60, 64, 69, 71, 84, 99, 101-102, 107, 110-111, 121-122, 129, 133-143, 151-153, 155, 158, 160-161, 163-164, 166, 174-175, 178, 180, 186, 188, 190-196, 198, 208, 210-217, 220-221, 225-231, 235-237, 239, 246-247, 249, 251-253, 262-263, 265, 267, 272-273, 277-280, 282, 284-289, 291, 293-295, 300
digital standardized patient 249, 261
distance learning 31, 41-44, 51, 210, 212, 224

E

educational milestones 57
Elaboration Theory 51
E-Mmediacy 141, 145
Entrustable Professional Activities 57, 59, 76
Entrustable Professional Activities (EPAs) 57, 76
epiglottis 105-106, 123-124, 126-129, 132
Epitome 51
evaluation 32, 35, 37, 40-42, 66, 83, 89, 99, 101-102, 107, 109-111, 120-123, 126, 128, 130, 133-134, 136, 138, 141-142, 145, 150, 158, 160, 165-166, 168, 178, 183, 196, 198-200, 210, 219-220, 232, 238-239, 247, 250, 262-264, 266-267, 286, 290-291, 300
evidence-based medicine 30, 43, 189, 234, 243, 291
experiential learning 150, 152-155, 161, 163, 170, 183, 245
extrinsic motivation 19-20, 27, 174

F

facilitation 79, 82, 86, 90-91, 99, 141, 167, 171, 192-193, 197, 199, 205, 282
faculty development program 192, 277, 280, 284, 286, 300
feedback 5-7, 10, 33, 44, 52, 55, 57-58, 60-61, 67, 69-71, 78-79, 88-90, 99, 121-122, 140, 142, 168, 174, 176-178, 193, 218-219, 232, 238, 249-252, 254, 260, 262-264, 266, 269-270, 273, 282, 286, 288, 290, 293, 295, 300
fidelity 79, 104, 123, 249, 260-261, 291
formal curriculum 129, 177, 229-230, 236, 238, 282
formal learning 226-227, 230-232, 236, 238-239, 243
formative assessment 69, 142, 145, 254

G

Group Presentation 51

H

healthcare 1, 20, 22, 42-43, 136, 143, 151-152, 156, 159, 186, 188, 190-191, 194, 199-200, 220, 230-231, 239, 245-247, 251, 254, 284, 287, 289-291, 293-294, 300
hidden curriculum 225, 229, 236, 238
High-Fidelity Simulation 249, 261
Human-Patient Simulator 99

I

Immersive Virtual Reality Simulation 261
implementation 31, 34, 37, 44, 55, 67-69, 71, 101-102, 107, 110-111, 119, 121, 129, 150, 160, 178, 186, 188, 192, 198-199, 208, 210, 212-219, 221, 232, 247, 252, 262-263, 271, 277, 280, 287, 292
informal curriculum 229, 236-239
Innovative Pedagogy 219, 224
instruction 1-6, 8, 10-18, 20-23, 27, 31-34, 36, 43-45, 47, 51, 54, 67, 69, 77-79, 91, 99, 101-102, 108, 111, 123-124, 130, 133-143, 145, 151, 153, 158, 164, 169-172, 177, 183, 210, 249-250, 252, 260, 273, 276, 278, 285, 293
instructional design 4, 21, 30-31, 33, 44, 53-54, 67-68, 71, 76-77, 79, 81, 90, 101, 105, 133-135, 140-143, 145, 150-155, 161, 164, 186, 212, 262-263, 267, 269-273
instructional strategies 5, 11, 19, 21-22, 30-32, 42, 51, 90, 99, 133, 138, 140, 151, 164, 166, 171, 174-175, 177-178, 180, 183
instructional strategy 16, 30-31, 34, 104, 140, 161, 170-171
interleaving 268-269, 276
interprofessional collaborative practice 188, 209, 220, 224
interprofessional education 186, 188, 200-201, 205, 208-209, 211-215, 217, 219-221, 224, 232, 244
Interprofessional Education and Practice 244
Interprofessional Education Collaborative (IPEC) 188, 205
intrinsic motivation 19, 27, 174, 178
intubation 101-104, 111, 114-115, 117, 123-125, 128-130, 132

L

laryngoscope 102, 105, 111, 123, 127-130, 132
learner analysis 1-2, 4-5, 8, 12-13, 19, 21-23, 27-28,

51, 109, 139
learner control 262-263, 267, 271, 273, 276
learning environment 3-4, 6, 10, 15, 18, 41-42, 45, 66, 78, 82-83, 86, 90, 133-136, 139-142, 155, 170, 173, 178, 180, 187, 226, 228-237, 239, 244, 250, 278
learning management system 44, 135, 140, 145, 156, 158, 215
learning objective 83, 120-121, 247
learning theory 2, 37, 42, 107, 134, 138-139, 152-153, 161, 164, 169, 171, 180, 183, 273
Liaison Committee on Medical Education (LCME) 58, 183, 226
lifelong learning 172, 178, 225-226, 230, 233-235, 239, 244, 277

M

Macro Strategies 32, 51
management strategies 31-32, 44-47, 51
meaningful learning 10, 42, 264-265, 269, 273, 276
medical education 30-32, 34-35, 42-47, 53-55, 57-58, 62-63, 66-70, 76-83, 90, 99, 164-166, 168-178, 180, 183, 225-226, 228-231, 233, 235-236, 238-239, 244, 246, 251, 264, 266, 272-273, 278, 280, 285, 289, 294-295, 300
medical schools 35, 37, 59, 61-65, 67, 71, 78, 165, 169, 180, 234, 239, 251, 278, 280, 291
medical students 2, 7, 12, 15, 33, 42-44, 65, 67, 76, 99, 107, 164-171, 173, 176, 178, 180, 183, 226, 229-230, 232-233, 251, 262, 264-265, 269-270, 272-273, 277-278, 282, 286, 291-292
Micro Strategies 31-32, 51
milestones 56-61, 63, 68-71, 76
modeling 85-90, 99, 175-176, 195, 233, 237, 247
Multimedia Instruction 273, 276

N

National League for Nursing (NLN) 133
neuropathology 262-264, 266-271
nursing education 133-135, 150-152, 155, 160, 163, 247, 251, 253

O

Objective Structured Clinical Examinations (OSCEs) 168, 183
One-Minute Preceptor Model (OMP) 166, 183
online 8, 13-15, 42, 44-45, 47, 51-52, 134-135, 138-142, 145, 150-156, 158-161, 163, 169, 174, 187, 208-210, 213, 217-218, 221, 224, 232-233, 235, 237, 245-246, 248-249, 261, 266, 271, 292
online education 151-152, 155, 160, 213, 224, 245
online learning 14-15, 44-45, 134-135, 138, 140, 142, 145, 151, 209, 217, 237, 271
Organizational strategies 31-33, 51

P

patient avatar 249-250, 254, 261
Pedagogical Skills 286, 300
pedagogy 4, 151-152, 172, 183, 192, 210, 218-219, 224, 252, 254
Performance Assessment 145
physicians 33, 55, 165-166, 225, 231-232, 238-239, 244-245, 251, 280, 288, 292-295
prior knowledge 2-3, 5, 8-11, 13, 21-22, 27, 30-31, 33, 51, 90, 196, 229-230, 271, 273
Problem-Based Learning (PBL) 31, 170, 183, 279
professional 1, 19, 31, 35-36, 45, 53, 57-59, 62, 76, 136, 143, 155-156, 161, 163, 169, 187, 189-194, 196, 198, 213, 225-226, 231-237, 239, 244, 248, 252, 278, 284, 291-292
program director 235

Q

quality management 286, 292, 294, 300

R

reflection 40, 44, 66, 152, 177, 190, 194-195, 227-228, 230-232, 235, 247, 281, 291-292
retrieval practice 262, 265, 269, 272-273, 276

S

scaffolding 85-91, 99, 176
scope 5, 31-33, 43, 51-52, 62-63, 85, 134, 142, 155, 188, 191-192, 197, 213, 218, 221
self-assessment 166, 231, 238, 262, 265-266, 269-270, 273, 276, 282
self-paced course 213, 217, 224
Self-Regulated Learning 15, 27
self-regulation 14-15, 20, 90
sequence 3, 10, 12, 31-32, 51-52, 79-80, 83, 85, 103-104, 138, 174, 267
simulation 22, 41, 64, 78-91, 99, 101-104, 107, 109-112, 114, 118-119, 121-123, 129-131, 152, 174, 176, 178, 187, 218, 245-254, 260-261, 278, 290-293, 300
simulation-based medical education 78, 82, 90, 99

SNAPPS 167, 183
sniffing position 115, 122, 132
SOAPS 168, 183
social media 42, 46, 52, 229, 232-233, 235-237, 244
Spatio-temporal Proximity 140, 145
standardized patient avatar 250, 254, 261
strategies 2, 5, 8, 10-11, 13, 15, 18-23, 30-34, 37, 40-47, 51, 53-54, 61, 65-67, 69-71, 82, 86-88, 90, 99, 107, 109-111, 133, 135, 138-142, 145, 151-153, 158, 161, 164, 166, 169-171, 174-178, 180, 183, 186, 193, 210, 213, 215, 225-226, 230, 235, 238-239, 253, 265, 273, 280-283, 285-286, 289, 293, 295
subcompetencies 59, 76
synchronous 13-15, 27, 61, 249-250, 261
Synchronous Instruction 13, 27
systematic design 133, 142
Systems Approach 145

T

Testing Effect 265, 276

V

vallecula 105-106, 111, 123-130, 132
videolaryngoscope 105-106, 123, 129, 132
virtual character simulation 249, 261
virtual human 250-251
virtual patient 245-254, 261
virtual reality 101, 123, 249-250, 261
Volition 20, 27

Purchase Print + Free E-Book or E-Book Only*

Purchase a print book through the IGI Global Online Bookstore and receive the e-book for free or purchase the e-book only! Shipping fees apply.

www.igi-global.com

Recommended Reference Books

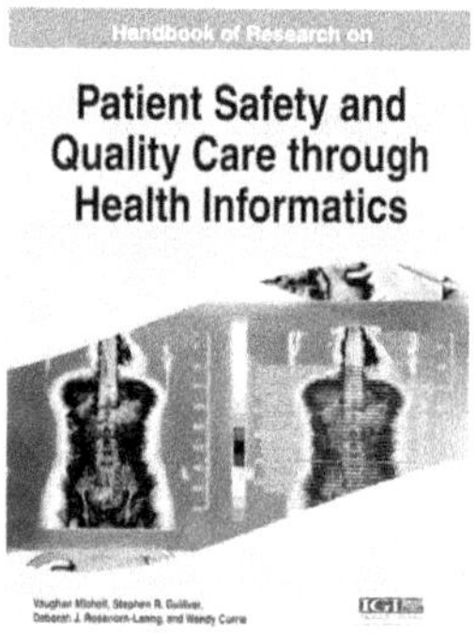

ISBN: 978-1-4666-4546-2
© 2014; 486 pp.
List Price: $292

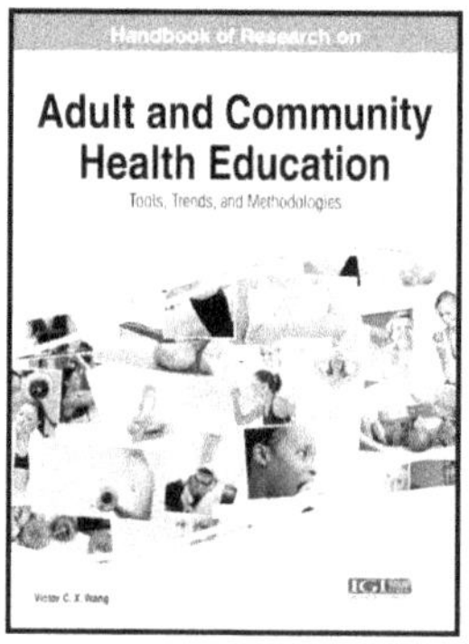

ISBN: 978-1-4666-6260-5
© 2014; 485 pp.
List Price: $260

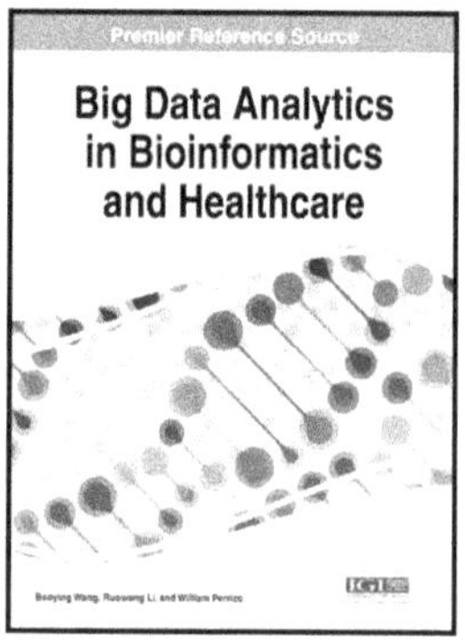

ISBN: 978-1-4666-6611-5
© 2015; 528 pp.
List Price: $204

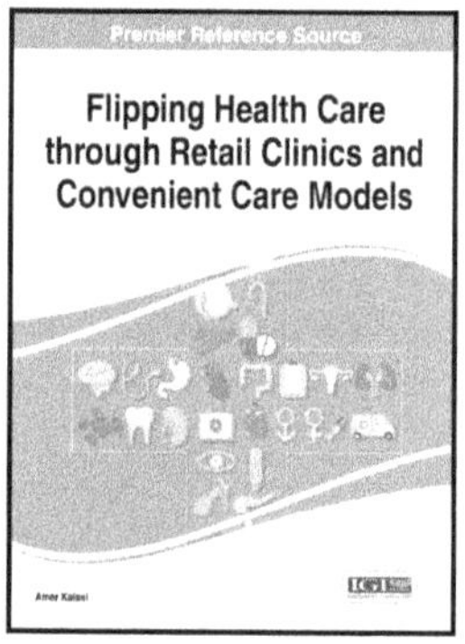

ISBN: 978-1-4666-6355-8
© 2015; 306 pp.
List Price: $196

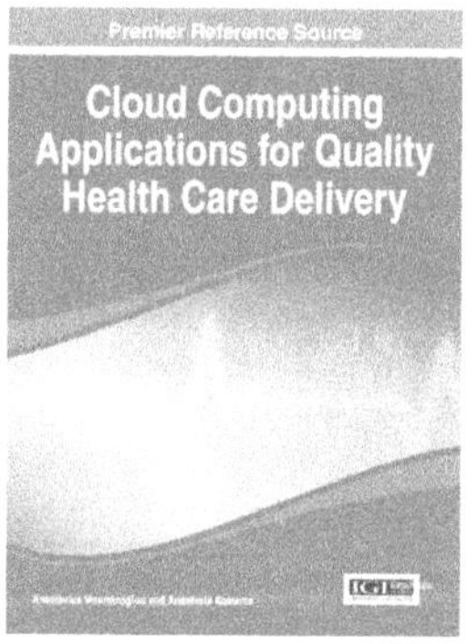

ISBN: 978-1-4666-6118-9
© 2014; 342 pp.
List Price: $196

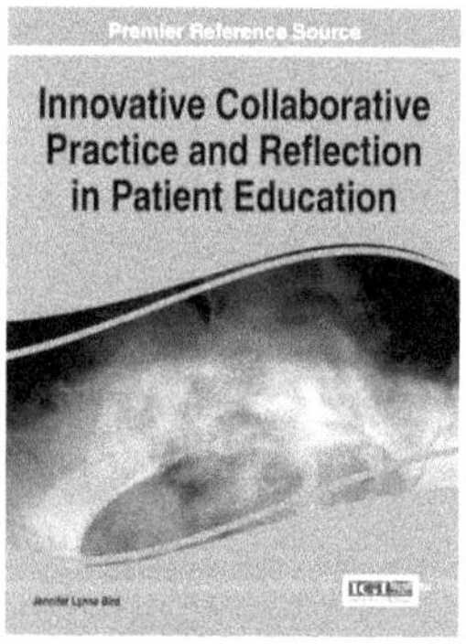

ISBN: 978-1-4666-7524-7
© 2015; 308 pp.
List Price: $180

*IGI Global now offers the exclusive opportunity to receive a free e-book with the purchase of the publication in print, or purchase any e-book publication only. You choose the format that best suits your needs. This offer is only valid on purchases made directly through IGI Global's Online Bookstore and not intended for use by book distributors or wholesalers. Shipping fees will be applied for hardcover purchases during checkout if this option is selected.

Should a new edition of any given publication become available, access will not be extended on the new edition and will only be available for the purchased publication. If a new edition becomes available, you will not lose access, but you would no longer receive new content for that publication (i.e. updates). The free e-book is only available to single institutions that purchase printed publications through IGI Global. Sharing the free e-book is prohibited and will result in the termination of e-access.

Publishing Information Science and Technology Research Since 1988

IGI Global DISSEMINATOR OF KNOWLEDGE

www.igi-global.com | Sign up at www.igi-global.com/newsletters | facebook.com/igiglobal | twitter.com/igig

upport Your Colleagues and Stay Current n the Latest Research Developments

3ecome a Reviewer

this competitive age of scholarly publishing, constructive and timely feedback gnificantly decreases the turn-around time of manuscripts from submission to ceptance, allowing the publication and discovery of progressive research at a much ore expeditious rate.

ne overall success of a refereed journal is dependent on quality and mely reviews.

everal IGI Global journals are currently seeking highly qualified experts in the field to vacancies on their respective editorial review boards. Reviewing manuscripts allows u to stay current on the latest developments in your ld of research, while at the same time providing constructive feedback to your peers.

eviewers are expected to write reviews in a timely, collegial, and constructive manner. I reviewers will begin their role on an ad-hoc basis for a period of one year, and upon ccessful completion of this term can be considered for full editorial review board atus, with the potential for a subsequent promotion to Associate Editor.

oin this elite group by visiting the IGI Global journal ebpage, and clicking on "**Become a Reviewer**".

pplications may also be submitted online at:
ww.igi-global.com/journals/become-a-reviewer/.

pplicants must have a doctorate (or an equivalent degree) as well as publishing and viewing experience.

you have a colleague that may be interested in this opportunity, e encourage you to share this information with them.

ny questions regarding this opportunity can be sent to:
urnaleditor@igi-global.com.

www.igi-global.com

InfoSci®-Books

A Database for Progressive Information Science and Technology Research

Maximize Your Library's Book Collection!

Invest in IGI Global's InfoSci®-Books database and gain access to hundreds of reference books at a fraction of their individual list price.

The InfoSci®-Books database offers unlimited simultaneous users the ability to precisely return search results through more than 68,000 full-text chapters from nearly 3,000 reference books in the following academic research areas:

Business & Management Information Science & Technology • Computer Science & Information Technology
Educational Science & Technology • Engineering Science & Technology • Environmental Science & Technology
Government Science & Technology • Library Information Science & Technology • Media & Communication Science & Technology
Medical, Healthcare & Life Science & Technology • Security & Forensic Science & Technology • Social Sciences & Online Behavior

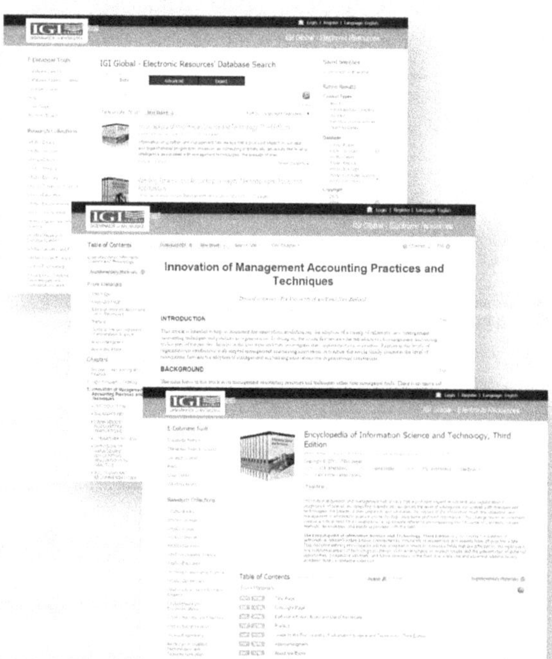

Peer-Reviewed Content:

- Cutting-edge research
- No embargoes
- Scholarly and professional
- Interdisciplinary

Award-Winning Platform:

- Unlimited simultaneous users
- Full-text in XML and PDF
- Advanced search engine
- No DRM

Librarian-Friendly:

- Free MARC records
- Discovery services
- COUNTER4/SUSHI compliant
- Training available

To find out more or request a free trial, visit: www.igi-global.com/eresources

IGI GLOBAL
DISSEMINATOR OF KNOWLEDGE
www.igi-global.com

IGI Global

Proudly Partners with

eContent Pro

eContent Pro specializes in the following areas:

Academic Copy Editing

Our expert copy editors will conduct a full copy editing procedure on your manuscript and will also address your preferred reference style to make sure your paper meets the standards of the style of your choice.

Professional Proofreading

Our editors will conduct a comprehensive assessment of your content and address all shortcomings of the paper in terms of grammar, language structures, spelling, and formatting.

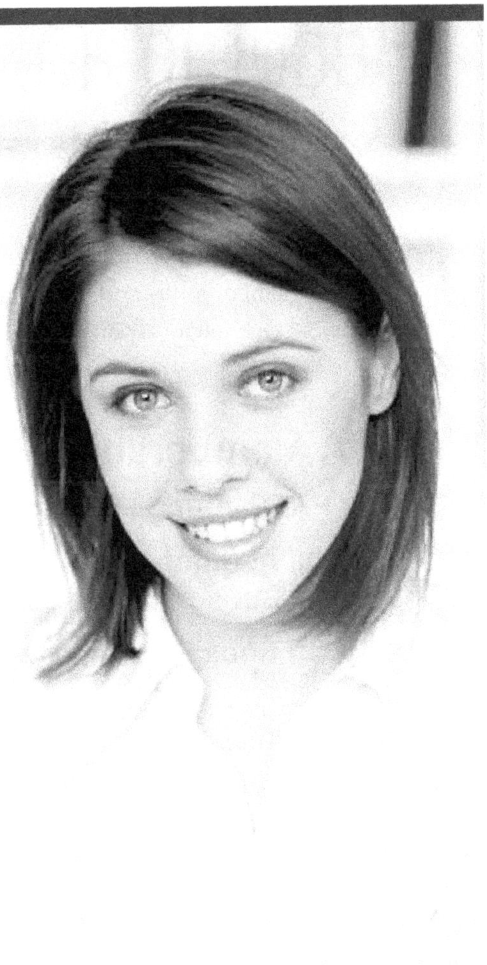

IGI Global Authors, Save 10% on eContent Pro's Services!

The IGI Global Editor/Author 10% discount promotion is applied directly to your eContent Pro shopping cart and may not be combined with any other sale, promotion, discount, code, coupon and/or offer. eContent Pro has the right to end or modify any promotion at any time.

Email: customerservice@mkptechnologies.com **econtentproediting.com**

IRMA INTERNATIONAL

Information Resources Management Association

Become an IRMA Member

Members of the **Information Resources Management Association (IRMA)** understand the importance of community within their field of study. The Information Resources Management Association is an ideal venue through which professionals, students, and academicians can convene and share the latest industry innovations and scholarly research that is changing the field of information science and technology. Become a member today and enjoy the benefits of membership as well as the opportunity to collaborate and network with fellow experts in the field.

IRMA Membership Benefits:

- **One FREE Journal Subscription**
- **30% Off Additional Journal Subscriptions**
- **20% Off Book Purchases**
- Updates on the latest events and research on Information Resources Management through the IRMA-L listserv.
- Updates on new open access and downloadable content added to Research IRM.
- A copy of the Information Technology Management Newsletter twice a year.
- A certificate of membership.

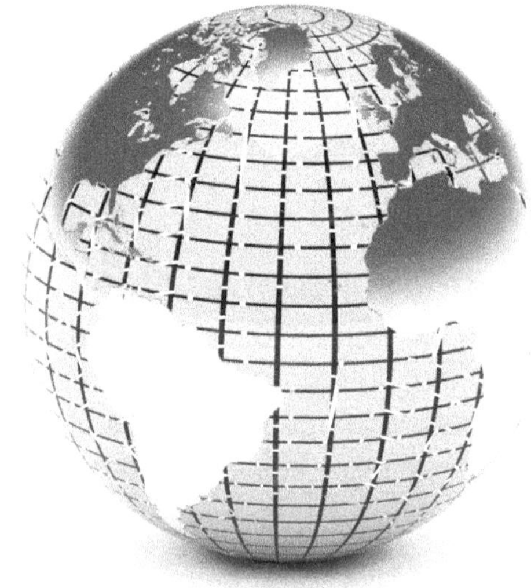

IRMA Membership $195

Scan code or visit **irma-international.org** and begin by selecting your free journal subscription.

Membership is good for one full year.

www.irma-international.org

Encyclopedia of Information Science and Technology, Third Edition (10 Vols.)

Mehdi Khosrow-Pour, D.B.A. (Information Resources Management Association, USA)
ISBN: 978-1-4666-5888-2; **EISBN:** 978-1-4666-5889-9; © 2015; 10,384 pages.

The **Encyclopedia of Information Science and Technology, Third Edition** is a 10-volume compilation of authoritative, previously unpublished research-based articles contributed by thousands of researchers and experts from all over the world. This discipline-defining encyclopedia will serve research needs in numerous fields that are affected by the rapid pace and substantial impact of technological change. With an emphasis on modern issues and the presentation of potential opportunities, prospective solutions, and future directions in the field, it is a relevant and essential addition to any academic library's reference collection.

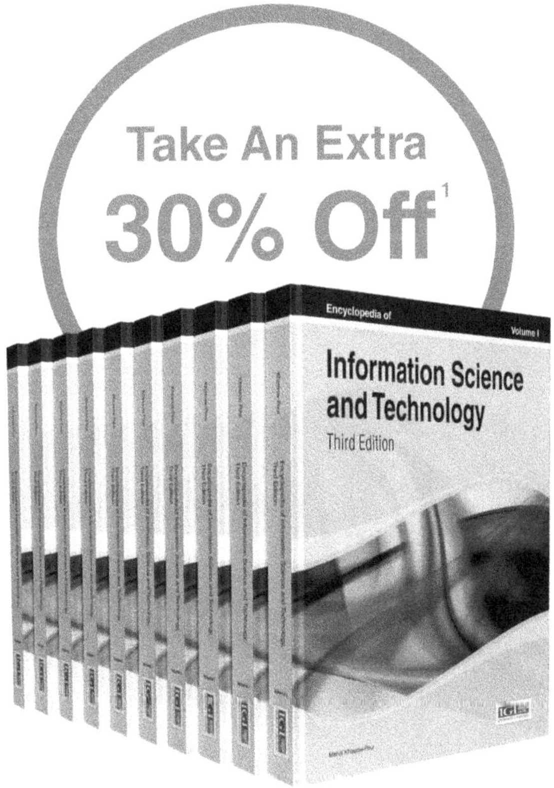

[1] 30% discount offer cannot be combined with any other discount and is only valid on purchases made directly through IGI Global's Online Bookstore (www.igi-global.com/books), not intended for use by distributors or wholesalers. Offer expires December 31, 2016.

Free Lifetime E-Access with Print Purchase

Take 30% Off Retail Price:

Hardcover with Free E-Access:[2] $2,765
~~List Price: $3,950~~

E-Access with Free Hardcover:[2] $2,765
~~List Price: $3,950~~

Recommend this Title to Your Institution's Library: www.igi-global.com/books

[2] IGI Global now offers the exclusive opportunity to receive free lifetime e-access with the purchase of the publication in print, or purchase any e-access publication and receive a free print copy of the publication. You choose the format that best suits your needs. This offer is only valid on purchases made directly through IGI Global's Online Bookstore and not intended for use by book distributors or wholesalers. Shipping fees will be applied for hardcover purchases during checkout if this option is selected.

The lifetime of a publication refers to its status as the current edition. Should a new edition of any given publication become available, access will not be extended on the new edition and will only be available for the purchased publication. If a new edition becomes available, you will not lose access, but you would no longer receive new content for that publication (i.e. updates). Free Lifetime E-Access is only available to single institutions that purchase printed publications through IGI Global. Sharing the Free Lifetime E-Access is prohibited and will result in the termination of e-access.

www.ingramcontent.com/pod-product-compliance
Lightning Source LLC
LaVergne TN
LVHW060413300926
849162LV00006B/1416